D0762043

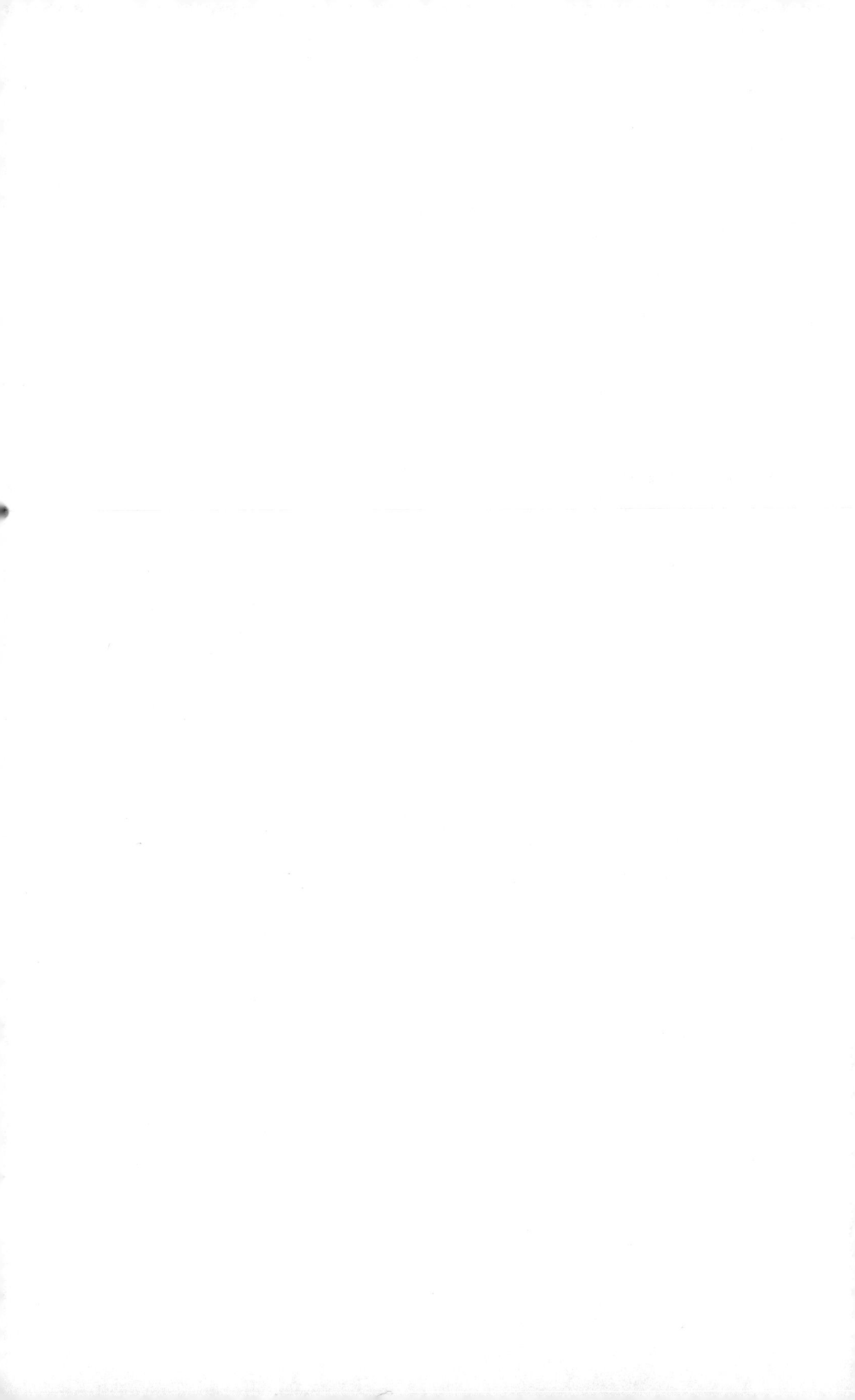

Differential Diagnosis in Speech-Language Pathology

Differential Diagnosis in Speech-Language Pathology

Edited by

Betty Jane Philips, Ed.D.

Professor, Research, University of North Carolina Craniofacial Center, School of Dentistry, Chapel Hill

Dennis M. Ruscello, Ph.D.

Professor of Speech Pathology and Audiology, West Virginia University, Morgantown; Adjunct Professor of Otolaryngology, Robert C. Byrd Health Sciences Center, Morgantown

Butterworth–Heinemann

Boston Oxford Johannesburg Melbourne New Delhi Singapore

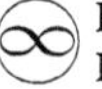

Recognizing the importance of preserving what has been written, Butterworth–Heinemann prints its books on acid-free paper whenever possible.

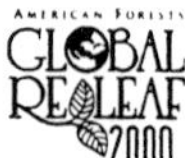

Butterworth–Heinemann supports the efforts of American Forests and the Global ReLeaf program in its campaign for the betterment of trees, forests, and our environment.

Library of Congress Cataloging-in-Publication Data

Differential diagnosis in speech-language pathology / [edited by]
Betty Jane Philips, Dennis Ruscello.
p. cm.
Includes bibliographical references and index.
ISBN 0-7506-9675-3 (alk. paper)
1. Speech disorders--Diagnosis. 2. Language disorders--Diagnosis.
3. Diagnosis, Differential. I. Philips, Betty Jane. II. Ruscello, Dennis M.
[DNLM: 1. Communicative Disorders--diagnosis. 2. Diagnosis, Differential. WL 340.2 D569 1997]
RC423.D536 1997
616.85'5075--dc21
DNLM/DLC
for Library of Congress 97–34816
CIP

British Library Cataloguing-in-Publication Data
A catalogue record for this book is available from the British Library.

The publisher offers special discounts on bulk orders of this book.

For information, please contact:
Manager of Special Sales
Butterworth–Heinemann
225 Wildwood Avenue
Woburn, MA 01801-2041
Tel: 781-904-2500
Fax: 781-904-2620

For information on all Butterworth–Heinemann publications available, contact our World Wide Web home page at: http://www.bh.com

10 9 8 7 6 5 4 3 2 1

Printed in the United States of America

"All cases are unique and similar to others."

—T. S. Eliot

Contents

Contributing Authors

Dolores E. Battle, Ph.D.
Professor of Speech-Language Pathology, Buffalo State College, Buffalo, New York

Gordon W. Blood, B.S., M.A., Ph.D.
Professor and Head of Communication Disorders, The Pennsylvania State University, University Park

Paul N. Deputy, Ph.D.
Dean of Education and Professor of Communication Disorders, School of Education, Northern State University, Aberdeen, South Dakota

Ashley S. Garber, M.S., CCC-SLP
Former Speech-Language Pathologist, Bill Wilkerson Center, Nashville; Former Clinical Instructor, Vanderbilt University Medical Center, Nashville

Lynne E. Hewitt, Ph.D.
Assistant Professor of Communication Disorders, The Pennsylvania State University, University Park

Alan G. Kamhi, Ph.D.
Professor of Audiology and Speech-Language Pathology, University of Memphis, Memphis, Tennessee

Jeri A. Logemann, Ph.D.
Ralph and Jean Sundin Professor of Communication Sciences and Disorders, Northwestern University, Evanston, Illinois; Director of Speech, Language, Voice and Swallowing Services, Northwestern Memorial Hospital, Chicago

Richard K. Peach, Ph.D.
Associate Professor of Otolaryngology, Neurological Sciences and Communication Disorders and Sciences, Rush University, Chicago;

Associate Scientist, Department of Otolaryngology, Neurological Sciences and Communication Disorders and Sciences, Rush-Presbyterian-St. Luke's Medical Center, Chicago

Sally J. Peterson-Falzone, Ph.D.
Clinical Professor, Department of Growth and Development, Center for Craniofacial Anomalies, University of California School of Dentistry, San Francisco

Betty Jane Philips, Ed.D.
Professor, Research, University of North Carolina Craniofacial Center, School of Dentistry, Chapel Hill

Dennis M. Ruscello, Ph.D.
Professor of Speech Pathology and Audiology, West Virginia University, Morgantown; Adjunct Professor of Otolaryngology, Robert C. Byrd Health Sciences Center, Morgantown

Teris Kim Schery, Ph.D.
Research Professor of Education and Human Development, Department of Special Education, Peabody College of Vanderbilt University, Nashville; Research Professor of Hearing and Speech Sciences, Vanderbilt University Medical Center

Joseph C. Stemple, Ph.D.
Director, Institute for Voice Analysis and Rehabilitation, Dayton, Ohio

Audrey D. Weston, Ph.D., CCC-SLP
Associate Professor of Speech Pathology and Audiology, Idaho State University, Boise

Differential Diagnosis in Speech-Language Pathology

1

Introduction

Betty Jane Philips and Dennis M. Ruscello

The purpose of this book is to provide a diagnostic reference text for speech-language pathologists. Many diagnostic assessments are routine and result in relatively predictable and common diagnoses. However, all clinicians encounter diagnoses that are unusual or that share symptoms similar to another possible diagnosis. The authors present information about some of these unusual and difficult diagnoses as well as information about assessment procedures to assist the clinician in the differentiation of a variety of diagnoses. These authors have expertise in specific types of speech-language and related disorders. The information is intended to supplement the knowledge and experience that the clinician brings to the diagnostic process and assist in identification of and differentiation among speech-language problems.

The diagnostic process requires the speech-language pathologist to make a number of sequential differentiations. For example, the clinician must differentiate among the types of communication problems and subtypes within those groupings, the possible etiologies for the delay or disorder, and the various treatment options. Even the selection of appropriate tests and measures requires that the clinician differentiate among them across a number of domains to find those that are most appropriate for the client. The diagnostic process leads to the development of a treatment plan based on the diagnosis that the clinician formulates. The diagnostic process then continues as the client's responses to treatment can provide additional information, indicating that the diagnosis has been correct, is questionable, or needs revision. The challenge for the practitioner is to make the differentiations that lead to the development of an appropriate treatment plan. Clinicians are referred to the decision trees, which define steps in assessment procedures—for example, assessment of swallowing disorders or assessment of dysarthria (Yoder and Kent 1988). This book provides helpful guidelines for practitioners.

When the diagnosis is used as a label, problems can arise. Lund and Duchan (1993) expressed concern about labels. A diagnosis, when treated as a label, can lead clinicians to the assumption that all clients who have a particular label have the same characteristics and degree of involvement. Moreover, labeling can foster stereotyped perceptions that lead to the recommendation of the same treatment for all clients within that diagnostic classification and to anticipation of similar responses to treatment for all clients so labeled. There also is a strong potential that others in the client's environment (e.g., family members, teachers, other professionals) have stereotyped perceptions of the diagnostic terminology. For example, a teacher may assume that all children with autism are retarded. A family who knows a person who has been diagnosed as aphasic may assume that the recovery and rehabilitation process for that person will be the same for their grandfather, who has aphasia. Careful discussion of the diagnostic information with those involved with the client can help to modify or eradicate such misconceptions. Despite the drawbacks of using the diagnosis as a label, there can be benefits, in that a label (classification) can result in acceptance of the client for treatment services by administrators of school and insurance programs.

Even the most experienced clinician encounters diagnostic dilemmas. These can occur at any time in the diagnostic process. The problems can occur for a number of reasons. The clinician may have used inappropriate evaluation procedures or may have simply overlooked or not seen some diagnostic clues or misinterpreted data. The family or client may have failed to provide or withheld important information. The clinician may encounter a problem that is outside the area of his or her usual practice. Difficulties can also develop when the diagnostic data are incomplete because information is needed from allied health care professionals. Sometimes the diagnostic situation is difficult because information provided from other sources is incorrect or misinterpreted in relation to the client's communication disorder.

When engaged in the diagnostic process, speech-language pathologists are urged to approach each diagnostic assessment with an open mind, regardless of prior diagnoses that others have provided and regardless of the seeming simplicity or complexity of the client's communication disorder. Diagnostic or treatment data available from other clinicians should be obtained and carefully studied. Referral to and consultation with other professionals may be needed. Data reported by other professionals, however, may require additional interpretation based on the knowledge and perspective of the speech-language pathologist. On occasion it is necessary to seek second opinions regarding data obtained from people in other disciplines. When a diagnosis is unclear, the clinician should consult with other speech-language pathologists, particularly those who have expertise in the area of concern. Longitudinal follow-up of a client's response to treatment recommendations can provide additional diagnostic information. The clinician must be willing to change diagnostic impressions. The speech-language pathologist's curiosity and inquisitiveness drive the process of differential diagnosis. The clinician who accepts diagnostic challenges, is curious about missing information and inconsistencies, constantly questions, and searches for possible answers is most likely to solve puzzles presented by difficult problems.

Interdisciplinary teams, in some cases, provide an ideal environment for diagnostic assessment and treatment planning. There are teams for special types of problems (e.g., developmental disabilities, neurologic disorders, cleft palate or craniofacial anomalies, auditory processing problems, learning problems). These teams bring together the knowledge and experience of a variety of specialists—for example, speech-language pathologists, ophthalmologists, pediatricians, audiologists, dentists, otolaryngologists, geneticists, psychologists, neurologists, orthopedists, teachers, and physical and occupational therapists. The makeup of the team depends on its purpose. Interdisciplinary teams provide an environment in which the members can share their expertise and questions. The team staffing helps to integrate the findings and recommendations, and facilitate referrals for special services. The interdisciplinary team thrives best when the members are willing to express opinions and represent their own profession. For example, a physician on the team may report that a child's developmental progress is good, but the speech-language pathologist may not agree because the child's language skills are significantly delayed. This situation requires that the speech-language pathologist listen carefully to the physician's opinions, comment on the parts of the opinion in which there is agreement, note exceptions to the opinions, and explain the basis for the exceptions. For example, in the area of language development, it would be important to provide data to support the view that there is language delay and make specific recommendations. The team is no place for the meek who routinely defer to the opinions of others. Neither is it the place to stand firm when others provide contradictory evidence. Sometimes there is no immediate answer, and only longitudinal follow-up treatment and assessments resolve issues that are before a team. Conflict in opinion also can occur when the client is seen by specialists in scattered environments. When there is little opportunity to discuss the differences of opinion concerning the client or the data obtained, diagnostic issues become more difficult to resolve. When an interdisciplinary team is not available for referral, the speech-language pathologist may want to take the lead in forming a team and asking other professionals to participate. Although many teams are organized for evaluation of specific types of disorders (e.g., dysphagia or cerebral palsy), teams can be formed for individual patients. When a team exists, the speech-language pathologist who provides treatment for the patient, if not a member of the team, should try to attend the team meeting. In such cases, the clinician should be prepared to provide information based on knowledge of the client's history, tests that have been conducted, and the client's response to treatment. The clinician should ask questions when needed to clarify information provided by the team members.

This book provides discussions of the need for referrals, consultation, interdisciplinary teams, tests and procedures, unusual cases, etiologies, speech-language characteristics, and problems that are unique but appear similar. Suggestions are also provided that can assist in the diagnostic process when the speech-language pathologist encounters clinical challenges. The authors of each chapter, having experience and specialization in each area, address the assessment of speech-language and related disorders from their perspectives of differential diagnosis.

REFERENCES

Lund N, Duchan J. (1993) *Assessing Children's Language in Naturalistic Contexts* (3rd ed). Englewood Cliffs, NJ: Prentice-Hall.

Yoder D, Kent R. (1988) *Decision Making in Speech-Language Pathology.* Philadelphia: Decker.

2

Differential Diagnosis of Communication Disorders in Multicultural Populations

Dolores E. Battle

The United States is becoming a nation of increasing cultural and linguistic diversity. Between 1980 and 1990, the white population of the United States increased by 6%, but all other racial and ethnic populations increased by considerably more, from 13.2% among African Americans to 107.8% among Asians and Pacific Islanders (U.S. Bureau of the Census 1996). According to the 1990 census, the minority population in the United States exceeded 60 million people, including 29.9 million African Americans, 22.3 million Hispanics, 7.2 million Asians and Pacific Islanders, and 1.9 million Native Americans (U.S. Bureau of the Census 1990). If current immigration trends continue, by the beginning of the next century more than one-third of the nation will be from historically cultural and linguistic minority groups. The early immigrants to this country were primarily from Europe. Since the 1980s, however, 80% of the legal immigrants to the United States have been from Asia and South and Central America (Robey 1985; Russell 1982; U.S. Bureau of the Census 1990).

Because language and communication are rooted in culture, the tremendous diversity of cultures and language in this country presents a challenge for the speech-language pathologist. The American Speech-Language-Hearing Association estimated that 10% of the population in the United States has a speech-language disorder unrelated to the ability to speak English as a native language (Cole 1989). The National Center for Health Statistics (1988) estimated that the greater prevalence of communication disorders is among racial and ethnic minorities rather than in mainstream groups, because of environmental, teratogenic, nutritional, and traumatic factors usually associated with lower socioeconomic status.

There is a significant relationship between socioeconomic status and language development (Ratusnik and Koenigsknecht 1975). Typical evaluation procedures tend to be biased against students from minority and low-income families. However, because there is a disproportionate distribution of racial and ethnic minorities among persons from lower socioeconomic groups, it is reasonable to assume that there is a disproportionate number of racial and ethnic minorities with communication disorders unrelated to the ability to speak Standard American English (SAE).

ASSESSMENT OF CULTURALLY AND LINGUISTICALLY DIVERSE CHILDREN

The Individuals with Disabilities Education Act (Public Law 107-15) requires that tests and other evaluation materials "be provided and administered in the client's native language or other mode of communication, unless clearly not feasible to do so" (Federal Register 1997). The Fifteenth Annual Report to the Congress on the Implementation of the Individuals with Disabilities Act (Office of Special Education Programs 1993) indicated that minorities are enrolled in special education in greater numbers than general population figures suggest. The reasons for overrepresentation of minority children in special education include overzealous referrals, inappropriate referrals, inappropriate testing and evaluation, and inappropriate consideration of normal, but culturally different behaviors.

To appropriately identify communication disorders in culturally and linguistically diverse clients, it is necessary to consider the triangulation of linguistic variables, cultural variables, and developmental variables. Linguistic variables require the distinction between the use of social dialects and second-language learning and language disorders. Cultural variables that affect the administration and interpretation of diagnostic techniques must be considered. Finally, a distinction must be made among normal communication and language development, normal second-language learning, and communication disorders.

Distinguishing Among Dialects, Development, and Communication Disorders

To appropriately provide differential diagnosis to culturally and linguistically diverse populations, communication disorders must be defined within the context of the client's cultural and linguistic community. They must be distinguished from social dialects and variables expected because of normal development. In a culturally sensitive definition of communication disorder, Taylor (1986, p. 13) stated that communication behavior can only be considered disordered if it

(a) deviates sufficiently from the norms, expectations and definitions of the indigenous culture or language group;
(b) is considered to be disordered by the indigenous culture or language group;
(c) operates outside of the minimal norms of acceptability of that culture or language group;
(d) interferes with communication *within* the indigenous culture or language group; or
(e) calls attention to itself within the indigenous culture or language group.

For example, the vocal patterns of Asian adults are usually of lower intensity than those of American speakers. People, especially women, in some Asian cultures, such as Chinese and Indian, are socialized to use lower vocal intensity. Use of low vocal intensity would be identified as a disorder on voice profiles for SAE speakers, yet as a culturally normal vocal parameter for some Asian speakers, low intensity should not be considered to be a voice problem. Cultural differences in vocal parameters differentially affect speakers of different languages dependent on the features of the language. In another example, speakers of tonal languages, such as Hmong and Chinese, are more impaired by the inability to alter vocal tone than speakers of atonal languages, such as Japanese or English (Cheng 1993). Assimilation nasality is frequently present in Korean speakers, since final stops are nasalized when they occur before nasal sounds (Cheng 1993).

Diversity in religion, sociopolitical background, and child-rearing practices affect the family's belief system concerning disability and communication disorders. Culturally sensitive assessment asks the following questions: (1) What is the language history of the client? (2) What is the cultural orientation of the client or family? (3) What language(s) is (are) spoken in the home? (4) What are the child-rearing and socialization practices of the family? (5) What is the family's perception of disability and approach to health and healing? (6) What is the family's perception of seeking help and intervention? (7) What is the culturally preferred mode of intervention for disabled persons—rehabilitation? prayer? herbs? acceptance? concealment? (8) What is the cultural view of the ideal speaker and the impaired speaker? (9) What is the community theory concerning how children develop language and about the cause and impact of disabilities? (10) What does the family or client expect from the speech-language assessment? and (11) What do they know about available resources and costs? All questions must be answered before attempting differential diagnosis with culturally and linguistically diverse clients.

The sociopolitical background of the client has an important influence on the client's perception of communication disorder. For example, the social and political history of Asian Pacific Americans is quite heterogeneous. The Asians who emigrated to the United States in the 1960s were largely educated professionals for whom knowledge and use of English was expected. During the 1970s and 1980s, a large percentage of Asians who came to the United States were fleeing war-torn rural Vietnam, Cambodia, and Laos. They have a higher rate of poverty and are less likely to be well educated. Many live in linguistic isolation, living in tightly knit communities where the use of English is limited. Social history affects the immigrant's interaction with English, so it is important to consider not only linguistic variables, but also cultural variables when obtaining information about a client (Cheng 1993).

Differentiating Social Dialects from Communication Disorders

A dialect is a variation within a specific language that characterizes a particular identifiable group. Dialects exist within every language in the world and are intrinsically valid for the group of persons who speak them (Taylor 1986). The use of a dialect is affected by geography, socioeconomic level, race and ethnicity, peer-group influence, and first- and second-language influence. Each dialect has its own unique phonologic, semantic, morphologic, syntactic, and pragmatic rule system that varies in some way from an ideal language standard. Dialects are mutually intelligible to all speakers of the language.

More than 200 different languages are spoken in the United States (U.S. Bureau of the Census 1990). Thirty-two million Americans speak a primary language other than English. The major racial and ethnic dialects in the United States are African American English (AAE) and Spanish-influenced English. It is estimated that at least 11 million Americans speak Spanish at home, and, of these, one-fourth either do not speak English well or do not speak English at all (Schick and Schick 1991). Of the 5.5% of students in American schools with limited English proficiency (LEP), 73% speak Spanish, 4% speak Vietnamese, 2% speak Hmong or Laotian, and 2% speak Cantonese Chinese, with the remaining 19% speaking a variety of other languages. Because Asian languages and English are not mutually intelligible, there is no specific Asian-English dialect. The Native American population is heterogeneous, with approximately 500 tribes speaking 250 different languages and dialects and as many different cultural beliefs among them.

According to the *Position Paper on Social Dialects* (American Speech-Language-Hearing Association 1982), no dialectal variety of English is a disorder or a pathologic form of speech or language. Therefore, a person who uses a social dialect that is appropriate to his or her indigenous community should not be identified as having a communication disorder.

Differentiating Between African American English and Communication Disorders

AAE is used by many, but not all, working-class African Americans in informal speaking situations. The primary characteristics of AAE are habitual *be* (e.g., "She *be* working since February"), triple negative (e.g., "*Nobody ain't* got *none*"), the deletion or weakening of the final consonants with prolongation of the preceding vowel, and the reduction of consonant clusters to single sounds in the final position (Moran 1993). In addition, intonation pattern, speaking rate, and a distinctive lexicon identify AAE (Owens 1995a).

Normal Language Development and African American English

A common error in diagnosis of phonologic and morphologic development in African American children is that all differences observed are related to the use of AAE. This is as much an error in diagnosis as is identification of dialectal features as features of disorders. It is necessary to consider normal development in the diagnosis of speech-language disorders in multicultural populations.

Communication ability develops with age, with significant changes occurring in the preschool and early elementary years. According to Labov (1972), there are three stages in the development of a dialect: birth to 5 years, 5–15 years, and 15 years to adulthood. Between birth and 5 years of age, the development of language and the development of dialect are greatly influenced by caretakers. Between 5 and 15 years of age, peer influence supersedes parental influence in the use of AAE.

The consonantal features that contrast AAE and SAE are undifferentiated in age-matched African American and white preschool children (Table 2-1). A number of phonologic variations that characterize AAE, including the deletion of final consonants, appear during later preschool years and kindergarten. Children gradually include more final consonants until they attain adult models in the middle elementary-school years (Haynes and Moran 1989; Light 1971; Seymour and Seymour 1981)

Table 2.1
Selected phonologic features of African American English

African American English Feature	*Examples*
Final consonant cluster reduction	"cold" → "col," "test" → "tes"
Use of *-es* plural with *-sk, -st,* and *-sp*	"tests" → "teses"
Omission of post-vocalic /r/, /l/	"help" → "hep," "their" → "they"
Final /n/ for /ŋ/	"sitting" → "sittin"
Initial /d/ for /ð/	"they" → "dey"
Medial and final /f/ for /θ/	"bathtub" → "baftub," "tooth" → "toof"
Medial /v/ for /ð/	"brother" → "brover"

There is considerable variation in the use of AAE among preschool and kindergarten children. For example, the use of /f/ for final /θ/ is a commonly recognized feature of AAE. Seymour and Seymour (1981) reported that while 54% of African American preschool children studied used final /f/ instead of /θ/, 46% used /θ/ (as in SAE). Because this feature of AAE is also among the later-developing consonant sounds in SAE, use of f/θ in the medial and final position of words is frequently misidentified as an articulation error in children who use AAE.

The type of articulation feature must also be considered when distinguishing normal development of dialectal features from articulation disorders. The substitution of f/θ in all positions of words may not be a dialectal feature. Seymour and Seymour (1981) found that African American children more frequently produce f/th in the medial and final word positions, b/v in the initial and medial positions, and d/ð in the initial and medial positions. SAE-speaking children more frequently produce f/θ in the initial word position; r/w in the initial word position; and t/ʧ, s/θ, and s/ʃ in all positions than African American children. If a child who uses AAE uses f/θ in the initial position of a word, the use should not be attributed to dialect. Because initial f/θ is not typically developed by speakers of SAE until 4.5 years of age (Sander 1972), a preschool child who uses f/θ in any position may either be using dialect or showing normal development. A 6-year-old child who is using f/θ in the initial position is most likely not using dialect and may be showing a true disorder.

Bleile and Wallach (1992) showed that adult AAE speakers distinguish normal from disordered speech in African American preschoolers by the child's use of more than one or two stop errors, initial word position errors, glide errors in children older than 4 years of age, more than a few cluster errors, and fricative errors other than /θ/. These characteristics are likely to be more reliable indicators of true phonologic and articulation disorders in African American children.

Since many contrasts between AAE and SAE are morphosyntactic, much study of the language development of African American children and the development of AAE has focused on morphosyntactic development. AAE-speaking children demonstrate the same range of early semantic categories and pragmatic functions as SAE-speaking children and develop the functions in the same sequence and at the same stages as other children (Blake 1984; Bridgeforth 1984; Reveron 1978; Stockman 1986; Stockman et al. 1982).

The morphosyntactic development of AAE-speaking children is similar to that of SAE-speaking children up to the age of 3 years, including the development of mean length of utterance (MLU) (Stockman 1986). Children learning AAE acquire the use of plural, possessive, past tense, and third-person singular in the same pattern as children learning the 14 morphemes described by Brown (1973). Thus, it is often difficult to distinguish between dialectal and developmental variation in children younger than the age of 3 years.

The dialectal features of AAE emerge as the child matures (Table 2.2). By the age of 3 years, AAE-speaking children are already demonstrating competency in the use of certain AAE variable grammar rules, particularly those involving use of the copula in declaratives (Wyatt 1991). There is a marked increase in the use of AAE or nonstandard English variants by children acquiring AAE between the ages of 3 and 5 years (Cole 1980; Kovac 1980; Reveron 1978). AAE equivalents produced by 90% of 3-year-old children include copula and auxiliary *be*, third person singular *-s*, past tense *-ed*, and remote time *been* (Cole 1980). The most consistent syntactic features found in the speech of African American preschoolers are the deletion of copula and the lack of the third-person marker (Craig and Washington 1994).

There is a marked increase in the use of nonstandard English variants by children acquiring AAE between the ages of 3 and 5 years, with social class differences becoming most pronounced after the age of 4 years (Kovac 1980; Reveron 1978; Stockman 1986). Ninety percent of the 4-year-old African American children studied by Cole (1980) produced features of AAE, including indefinite articles and multiple negation. Demonstrative and reflexive pronouns were produced by 90% of the 5-year-old African American children. AAE equivalents produced by less than 90% of the 5-year-old children included possessive *-s*, plural *-s*, use of *at* in questions, *go* copula, distributive *be*, first-person future, embedded questions, past-tense copula, present copula, and second-person pronoun. Some AAE features, such as habitual (invariant, distributive) *be*, developed at a much later age than others.

Table 2.2
Selected grammatical features of African American English

African American English Feature	*Examples*
Absence of regular past-tense marker	"played" → "play," "missed" → "miss"
Past-tense form as past participle	"I *had went* there."
Past-tense participle as past	"He *seen* it."
Habitual *be*	"Sometimes she *be* here."
Remote time *been*	"I *been* had this."
Absence of auxiliary and copula *be*	"You a boy." "He eating."
Nonstandard subject-verb agreement	"He *sit* right there."
Multiple negation	"I *didn't* do *nofin*."
Absence of plural *-s* in measure nouns	"He got five *cent*."
Regularization of irregular plurals	"De *childrens* goin home."
Absence of possessive *-s* marker	"Give me *Mary hat*."
Regularization of possessive pronouns	"Dat *mines*."
Pronominal differences	"He hurt *hissef*."
Nonstandard relative pronouns	"Sat the one *what* I tellin you 'bout."

Source: Adapted from T Wyatt. (1991) Linguistic constraints on copula production in black English child speech, Ph.D. diss., University of Massachusetts.

Preschool African American children from the age of 4.0 to 5.4 years studied by Craig and Washington (1994) produced complex sentences in their utterances. Because the forms of *be* that are characteristic of AAE are among the later developing morphosyntactic forms in SAE, it is difficult to identify whether young children 3–5 years of age are showing the use of AAE morphology or are in the process of normally developing SAE.

Code Switching in African American English

Some speakers of AAE are bidialectal, using AAE at home and in informal settings and switching to SAE or the dominant regional dialect in more formal settings. The ability to code switch within the phonologic and morphologic systems increases with age. According to a study by Seymour and Ralabate (1985), first- and second-grade AAE speakers used f/θ in both a spontaneous conversation and a structured picture-labeling task. Third- and fourth-grade AAE speakers used f/θ in spontaneous conversation; however, they used /θ/ in a structured picture-labeling task, demonstrating the ability to code switch between the phonologic features of AAE and SAE depending on the communication situation during the school years.

Wyatt and Seymour (1990) reported differences in code switching of a 5-year-old African American girl in communication situations while speaking on various topics, to different listeners, and with different communication intents. When repeating sentences presented by the examiners, she used 5% AAE features. While describing action in pictures, she used 9% AAE features. However, when spontaneously expressing feelings or making comments to other children, she used 47% AAE features. Her use of AAE features also varied with the listener. When speaking to her classroom teacher, an adult white woman, she used 0% AAE features. When speaking to the examiner, an African American woman who speaks SAE, she used 15% AAE features. However, when speaking to her African American peers she used 47–53% AAE features. A similar pattern was shown in the use of AAE according to her intent. When requesting clarification, she used 11% AAE features. When reporting her personal feelings about others, she used 25% AAE features. When protesting or complaining, however, she used AAE features 56% of the time. Code switching morphosyntactic features of AAE by school-age children is a function of the social situation and communication function rather than a lack of knowledge of SAE.

There is a significant decline in the use of AAE in school-related tasks as children progress through the elementary school years (DeStefano 1972; Melmed 1971). This indicates that the AAE speakers learn more standard forms over time and learn to use them in appropriate contexts. As children approach late adolescence, they become aware of the social significance of the use of SAE for educational and occupational access and begin to use more SAE forms in social situations. They may, however, be unable to maintain consistent use of the SAE in all contexts, particularly where more formal use of English is expected (Labov 1972; Wolfram and Fasold 1974). It can be expected that clients who use the features of AAE in informal conversation may use SAE phonologic and syntactic forms during formal testing situations, including sentence imitation and picture-naming tasks.

CASE 1

The following is a transcript of a narrative account presented by a 4-year-old African American girl:

This how I broke my toof.
I runnin and the ice was slipi.
My momma say watch the ice.
And I say I don see no ice.

Then I runnin an I fall down and broke my toof and cut my leg.
Then I was bleedin ebriwhere.
And my momma come and hep me.
And dat's all.

An analysis shows that most of these variations are within the norms for the development of articulation in SAE (f/θ, d/ð, b/v). Others could be reflective of AAE, notably the reduction of the final consonant cluster (e.g., "hep"/"help"); however, final consonant clusters are often reduced by 4-year-old children speaking SAE.

This child's morphology also shows features of later developing morphologic features (e.g., "this how"/*this is how* [omits copula]) and irregular past-tense verbs (e.g., "fall"/"fell," "come"/"came," "say"/"said"). Although they could be identified as features of AAE, it is not uncommon for these forms also to be omitted by 4-year-old children using SAE (Shipley et al. 1991; Brown 1973). The child's articulation and morphology are within normal limits for 4-year-old speakers of both AAE and SAE.

Differentiating Between Spanish-Influenced English and Communication Disorders

One of the most rapidly growing populations in the United States is the LEP population, consisting of people whose native language is other than English. The largest group of LEP students are those whose first language is Spanish. In the United States, the primary groups of Spanish speakers are from Puerto Rico and other Caribbean islands, Mexico, and Central America. Although there are differences in vocabulary and some pronunciation, the dialects are mutually intelligible. Differential diagnosis of communication disorders from dialects and normal development are further complicated by the development of second-language acquisition in Spanish-influenced English. There are few scientifically controlled studies on phonology of bilingual children. Most of the research information has come from case studies.

As shown in Table 2.3, there are several sound features of Spanish that are different from the sounds of English. Spanish has five vowels and four diphthongs, while English has 12–14 vowels (Cheng 1993; Langdon 1992). While English vowels can be produced in the front, mid, or back positions and can show variations in duration and stress patterns, Spanish vowels are usually produced in the front or back positions and have little duration difference, full pronunciation, and only strong and weak stress patterns. The English vowels /æ/, /ʌ/, and /ɪ/ do not exist in Spanish. These differences influence the production of vowels spoken by native Spanish speakers. For example, because there is no /ɪ/ in Spanish, /bɪt/ ("bit") is pronounced as /bit/ ("beat").

Table 2.3
Common phonetic differences between Spanish and English

Substitution	*Example*
s/z	"sebra"/"zebra"
ʃ/ʧ	"shair"/"chair"
tʃ/ʃ	"chip"/"ship"
d/ð	"den"/"then"
t/θ	"tief"/"thief"
f/v	"fan"/"van"
b/v	"berry"/"very"
ʊ/u	"pull"/"pool"
i/ɪ	"cheap"/"chip"
ə/ou	"call"/"coal"
esp/sp	"Espanish"/"Spanish"
s/st	"sove"/"stove"
esn/sn	"esnow"/"snow"
Omission of final /s/	"bu"/"bus"

Source: Adapted from H Langdon. (1992) *Hispanic Children and Adults with Communication Disorders*. Gaithersburg, MD: Aspen.

The consonant systems of Spanish and English also differ. English sounds that do not exist in Spanish include /θ, ð, z, ʃ, ʒ/. The /s/ clusters (e.g., *st, sp*, and *sk*) are used only in the medial position in Spanish; /e/ plus the cluster is used in the initial position (e.g., *esp/sp*) (Langdon 1992). Unvoiced consonants /p, t, k, f/ are omitted or weakened in the final position. Some voiced consonants are devoiced, especially in the final position. Alveolar /d, t, n, l/ are often produced as linguadentals, and /θ/ is produced as /d/. The phonemes /ʃ, ʤ, ʧ/ are produced with fronting, and /h/ is often palatalized. Two Spanish consonants do not exist in English: trilled /rr/ as in *perro* and /ñ/ as in *mañana*.

The development of phonology in monolingual Spanish speakers between 3 and 6 years of age is similar to that of SAE speakers. By the age of 4 years, all but /rr, b, p, s, w/ were mastered in a study reported by Linares (1981). By the age of 6 years, all of these later-developing phonemes were developed. Eblen (1982) and Acevedo (1989) reported that by the age of 4 years, Mexican American monolingual Spanish speakers acquired all but the liquids and glides /j, l, rr/, /d, ʧ/, and /s/. The sounds /g, d, f, x, r, ñ/ were mastered after the age of 4 years, with /j, r, rr, s/ and /ʧ/ being more difficult. In differentiating use of dialect from normal speech-sound development, the clinician must consider the normal development of articulation in the language spoken by the child.

In general, the morphologic markers of English are often omitted or overgeneralized by speakers of Spanish dialects, because the Spanish does

Table 2.4
Common morphologic and syntactic features of Spanish and their influence on English

Feature	*English*	*Example of Spanish-Influenced English*
Possessive noun	This is the mother's house.	This is the house of the mother.
Nonobligatory plural *-s*	The girls are playing.	The girl are playing.
Nonobligatory past *-ed*	I talked to her yesterday.	I talk to her yesterday.
Nonobligatory article	I am going to the store.	I am going to store.
Nonobligatory auxiliary	He is going.	He going to store.
Nonobligatory third person singular	The boy eats dinner.	The boy eat dinner.
Future go + to	I will go to the store.	I go to store.
Nonobligatory infinitive *to*	I go to school.	I go school.
Nonobligatory pronoun	Then she came back.	Then came back.
Addition of pronoun	The cow came.	The cow he came.
Double negatives	I don't want any.	I don't want no one.
Negative before verb	The man is *not* tall.	The man no is tall.
No used for *don't*	Don't throw stones.	No throw stones.
Adjective after noun	The green tree.	The tree green.
No question inversion	Is Maria going?	Maria is going?
Nonobligatory *do* insertion	Do you like ice cream?	You like ice cream?

not have a comparable English form, the English morphologic system is more complex, or the form is marked in another way. For example, as shown in Table 2.4, articles, auxiliaries and modals, contractions, copula, the gerund *-ing* ending, the plural *-s*, the possessive *-s*, the past regular *-ed*, and the third person *-s* are often omitted or overgeneralized by LEP speakers. Prepositions and pronouns are often substituted or show agreement error because of the complexity of the systems in English (Owens 1995a). As shown in Table 2.5, the order for the acquisition of grammatical morphemes in the dialects of Spanish is similar to that for the development of English. The natural order may not surface during the administration of sentence-completion grammatical tests and is more likely to appear in conversation. As with AAE, the natural features of Spanish-influenced English must be distinguished from the normal development of dialect.

Speech-Language Disorders Versus Normal Second-Language Acquisition

The combination of a possible communication disability, the effects of second-language acquisition, and LEP makes differential diagnosis of com-

Table 2.5
Comparison of order of acquisition of grammatical morphemes between English as a second language and English as first language

English as a second language	*English*
-ing	*-ing*
Plural	Plural
Copula (*to be*)	Irregular past
Auxiliary (progressive)	Article
Article (*a, the*)	Regular past
Irregular past	Singular *-s*
Regular past	Possessive
Third-person singular *-s*	Copula
Possessive *-s*	Auxiliary

Source: Adapted from H Langdon. (1992) *Hispanic Children and Adults with Communication Disorders*. Gaithersburg, MD: Aspen.

munication disorders in LEP extremely challenging. Some speakers of Spanish are bilingual with equal proficiency in two languages. Others are considered LEP because they are proficient in their native language (L1) but not in the second language (L2). Some speakers, however, are limited in both L1 and L2. The LEP speaker may be in the process of learning the second language. The effects of language interference, language loss, and language mixing can render the client less proficient in L1 than in L2 at the time of testing. These effects often lead erroneously to the conclusion that the client has a speech-language disorder, because neither L1 nor L2 is developing appropriately. It is important for the speech-language pathologist to understand the effects of second-language learning on both L1 and L2 to identify true language disorders in bilingual individuals.

Simultaneous Versus Sequential Bilingual Language Development

Simultaneous bilingualism occurs when young children develop two languages, usually younger than the age of 3 years. Since they are learning both languages simultaneously, they are usually able to learn each language equally well, particularly if significant caretakers or parents are consistent in the use of the two languages. The children are usually able to code switch or alternate the use of the two languages with a complete separation between the two languages (Kayser 1993, 1995).

Sequential or consecutive bilingualism occurs when the speaker acquires L2 after basic linguistic acquisition of L1 has been achieved (Langdon 1992). Children who are learning L2 sequentially can be at various stages of acquisition of both L1 and L2.

The monolingual age-stage model of development is inappropriate in describing L2 because of the many variables that affect second-language learning, according to Cummins (1984, 1994). The acquisition of first and second languages is interdependent. In general, competence in L2 is related to the maturity of L1. If L1 is not well developed before learning L2, it is possible that neither language will reach proficiency. The more mature the child's use of L1, the easier it is to learn L2. A synthesis of research conducted by Collier (1989) on second-language acquisition found that it does not matter when before puberty children begin to learn a second language, as long as the first language is developed before L2 is introduced. If the child stops development of L1 before it is sufficiently developed, the child will experience negative cognitive effects on second-language development. Research also suggests that older children (ages 8–12 years) who have had several years of education in the first language are most efficient in the second language.

Research on second-language acquisition indicates that when children are exposed to two languages, both language minority and language majority children generally reach language competence sufficient for social language, mathematics, and language arts in 2–3 years. They may require from 4 to 7 years to reach language competence sufficient for academic success in verbal tasks, such as social studies, reading, and science. The data also indicate that adolescents who have had no second-language exposure, and who are not able to continue academic work in their first language while they are acquiring the second language, may never reach the fiftieth percentile on standardized tests. LEP students are often misdiagnosed as having a language or learning disorder because of the discrepancy between their ability in L1 and L2 in various subjects when they are in the normal process of second-language learning (Baca 1990). This misdiagnosis is often due to unrecognized effects of language loss, language mixing, and language interference.

Language Loss

Language loss is the loss or decline of a first or second language because of lack of use. Language loss is a natural phenomenon as speakers become more proficient in one language and prefer its use in settings out of the home (Langdon 1992). As the speaker becomes more involved in the monolingual environment, he or she uses English (L2) more often than his or her first language (L1) and becomes less proficient in L1. While he or she is developing competence in the second language, the speaker is often identified as having a language disorder, because neither the first language nor the second language is used well. It is important to take a careful history of language use in the school, work, and home environments and a history of language development in both languages. This will allow the clinician to distinguish normal second-language acquisition from the effects of language loss.

Language Mixing

Language mixing occurs when entire linguistic units from one language are attached to units of another language, resulting in speech patterns not common to either language. Language mixing is illustrated in the sentence, "Pero verdad que it was worth it" ("But the truth is that it was worth it"). Words of the dominant language are more frequently used in the sentences of the nondominant or weaker language. The speaker may also use pronunciation, rhythm, intonation, and other suprasegmental features of the dominant language while speaking the other language (Kayser 1995). The normal characteristics of language mixing are often misidentified as language disorders by persons not familiar with the languages being used.

Language Interference

Language interference occurs when the sounds of one language interfere with the production of the sounds of the other language, giving the appearance of a speech disorder. It is common for speakers of Spanish to use the following sounds in place of the SAE sounds, because of the effects of language interference (Langdon 1992):

s/z
/"*s*ebra"/"*z*ebra"

ʃ/ʧ
/"*sh*air"/"*ch*air"

ʧ/ʃ
"*ch*ip"/"*sh*ip"

d/ð
"*d*en"/"*th*en"

t/θ
"*t*ief"/"*th*ief"
"ba*t*"/"ba*th*"

f/v
"*f*an"/"*v*an"

b/v
"*b*erry"/"*v*ery"

u/ʊ
"p*u*ll"/"p*oo*l"

i/ɪ
"ch*ea*p"/"ch*i*p"

ʌ/ou
"c*a*ll"/"c*oa*l"

esp/sp
"*Es*panish"/"*S*panish"

Language interference can also be present in morphology and syntax. As a child acquires the second language, he or she may use the word order from L1 and the semantics or words from L2. Because flexibility in syntax is permissible in Spanish, for example, it is acceptable to say "The moon looks pretty" as either "Se ve linda la luna" (Looks pretty the moon) or "La luna se ve linda" (The moon look pretty). Variations in SAE word order within noun phrases should not be confused with language disorder by speakers of Spanish-influenced English.

Differentiating Code Switching and Language Impairment in Bilingual Adults

Code switching is a socially and grammatically rule-governed alternation between languages across and within contexts (Aquirre 1988). Poplack (1982) delineated four characteristics of code switching in normal bilingual adults: (1) smooth transition between L1 and L2 without false starts, hesitations, or lengthy pauses; (2) seamless transition or alternation between the two languages; (3) segments of larger than single nouns in one language inserted in a sentence of the other language; and (4) code switching used for expressing otherwise untranslatable items. Clinicians should be familiar with the code switching patterns of adult bilinguals in determining the presence of a disorder, so that normal code switching is not misidentified as characteristics of disfluency or language difficulty.

All adult bilingual speakers are not proficient in code switching in all circumstances. Some speakers code switch only when speaking the second language to add information or emphasis in the stronger language or when a concept or lexical item is more explicit in one language than the other. Others code switch when they find difficulty expressing a concept in the weaker language (Lipski 1985). According to Valdes-Fallis (1978), it is rare for Mexican American adult bilinguals to code switch in conversations with English-speaking monolinguals.

Certain causes of neurologic impairments, such as cardiovascular disease and stroke, trauma, and infectious disease, disproportionately affect minority individuals, including Hispanic adults (Reyes 1995; Wallace 1993). Differential diagnosis of speech-language disorders in bilingual adults with neurologically based language disorders is more challenging than that among monolingual adults. There have been few studies of the effect of aging or aphasia on bilingual adults. Albert and Obler (1978) reviewed 107 cases of bilingual aphasics selected from the literature and reported that individuals who had acquired aphasia before the age of 65 years first reacquired the language used at the time of the injury, regardless of their principal language. In patients older than 65, there was no clear parameter of recovery. Research examining the use of language following stroke or neurologic disease in bilingual adults is limited. Albert and Obler (1978) and Hamers and Blanc (1989) indicated that bilinguals rarely produce language mixing qualitatively different from the code-switching patterns that they used premorbidly. In some cases, however, the symptoms of aphasia observed in one language were different from the symptoms observed in the other language. Paradis (1995), however, believes that code switching is potentially impaired in bilinguals with aphasia. Muñoz et al. (1997) showed that code switching among bilinguals with aphasia was qualitatively and quantitatively different from that of normal bilinguals in the same community. The aphasic bilinguals code switched more frequently than the normal bilinguals; and the aphasic bilingual experiences communication breakdowns associated with code switching. In assessing the language performance of posttraumatic aphasic bilingual clients, it is important to consider the language history of the client, their manner of second-language acquisition, and their premorbid pattern of language attrition, code switching, and language mixing.

Differentiating Language Disorders from Second-Language Learning

There are many verbal and nonverbal behaviors specific to various cultures that can be misidentified as behaviors indicating a communication disorder. Nonverbal and verbal behaviors of children who are culturally or linguistically diverse can be and often are misidentified as indicators of communication disorders (Hoover and Collier 1985). Children who are culturally different may be withdrawn and nonverbal in the classroom. They may not interact verbally with their peers and prefer to be alone. They may not respond or may make a minimal verbal response when spoken to by the teacher, because they are unsure of their ability to use appropriate language skills. This is particularly true of students learning a second language and adapting to a new culture. It may also be culturally appropriate for the child not to respond when unsure of the response. For example, Native American children are taught to observe behaviors before attempting to respond in new situations. The lack of response can be misinterpreted as a communication disorder (Harris 1993).

A preschool child may be silent for a while when initially exposed to L2, giving the impression of language disorder. Older children may have difficulty with L2 in the decontextualized, cognitively demanding academic environment, yet they may have good basic communication skills. Their competence in basic interpersonal communication skills may mislead the clinician to believing that the client has the ability to deal with decontextualized, cognitively demanding language skills required for academic success. The child may be diagnosed as having a communication or language disorder, when he or she is actually in the process of acquiring cognitive academic language proficiency (Cummins 1984).

When exposed to the unstructured environment of American schools, Asian children may exhibit a range of reactions from withdrawal to overexuberance due to a lack of understanding limits (Olion and Gillis-Olion 1984). During a one-on-one testing situation, Asian students may exhibit stress because of a cultural difference in the reason for testing. In many Asian countries, testing is used to screen out students from programs. One-on-one relationships with teachers and educators are not common in Asian countries. These cultural differences create tremendous pressure and can reduce performance ability.

New immigrant, culturally different children may appear to be disorganized in school, because they have difficulty keeping their belongings or bringing required materials from home. The child may not be familiar with the supplies necessary for school and may not have the requested materials in the home. The child may appear to waste time, fail to keep schedules, or not complete assignments within the prescribed time period. Such behavior may be caused by the concept of time in the child's home culture, which may be different from the concept of time used in school.

Just as it is unacceptable to identify speakers with the effects of language loss, language mixing, or language interferences as having a language disorder, it is also unacceptable to fail to identify persons with LEP who have a true communication disorder. Among the indicators of language-learning disabilities that are also characteristic of students in the process of learning English are significant discrepancies between verbal and performance measures on intelligence tests; academic learning difficulty; social and emotional problems; attention and memory problems; and hyperactivity, hypoactivity, and impulsivity (Mercer 1987).

Mattes and Omark (1991) and Kayser (1990) identified observable communication behaviors for Spanish- and English-speaking language-impaired clients that can be useful in distinguishing between the effects of second-language learning and true disorders. These observable behaviors include the following:

1. Client rarely initiates verbal interactions or activities with peers or family members.
2. Client does not respond verbally when verbal interactions are initiated by peers or family members.
3. Client does not engage in dialogue or conversation with peers or family members outside the classroom.
4. Client uses gestures rather than speech to communicate with peers.
5. Peers indicate that they have difficulty understanding the client's oral communications, nonverbal communications, or both.
6. Peers rarely initiate verbal interactions with the client.
7. The client's nonverbal aspects of communication are perceived by peers as being inappropriate.
8. Client does not attempt to repair communication failures.
9. Client does not comment on his or her actions or the actions of others, express feelings, or express needs like age peers.
10. Client does not follow directions or attend to the speaker.
11. Client does not take turns during conversations or maintain topic.
12. Client does not request information or clarification.

Suggestions for Assessment of Clients with Limited English Proficiency

Special care is necessary to assure unbiased assessment for LEP students. Under the Individuals with Disabilities Education Act (PL 107-15), all tests and materials are to be provided and administered in the client's native language unless it is clearly not feasible to do so. In assessing the speech-language ability of LEP clients, the speech-language pathologist should observe the client in several settings with different conversational partners, topics, and activities. Communication ability in both L1 and L2 should be assessed. Testing in the stronger language first, followed by testing in the weaker language, usually results in the best performance, especially for children from monolingual homes. Simultaneous testing can be best for children with poor performance in both L1 and L2 (Cummins 1984).

When the speech-language pathologist does not have native or near-native proficiency in the use of both languages, speech-language assessment can be assisted by the use of interpreters. Damico (1991) suggested several questions to ask in interpretation of assessment data for bilingual or LEP clients:

1. Are there variables, other than disorder, that could explain difficulties with English, such as limited exposure to English, infrequency of the error, procedural mistakes, or differences in exposure to testing situations?
2. Are similar problems exhibited in both L1 and L2?
3. Are the problems related to second-language acquisition, including language loss, language mixing, or language interference?
4. Are the problems related to dialectal differences?
5. Can the problems be explained by cross-cultural interference or related cultural phenomena?
6. Can the problems be related to bias in the materials or procedures?
7. Is there any system or consistency to the linguistic problems exhibited that could suggest an underlying rule?

CASE 2

Anna, a 3½-year-old child, relocated from Puerto Rico to New York City with her parents and older sister. The parents attended English classes and began to use some English at home, although their primary language was Spanish. Her sister attended elementary school and, with her family's encouragement, began to use English at home. Anna was enrolled in an English-only Head Start program. Immediately on enrollment, she was given a speech-language screening test in English. Because she did not pass the screening test, she was referred to a local speech-language program.

During the evaluation, Anna was observed at play with her older sister. During play she spoke freely using long sentences in Spanish using age-appropriate syntax. Neither her sister nor the interpreter had any difficulty understanding her. Occasionally, while they played, her sister reminded her to speak English, at which time Anna would switch to English. There was no alteration in her use of syntax or her ease in communicating when she used English. The following is representative of her performance on the Goldman-Fristoe Test of Articulation (Goldman and Fristoe 1986):

Target	Production	Analysis
telephone	"telefo"	final /n/ omission
scissors	"tis s"	t/s, s/z
matches	"mæshis"	ʃ/θ, s/z
feather	"fweder"	d/ð
this	"dis"	d/ð
bathtub	"bæ tup"	θ omitted
bath	"bæf"	f/θ
thumb	"tum"	t/θ
brush	"bluch"	bl/br, θ/ʃ
drum	"klum"	kl/dr
Christmas tree	"slima trri"	sl/kr, /s/ omitted, trr/tr
squirrel	"ekwowo"	ek/sk, w/r, final /l/ omitted
shovel	"chobo"	t/ʃ, b/v, final /l/ omitted
stove	"tob"	t/st, b/v

Analysis of the pattern shows that most errors can be accounted for by either development (i.e., f/θ) or dialectal differences—notably, ʧ/ʃ, d/ð, t/θ, s/z, t/st, rr/r, l/r, and ek/sk. Anna's articulation was showing the influence of Spanish on her English articulation and should not be considered a disorder.

Differentiating Communication Disorders from Verbal and Nonverbal Variables in Assessment

Nonverbal Aspects of Testing

Because culturally and linguistically diverse students have been found to perform better on nonverbal tests than on verbal ones (Gerken 1978), nonverbal ability should be stressed with culturally and linguistically diverse clients. Although nonverbal tests do not require verbal expression, there are cultural variables that affect the testing situation.

Perception and Use of Time

Cultures vary in their perception of time. In Western cultures, time perception is rigid or linear. Clients start and finish tasks without interruption and attempt to complete the task quickly. Clients begin tasks on time, finish tasks in the appropriate time, and, thus, do well on timed tasks.

In non-Western cultures, such as Hispanic and Middle Eastern cultures, time markers are not rigid. Clients are not pressed by time constraints. These clients are at a disadvantage in timed tests. They may not progress quickly through items, may leave items uncompleted for lack of time, or they may not attend to the uncompleted task for the duration of the testing period.

Clients who have a cognitive style that requires a longer contemplative response time may be penalized in test items that require a quick response. If the tester believes that the longer response time indicates that the client does not know the answer, the tester may penalize the client. For example, Navajo and Pueblo Indian clients prefer a longer wait time before responding and prefer a longer time following a response before speaking again. What clinicians perceive as a completed response is often a contemplative pause by a Navajo client (Harris 1993).

In some Asian cultures, speed and accuracy in tasks are reinforced. The clients may sacrifice speed for accuracy. The clinician must remind the client that accuracy is at least as important as speed, if not more so (Kitano and Chinn 1986).

Learning and Display Learning

Clients from Western European cultures are encouraged to display what they know and to guess, rather than let it be thought that they do not know an answer. They are willing to attempt unfamiliar test items or test formats, are willing to guess when they are uncertain, and are willing to change their response if necessary.

Clients from non-Western cultures, such as African American, Asian and Pacific Islander, or Native American, prefer not to display what they know until they are certain that they are correct. They are socialized to observe before attempting a task, are hesitant to attempt unfamiliar tasks, resist trial-and-error approaches to test items, resist guessing, and are reluctant to change their answer after they have made a response.

Group Versus Individual

Clients from Western cultures are competitive and strive for individual recognition and achievement. In test situations, they strive to obtain a high score to earn individual recognition. They are concerned about their number of correct answers and are often overly concerned when they are not correct. This is especially true as they reach a ceiling and become aware that their responses may not be correct.

Non-Western clients strive for recognition and to bring honor to the group or family. Assurance that family members will be pleased at the success serves as a motivator during testing. The perception of failure can result in a lack of response or willingness to continue the task for fear of bringing shame to the family.

Sociolinguistic Dimensions

Multicultural clients are also affected by the social relationship between themselves and the clinician. Clients from some cultures have a conflict between their race and gender and that of the clinician. Terrell and colleagues (1996) showed that, in general, African Americans across educational, socioeconomic, gender, and geographical strata do not trust whites. African American children who had a high level of mistrust of whites obtained lower test scores on intelligence tests than persons with low levels of mistrust (Terrell and Terrell 1983). It can be expected, then, that clients who have mistrust of the clinician will not do well on speech-language tests in cross-racial testing situations (Terrell and Terrell 1993).

Normal language development is significantly related to the socioeconomic status of the family, as determined by combinations of factors, including occupation, education of the parents (especially the mother), income, and lifestyle (Ratusnik and Koenigsknecht 1975). The literature highlights differences in the language environment of young children in working-class and middle-class homes according to the particular values and beliefs of their language community (Heath 1982; Lynch and Hanson 1992). Failure to consider the socioeconomic status of children and the opportunity of children to learn the characteristics of language considered to be important by the dominant culture can result in overidentification of disorders in culturally and linguistically diverse children.

Verbal Aspects of Testing

There are several aspects of testing that are directly related to verbal language use. These differences affect the ability of the culturally and linguistically diverse clients to perform in the test situation.

Language Function

The rules for language function across cultures affect the client's manner of responding in the testing situation, particularly among young children. In assessing speech-language disorders in culturally and linguistically diverse students, functional or pragmatic criteria are more indicative of a disability than surface-oriented criteria such as syntax, morphology, or phonology. Clients who have difficulty in functional and pragmatic skills, such as excessive pauses, delays before responding, use of inappropriate responses, use of nonspecific vocabulary, and poor topic maintenance, are more likely than clients who have difficulty with syntactic form to have a disability. In a study reported by Cummins (1984), children identified as normal according to pragmatic criteria seemed to make substantial gains in academic achievement, while those judged abnormal by syntax and morphologic criteria failed to make comparable gains. Further, children identified as having language disorders according to the pragmatic criteria failed to make substantial academic gains, while some children who probably would have been identified as disordered according to syntax-morphology criteria made normal gains in school achievement (Hamayan and Damico 1991).

Preparation for testing situations is a cultural phenomenon. The child's preparation for testing is largely a factor of the type, quality, and quantity of interactions that vary as result of parents' educational level, home language, ethnicity, and socioeconomic status (Erickson and Iglesias 1986).

Much of speech-language evaluation depends on the client's ability to interact with the evaluator in a variety of discourse forms, including conversations, recounts or verbalized memories of past events, story telling, and other narrative genres. However, the use of discourse differs across cultures. Clinicians should be aware of cultural variation in discourse styles to differentiate between culturally appropriate discourse patterns and disorders.

There are cultural differences that affect the child's ability to engage in discourse. In mainstream homes, children are active verbal participants in sustained conversations. Parents encourage their children to look at books and pictures and to label pictures, answer questions, and retell stories assisted by scaffolding provided by adults. In other homes, children are passive participants in conversations. They have little experience in looking at pictures in books with verbal input from caretakers, are rarely read fantasy or fiction stories, and do not engage in story retelling or recounts of past events (Farran 1982; Heath 1982, 1983, 1986a). When children from passive homes are asked to engage in picture naming or picture identification test items, there is a communicative mismatch between the child's communication skills and those expected in the testing situation. The child may not do well on items that depend on his or her previous preliteracy skill development with picture identification, picture naming, story telling, and recounts.

Cultural differences in question function must also be considered in testing situations. According to Heath (1982), in mainstream homes, questions are used to engage children in question-answer routines that are intended to teach picture-identification and picture-naming tasks. These questions are used for instruction and are common activities in homes in which the development of literacy is important. Such families challenge their children to expand on answers and ask for clarification, explanations, event casts, and recounts. Children from such homes come to the testing situation able to identify pictures and to respond to questions as demanded in most standardized tests.

In the homes of working-class families, children are asked genuine questions (i.e., those to which the adult does not know the answer), such as "Where are your shoes?" The children are encouraged to provide only the direct answer to the question without elaboration. These children have less practice and experience with the tasks that are needed to be successful in testing situations and are more likely to obtain a lower score because of their unfamiliarity with the task (Heath, 1983).

Children from cultures that do not encourage students to ask questions of adults or authority figures do not ask questions for clarification during test situations. To ask a question is considered disrespectful, implying that the clinician did not give adequate instruction. This is a particular problem when children are exposed to an unfamiliar test format with unfamiliar directions. Test takers may not perform the test item correctly and thus be penalized by obtaining a score that does not reflect true ability.

Finally, persons from non-Western cultures often do not respond to questions when they are not sure of the answer or if they believe the question is personal. This also impacts the clinician's perception of the client's ability to answer questions.

Language Content

There is cultural variation in the concepts taught to children. Preacademic skills, such as color names, shapes, numbers, object names, reading routines, and prewriting skills, are important parts of Western middle-class homes. In non-Western and impoverished homes, children are expected to learn such concepts in school. These homes focus on socialization skills, group cooperation, and family roles, rather than on specific content. Children from these homes do not do well on tests that have heavy content in preacademic skills, such as the Preschool Language Scale–III (Zimmerman 1992). If color words are not important in a culture, a child's response when asked to define *brown*, as on the Test of Language Development P:2 Oral Vocabulary Subtest (Newcomer and Hammill 1988), is influenced by the child's lack of exposure to the term rather than his or her ability to describe concepts orally.

There is bias in the way words and concepts are represented on vocabulary tests and in application of norms. There are few norms available to establish what is appropriate lexical development for culturally and linguistically diverse children. For example, there are no appropriate tests to determine appropriate lexical or vocabulary development for Native American children living on reservations. What is appropriate lexical development for recent Chinese immigrants from Beijing or Taiwan versus those from Hong Kong? Tests that purport to provide assessment of vocabulary or concepts in a particular language or dialect fail to account for the tremendous difference in language experiences across cultures and the lack of developmental norms for the particular group being tested.

Certain vocabulary words do not translate easily from one language or dialect to another. For example, in Navajo *construction* is translated as *there is a man hitting a board with a hammer*. If a child gave this response, he or she would be misidentified as using circumlocution or having a word-finding problem.

Certain vocabulary items can be easily represented in a particular culture. Some concepts develop early in one culture but do not develop until a later age or develop differently for a child in another culture. For example, a child living in the rural Midwest may not develop an understanding of vocabulary items more common in cities, such as *hydrant* or *curb*. A child reared in Nebraska may develop the concept *ocean* later than a child reared in Florida or California. There is no word for *crib* in Korean. *Hitting with a stick* in English is translated as *sticking* in Spanish; however, one cannot *stick* a ball in Spanish. Even items on articulation tests are subject to cultural bias in selection of vocabulary. For example, the use of Santa Claus and Christmas tree on the Goldman-Fristoe Test of Articulation (Goldman and Fristoe 1986) is culturally biased against children from non-Christian homes and cultures where Christmas is not observed. These differences in vocabulary and semantic meanings make the use of vocabulary tests a questionable practice for the identification of communication disorders in culturally and linguistically different children.

Language Organization

The way language is organized differs across languages. The narrative style of children from lower- or working-class families is organized differently from that of children from middle-class families (Campbell 1994; Heath 1982; Michaels 1981). Middle-class children produce topic-centered linear narratives tightly structured on a single topic or a series of closely related topics with no major shifts in perspectives. Because there is a lack of shared knowledge, their narratives contain precise detail and a high degree of temporal organization, with a temporal or sequential organization that begins with a temporal grounding and statement of focus; followed by the introduction of key agents, developed through elaboration of the theme or topic; and ending with a resolution of the problem.

According to Heath (1986b), children from working-class families produce associative narratives consisting of a series of associated segments implicitly linked by topic, theme, or event. The topics are marked by shifts across segments often marked by changes in pitch and tempo.

Because there is a presumed shared knowledge, there is less detail. Narratives are longer because of the increased number of themes. Topic-associated narratives can be interpreted as lacking cohesion, sequence, and focus, rather than a well-developed, culturally appropriate narrative style. Differences in organization or structure of language across cultures must be considered when evaluating whether the observed behavior is a speech-language disorder, the reflection of normal development, or a reflection of cultural organization of language.

ETHNOGRAPHIC PROCEDURES

Using Ethnographic Procedures in Differential Diagnosis

The more superficial and limited the scope of language capability tapped in a testing instrument, the greater the likelihood that the instrument will be inappropriate for speakers beyond the immediate population on which it was normed (Westby 1997; Wolfram 1983).

Standardized and norm-referenced tests produce test results that are biased against culturally and linguistically diverse clients, those of low socioeconomic status, and those with existing disabilities. To be used appropriately, standardization criteria of normative tests must be representative of the various cultures, including racial and ethnic groups, social class, and geographical regions, in addition to such variables as age and gender. Standardized tests usually do not account for the verbal and nonverbal variables related to testing, nor do they account for cultural and linguistic variables.

The following guidelines, adapted from Vaughn-Cooke (1983), are useful for evaluating assessment instruments for use with cultural and linguistic minority clients:

1. Can the procedure account for verbal and nonverbal cultural and linguistic variations?
2. Will the sociologic assumptions underlying the social occasion of the testing and the particular elicitation techniques influence the results of the test?
3. Are the assumptions about language and communication that underlie the procedure valid?
4. What is the relationship of the norming population and the client?
5. What is the client's experience with the content area of the test? Has the client had an opportunity to learn the content?
6. Does the procedure include a culturally based analysis of a spontaneous speech sample?

7. Does the procedure allow the reliable determination of whether the system is developing normally? What is the relationship of the language, dialect, or both being tested and the client's language, language dominance, or both? How does the client function within his or her linguistic or dialectal community?
8. Can the test distinguish between those differences that can be attributed to dialect and cultural differences? Can the results of the test be adjusted to account for dialect differences? Would the test be able to distinguish those speakers with a true pathology from those that use indigenous community dialect?
9. Can the procedure provide an adequate description of the client's knowledge of language?
10. Do the results provide principled guidelines for culturally based recommendations?

Ethnographic Assessment of Speech and Language in Culturally and Linguistically Different Clients

Ethnographic assessment techniques facilitate the diagnosis of communication disorders in culturally and linguistically diverse clients by enabling the evaluator to collect data through behavioral descriptions in naturalistic contexts. This increases the representativeness, reliability, and validity of the data used to determine possible communication difficulties (Cheng 1990). Through triangulation of cultural, linguistic, and experiential factors, ethnographic assessment increases the validity of the data and reduces potential biases that frequently arise when assessing culturally and linguistically diverse clients. Finally, because data collected in ethnographic assessment are filtered through the client's culture, the interpretation of the assessment data is less biased and more valid.

In spite of the acknowledged difficulty with the use of standardized test procedures to document a client's disability, standardized tests are often required to verify that a disability exists. The client's performance on standardized tests must be interpreted against the sources of cultural bias, lack of opportunity to learn the required material, unfamiliarity with the test item or test format, and difficulty in the social situation of testing. Several methods in the numbered paragraphs that follow are suggested to employ ethnographic assessment techniques and to modify tests to make them more useful; however, caution must be taken not to assume that the use of any or all of these procedures eliminates the bias present in the testing situation itself (Erickson and Iglesias 1986; Hamayan and Damico 1991; Vaughn-Cooke 1983; Westby 1990). It is important that the clinician:

1. *Understand the cultural parameters associated with the particular client being evaluated.* All judgments and decisions must be made within the cultural context. Before the session, the clinician should review the cultural and linguistic variables associated with the client and review all materials and procedures for their appropriateness with the client. Clinicians should not make assumptions about the cultural background or beliefs of clients based on their biological race or country of origin. African American people may have their cultural roots in the Caribbean, any one of the African nations, or from any nation in the world. Asians from Hong Kong, Vietnam, and the Philippines have a strong European influence and are more likely to hold Western beliefs than other Asian groups.

Because socioeconomic status has been linked to language development, clinicians should also not make assumptions about the socioeconomic status of clients. Clear distinctions should be made between race, ethnicity, and socioeconomic status when learning about a client's culture. Each client should be considered from his or her individual, personal culture rather than preconceived cultural notions or racial stereotypes.

2. *Observe the client in multiple contexts with multiple communication partners.* The clinician should become familiar with the verbal and nonverbal aspects of communication relevant to the client's culture. The clinician should observe the client in a variety of communication settings, recording who the client talks to, what he or she talks about, and how the client interacts. Observation of what is difficult and what is successful for the client provides a universal evaluation of the client's ability to communicate in low-anxiety, high-motivation naturalistic environments. The lack of developmental data and data on appropriate cultural communication behavior and expectations within cultural groups makes the evaluation of language samples and other observational data difficult. Without information on acceptable communication behavior within a cultural group, it is not possible to make reliable judgments about the normalcy of a client's communication behavior within the cultural community.

3. *Focus on the universal aspects of language.* Since the parameters of phonology and vocabulary are greatly influenced by dialect and second language, language assessment of the culturally and linguistically different client should focus on the client's ability to communicate using semantically and pragmatically appropriate strategies. Family members or age peers can be helpful in creating a more natural communication environment to observe more universal aspects of language.

Dynamic tasks, such as narration and conversation on culturally relevant topics, are appropriate for the speech-language assessment of culturally and linguistically diverse clients as they de-emphasize grammar in favor of ability to communicate (Butler 1993; Damico 1991). Assessment, however, must take into account cultural differences in discourse and narrative style.

4. *Involve families in the assessment.* Family involvement is particularly important in speech-language evaluation of culturally and linguistically diverse children and adults. Because the dynamics and social roles within families are diverse, it is important that the clinician become familiar with the family of the client so that ethnographic procedures can be used in interviewing, assessment, and intervention.

Cultural factors can impede full parental involvement with culturally and linguistically diverse clients. Asian parents may not be accustomed to participating in decisions related to their child's schooling (Kitano and Chinn 1986). Parents may be reluctant to discuss the disability of a family member because of a stigma associated with disabilities (Olion and Gillis-Olion 1984). To some families, the disability can be explained by punishment for sins committed by the parents or their ancestors, or that the client is possessed by evil spirits. In other cultures, a *disabled* person may be considered imperfect or inferior.

Hispanic parents tend to be trusting of school personnel and feel that they are intruding into the school's domain if they express concerns about their child's education (Ortiz and Yates 1983). Ethnographic procedures have the goals of assisting the clinician in understanding the social situation in which the client lives, how the family perceives and understands the problem, and the family's role in the treatment process (Westby 1990).

5. *Interview clients in the language they are most comfortable using, using an interpreter if necessary.* Caution must be taken, however, to prepare the interpreter for the testing situation. This involves briefing the interpreter before the session concerning the nature of the session and cautioning the interpreter to avoid unnecessary rephrasing or radically changing items. When an exact translation is not possible, the translator or interpreter should inform the clinician. Interpreters must also watch their use of gestures, voice patterns, and body language, so as not to inadvertently provide cues to the client. Any nonverbal cues from the client or the interpreter should be noted during the session and should be discussed with the interpreter after the session. After the session, the clinician should review the session with the interpreter and discuss any difficulties that are relevant to the testing process, to the interaction, or to the interpretation of data (Bernstein 1989; Medina 1982).

6. *Use caution when translating tests.* Using interpreters or translating a test into a client's dominant language is a frequently used method to accommodate cultural differences. However, using trans-

lations or interpreters in test administration does not solve the problem of inappropriate test standardization or inappropriate test content (Kayser 1989). The linguistic differences in languages and differences in specific dialects within a language often make translations inappropriate. For example, in Spanish, there are differences in honorifics (e.g., formal *usted* versus familiar *tu*), gender markers (e.g., *el* versus *la*), semantics (e.g., *arroz,* tomato-based and spicy grain, versus *rice,* white or brown grain), structural rules, and registers (e.g., Cuban versus Mexican), as well as social discourse rules. In Spanish, there are few single-syllable words and no spondee words. In Vietnamese, there are plurals and no possessives. Many Native American languages do not have gender pronouns, future tense verbs, or a word for time (Roseberry-McKibbin 1995). These differences in languages make translations equivalent to the original test item impossible. In a study using a Spanish version of the Wechsler Intelligence Scale for Children, Revised (WISC-R) adapted for Puerto Rican students, researchers found that Puerto Rican students in the United States showed a verbal performance discrepancy of 20 points on both English and Spanish versions when compared with their native English-speaking and Puerto Rican peers. The students were not only unfamiliar with some of the English terms but were also unfamiliar with some of the Puerto Rican terms on the Spanish verbal scale, despite being familiar with the English equivalent terms (Cummins 1984).

Few tests are normed for Asian students. Those tests that are normed do not take into account the cultural and linguistic diversity among Asian groups. Attempts to translate intelligence tests for recent Hong Kong and Taiwanese immigrants require a level of Chinese proficiency that few speech pathologists in the United States possess (Kitano and Chinn 1986).

Interpreters may not accurately reflect the intent of the test item, preferring to explain their perceived meaning rather than to directly translate the test item or the response. In addition, translations may not take into account differences in the development of linguistic or semantic concepts, nor do they take into account the linguistic complexity differences between languages.

7. *Use caution in standardizing existing tests for culturally and linguistically diverse populations.* Most commercially available tests are standardized on mainstream cultures. Attempts to standardize tests on particular racial and ethnic or cultural groups usually is not feasible because of the cost involved in developing a large enough representative sample within a particular cultural group. Because there is such heterogeneity among and across cultural groups, any attempt to stan-

dardize a test on "minority populations," in general, results in the same problems that occur with standardization of the test on the mainstream population.

8. *Use tests that include only a representative sample of minorities in the standardization sample with caution.* Some tests attempt to include a representative sample of minorities within the standardization sample. The resultant standardization sample is representative of the group that participated in the standardization. It is not representative of a particular culture or the particular client being tested. The results can only be used to compare the client's performance against the group and cannot be used to indicate whether the client has a speech-language disorder within his or her cultural or linguistic community. Tests used to determine severity and prognosis in aphasia and other adult neurological disorders may also be culturally biased. Most tests for aphasia were developed on educated middle-class whites and may not have considered the linguistic variations used by some African Americans (Kimbarow et al. 1994). James et al. (1997) suggest examining cultural bias in aphasia tests by administering the test to normal samples of African American and white subjects who are equated for age, gender, education, and socioeconomic status. Any difference in performance could be considered to be due to cultural bias.

9. *Modify existing tests and test procedures.* The difficulty with modification of existing tests is similar to the problems involved with translators or interpreters. Lack of equivalency across languages and cultures makes test modification difficult. In addition, the sociolinguistic, verbal, and nonverbal factors in testing itself cannot be modified within the paradigm of the test.

It can be helpful to modify the test administration process by allowing extra time for responding, increasing the number of practice items, removing or adapting potentially culturally biased items, rewording or modifying instructions, continuing beyond the ceiling, or asking the client to explain his or her answer, particularly when the client changes an answer, explains, comments, or demonstrates the answer. The clinician should accept responses that would be appropriate within the client's dialect. The clinician should support the test results with nonstandardized elicitation and criterion-referenced measures. When possible, the clinician should use a dynamic test-teach-retest assessment approach to evaluate the client's learning potential. When reporting results, the clinician should indicate the adjustments that were made and the impact that the modifications made on the client's score.

10. *Obtain a language sample.* If a language sample is used, however, caution must be taken to assess language in a variety of communica-

tion situations, since it has been demonstrated that speakers code switch between their dialect and SAE dependent on the speaking situation and the communication partner.

When calculating the mean length of utterance, the clinician should consider the distribution of morphemes in the client's language (Linares-Orama 1975). For example, in Spanish, one morpheme can have a generic ending (e.g., *-a* [feminine] or *-o* [masculine]), only when the root can have different generic endings. For example, in Spanish *gato* (cat) has two morphemes: *gat* (cat [masculine]) and *-o* (singular). *Luz* (light) has one morpheme, *luz* (no gender and singular). The adjective *alto* (tall) has two morphemes: *alt* and *-o* (masculine and singular). *Grande* (big) has one morpheme: *grande* (no gender and singular). This affects the use of normative data for interpreting the expected age for speakers of Spanish.

11. *Focus on nondialect-specific phonologic features.* Focusing on nondialect-specific errors can help distinguish those persons who have a true disorder from those who are using features of a dialect or are developing phonologic skills.

12. *Focus on nondialect-specific morphologic features.* When assessing the morphologic competence of young speakers, the clinician should focus on those features that are known to be nondialect specific and on those features that are produced in obligatory contexts as defined by the rules of the dialect. In AAE, nondialect specific features include the articles *a* and *the*, past tense auxiliary *be*, relative clauses, infinitive clauses, and adjective and noun word order (Wyatt 1995).

13. *Use criterion-referenced measures.* Criterion-referenced measures are designed to ascertain the client's performance in relation to a specific standard or criterion. The test scores are thus interpreted by comparison with predetermined performance criteria, rather than by comparison with scores of a reference group.

Criterion-referenced testing requires the establishment of a standard against which to compare the client's performance to determine whether it is minimally adequate. The difficulty comes in determining what the criterion should be and the importance of the criterion to effective communication in the particular culture or linguistic community. To determine whether a child has met the criterion, it may be necessary to determine whether the tasks are performed at levels acceptable to his or her culture, by comparing his or her performance with that of age peers in his or her culture or family members rather than with a general norm-referenced test. It may be necessary to observe normal age peers in natural settings to determine criteria for culturally appropriate communication behaviors. The following are examples of criterion-referenced assessment questions (Lee 1989):

- Are the client's receptive skills greater than his or her expressive skills? Are the client's receptive and expressive language skills in the native language appropriate?
- Is the client demonstrating signs of neurologic disability? Does he or she have difficulty retaining concepts that are culturally appropriate? Is he or she able to remember culturally relevant events? Does he or she follow directions in the proper sequence? Does the client show evidence of difficulty with oral motor functioning?
- Is the client functioning at the same level as others in his or her cultural or language group who have similar histories of exposure to the mainstream culture and language?
- Is the client struggling to communicate in his or her native language? With same-language peers? With family members? With siblings?
- How does the client attempt to communicate with peers? Does the client attempt to adapt and revise or repair his or her communication attempt to express his or her ideas?
- Does the client use language to attract attention? Does the client make requests? Does the client initiate communication? Are attempts or lack of attempts to communicate explainable by cultural communication rules?
- Does the client ask questions or request clarification when he or she does not comprehend the message? Is his or her use of questioning appropriate for cultural expectations?
- Has the client learned language and literacy at the same rate as same-culture and same-language age peers?
- How does the client deal with concepts that he or she has had an opportunity to learn versus concepts he or she has had no opportunity to learn? Is the material that the client is able to learn context embedded or context reduced? Are there cues in the environment, or must the client rely on verbal cues alone?
- Is there a difference between the client's ability with basic interpersonal communication skills (i.e., familiar conversation with peers) and his or her cognitive academic language proficiency (i.e., the ability to use language to analyze, synthesize, and evaluate information)?

CONCLUSION

Taylor and colleagues (1987) suggested guidelines for interacting with clients from different cultures. Each clinical encounter should be viewed as a socially situated communicative event subject to cultural rules governing such events. Clients perform differently under differing conditions because of their unique cultural and linguistic backgrounds. Different modes, channels, and functions of communication can evidence differing levels of linguistic and communicative performance. Ethnographic techniques and cultural norms should be used for evaluating behavior and making determinations of language impairment. Possible sources of cultural conflict in assumptions and norms should be identified before interaction and action are taken, to prevent them from influencing the diagnostic situation. Learning about culture is ongoing and should result in constant reevaluation, revision of ideas, and greater sensitivity

REFERENCES

Acevado M. (1989) Typical Spanish Misarticulations of Mexican-American Preschoolers. Presented at the annual meeting of the American Speech-Language-Hearing Association, St. Louis.

Aguirre A. (1988) Code Switching: Intuitive Knowledge and the Bilingual Classroom. In H Garcia, R Chavez (eds), *Ethnolinguistic Issues in Education* (pp. 28–38). Lubbock, TX: Texas Tech University.

Albert ML, Obler LK. (1978) *The Bilingual Brain*. New York: Academic Press.

American Speech-Language-Hearing Association. (1982) Position paper on social dialects. *Asha* 25, 23–24.

Baca L. (1990) *Theoretical and Applied Issues in Bilingual/Cross-Cultural Special Education: Major Implications for Research, Practice, and Policy*. Boulder, CO: BUENO Center for Multicultural Education.

Bernstein DK. (1989) Assessing children with limited English proficiency: current perspectives. *Topics in Language Disorders* 9, 15–20.

Blake I. (1984) Language development in working-class black children: an examination of form, content and use, Ph.D. diss., Columbia University.

Bleile K, Wallach H. (1992) A sociolinguistic investigation of the speech of African-American preschoolers. *American Journal of Speech-Language Pathology* 1, 54–62.

Bridgeforth C. (1989) The Development of Language Functions Among Black Children from Working-Class Families. Presented at the pre-session of the 35th Annual Georgetown University Round Table on Language and Linguistics, Washington, DC.

Brown R. (1973) *A First Language: The Early Stages*. Cambridge, MA: Harvard University Press.

Butler KA. (November 1993) Toward a Model of Dynamic Assessment: Application to Speech. Presented at the Annual Convention of the American Speech-Language-Hearing Association, Anaheim, CA.

Campbell L. (1994) Discourse Diversity and Black English Vernacular. In D Ripich, N Creaghead (eds), *School Discourse Problems* (pp. 93–131). San Diego: Singular Publishing Group.

Cheng L. (1990) Identification of communication disorders in Asian-Pacific students. *Journal of Communication Disorders* 13, 113–119.

Cheng LL. (1993) Asian-American Cultures. In DE Battle (ed), *Communication Disorders in Multicultural Populations* (pp. 38–77). Boston: Butterworth–Heinemann.

Cole L. (1980) A developmental analysis of social dialect features in the spontaneous language of preschool black children, Ph.D. diss., Northwestern University.

Cole L. (1989) E pluribus unum: multicultural imperatives for the 1990's and beyond. *Asha* 31, 65–70.

Collier V. (1989) How long? A synthesis of research on academic achievement in a second language. *TESOL Quarterly* 23, 509–531.

Craig H, Washington H. (1994) The complex syntax skills of poor, urban African American preschoolers at school entry. *Language Speech and Hearing Services in Schools* 25, 181–190.

Cummins J. (1984) *Bilingualism and Special Education: Issues in Assessment and Pedagogy*. Austin, TX: PRO-ED.

Cummins J. (1994) Interdependence of First and Second Language Proficiency in Bilingual Children. In E Bialystok (ed), *Language Processing of Bilingual Children* (pp. 87–105). Cambridge, MA: Cambridge University Press.

Damico JS. (1991) Descriptive Assessment of Communicative Ability in LEP Students. In EV Hamayan, JS Damico (eds), *Limiting Bias in the Assessment of Bilingual Students* (pp. 157–218). Austin, TX: PRO-ED.

DeStefano J. (1972) Social Variation in Language: Implications for Teaching Reading to Black Ghetto Children. In JA Figurel (ed), *Better Reading in Urban Schools* (pp. 18–24). Newark, DE: International Reading Association.

Eblin RE. (1982) A study of the acquisition of fricatives by three-year-old children learning Mexican Spanish. *Language and Speech* 25, 201–220.

Erickson JG, Iglesias SA. (1986) Speech and Language Disorders in Hispanics. In O Taylor (ed), *Nature of Communication Disorders in Culturally and Linguistically Diverse Populations* (pp. 181–218). San Diego: College-Hill Press.

Farran D. (1982) Mother-Child Interaction, Language Development and School Performance of Poverty Children. In L Feagans, D Farran (eds), *The Language of Children Reared in Poverty: Implications for Evaluation and Intervention*. New York: Academic Press.

Federal Register. (1997) Education of the Handicapped Act Amendments of 1997, PL 107-15.

Gerken KG. (1978) Language dominance: a comparison of measures. *Language, Speech, and Hearing Services in Schools* 9, 187–196.

Goldman R, Fristoe M. (1986) *Goldman-Fristoe Test of Articulation*. Circle Pines, MN: American Guidance Services.

Hamayan EV, Damico J. (1991) *Limiting Bias in the Assessment of Bilingual Students*. Austin, TX: PRO-ED.

Hamers JF, Blanc MH. (1989) *Bilinguality and Bilingualism*. Cambridge, MA: Cambridge University Press.

Harris G. (1993) American Indian Cultures: A Lesson in Diversity. In DE Battle (ed), *Communication Disorders in Multicultural Populations* (pp. 78–113). Boston: Butterworth–Heinemann.

Haynes W, Moran M. (1989) A cross-sectional developmental study of final consonant production in southern black children from preschool to third grade. *Language, Speech, and Hearing Services in Schools* 21, 400–406.

Heath SB. (1982) What no bedtime story means: narrative skills at home and school. *Language in Society* 11, 49–76.

Heath SB. (1983) *Ways with Words*. Cambridge, MA: Cambridge University Press.

Heath SB. (1986) Taking a cross-cultural look at narratives. *Topics in Language Disorders* 7, 84–94.

Hester EJ. (1994) The relationship between narrative style, dialect, and reading ability of African-American children, Ph.D. diss., University of Maryland.

Hester EJ. (1996) Narrative of Young African-American Children. In AG Kamhi, KE Pollack, JL Harris (eds), *Communication Development and Disorders in African-American Children* (pp. 227–245). Baltimore: Paul Brookes.

Hicks D. (1991) Kinds of Narrative: Genre Skills among First Graders from Two Communities. In A McCabe, C Peterson (eds), *Developing Narrative Structure* (pp. 55–87). Hillsdale, NJ: Erlbaum Associates.

Hoover JJ, Collier C. (1985) Referring culturally different children: sociological considerations. *Academic Therapy* 20, 503–509.

Hyon S, Sulzby E. (1992, April) Black Kindergarteners Spoken Narrative: Style, Structure, and Task. Paper presented at the annual meeting of the American Educational Research Association, San Francisco.

James TD, Burch-Sims JG, and Wertz RT. (1997) Aphasia testing in African American and Caucasian populations. *Communication Disorders and Sciences in Culturally and Linguistically Diverse Populations* 3(2), 6–7.

Kamhi AG, Pollack KE, and Harris JL (eds). (1996) *Communication Development and Disorders in African-American Children: Research, Assessment, and Intervention* (pp. 19–34). Baltimore: Paul Brookes.

Kayser H. (1989) Speech and language assessment of Spanish-English speaking children. *Language, Speech, and Hearing Services in Schools* 20, 226–244.

Kayser H. (1990) Social communicative behaviors of language disordered Mexican-American students. *Child Language Teaching Therapy* 6, 255–569.

Kayser H. (1993) Hispanic Cultures. In DE Battle (ed), *Communication Disorders in Multicultural Populations* (pp. 114–157). Boston: Butterworth–Heinemann.

Kayser H. (1995) *Bilingual Speech-Language Pathology: An Hispanic Focus*. San Diego: Singular Publishing Group.

Kimbarow ML, Vangel SJ, and Lichtenberg PA. (1994, April) The influence of demographic variables on normal elderly subjects' performance on the Boston Naming Test. Paper presented to the Clinical Aphasiology Conference, Travers City, MI.

Kitano MK, Chinn PC. (1986) *Exceptional Asian Children and Youth*. Reston, VA: The Council for Exceptional Children.

Kovac C. (1980) Children's acquisition of variable features, Ph.D. diss., Georgetown University.

Labov W. (1972) *Language in the Inner City*. Philadelphia: University of Pennsylvania Press.

Langdon HW. (1992) *Hispanic Children and Adults with Communication Disorders*. Gaithersburg, MD: Aspen.

Lee A. (1989) A socio-cultural framework for the assessment of Chinese children with special needs. *Topics in Language Disorders* 9(3), 38–45.

Light R. (1971) Some Observations Concerning Black Children's Conversations. In R Jacobson (ed), *The English Record (Special Anthology Issue and Monograph)* 14, 155–167.

Linares TA. (1981) Articulation Skills in Spanish-Speaking Children. In RV Padilla (ed), *Ethnoperspectives in Bilingual Education Series (Vol. III). Ethnoperspectives in Bilingual Education Research: Bilingual Education Technology* (pp. 363–367). Ypsilanti, MI: University of Michigan Press.

Linares-Orama N. (1975) The language evaluation of preschool Spanish-speaking Puerto-Rican children. Ph.D. diss., University of Illinois, Urbana.

Lipski JM. (1985) *Linguistic Aspects of Spanish-English Language Switching*. Tempe, AZ: Center for Latin American Studies.

Lynch EW, Hanson MJ. (1992). *Developing Cross Cultural Competence: A Guide for Working with Young Children and Their Families*. Baltimore: Brookes Publishing.

Mattes LJ, Omark DR. (1991). *Speech and Language Assessment for the Bilingual Handicapped* (2nd ed). Oceanside, CA: Academic Communication Associates.

Medina V. (1982) *Interpretation and Translation in Bilingual B.A.S.A.* San Diego: Superintendent of Schools, Department of Education.

Melmed PJ. (1971) Black English phonology: the question of reading interference. *Monographs of the Language-Behavior Research Laboratory* 1.

Mercer CD. (1987) *Students with Learning Disabilities* (3rd ed). Columbus, OH: Merrill.

Michaels S. (1981) "Sharing time": children's narrative styles and differential access to literacy. *Language in Society* 10, 423–442.

Moran M. (1993) Final consonant deletion in African American children speaking black English: a closer look. *Language, Speech, and Hearing Services in Schools* 24, 161–166.

Muñoz ML, Copeland G, and Marquard T. (1997) A comparison of the code switching abilities of aphasic and neurologically intact bilinguals. *Communication Disorders and Science in Culturally and Linguistically Diverse Populations* 3(2), 10–11.

National Center for Health Statistics. (1988) *Current Estimates from the National Health Interview Survey*. United States Vital and Health Statistics Series 10, No. 173. DHSS Publication No. 88-1588. Washington, DC: Government Printing Office.

Newcomer, H. (1988) *Test of Language Development*. San Antonio, TX: PRO-ED.

Office of Special Education Programs. (1993) Limited English Proficient Students with Disabilities. Fifteenth Annual Report to Congress on the Implementation of the Individuals with Disabilities Education Act, Appendix F (pp. F-1–F-35). Washington, DC: Office of Special Education.

Olion L, Gillis-Olion M. (1984) *Assessing Culturally Diverse Exceptional Children. Early Childhood Development and Care*. United Kingdom: Science Publishers.

Ortiz A, Yates JR. (1983) Incidence of exceptionality among Hispanics: implications for manpower training. *ABE Journal* 7, 41–51.

Owens RE. (1995a) *Language Development: An Introduction* (4th ed). Boston: Allyn & Bacon.

Owens RE. (1995b) *Language Disorders: A Functional Approach to Assessment and Intervention* (2nd ed). Boston: Allyn & Bacon.

Paradis M. (1995) Introduction: The Need for Distinctions. In M Paradis (ed), *Aspects of Bilingual Aphasia* (pp. 177–205). New York: Elsevier Science.

Poplack S. (1982) "Sometimes I'll start a sentence in Spanish y termino en español": Toward a Typology of Code Switching. In J Amastae, L Elias-Olivares (eds), *Spanish in the United States: Sociolinguistic Aspects* (pp. 230–263). Cambridge, MA: Cambridge University Press.

Ratusnik D, Koenigsknecht R. (1975) Influence of certain clinical variables on Black preschoolers' nonstandard phonological and grammatical performance. *Journal of Communication Disorders* 8, 281–297.

Reveron W. (1978) The acquisition of variable features. Ph.D. diss., Ohio State University.

Reyes BA. (1995) Considerations in the Assessment and Treatment of Neurogenic Communication Disorders in Bilingual Adults. In H Kayser (ed), *Bilingual Speech-Language Pathology: An Hispanic Focus* (pp. 153–182). San Diego: Singular Publishing Group.

Robey B. (1985) America's Asians. *American Demographics* 53, 22–29.

Rosenberry-McKibbin C. (1995) *Multicultural Students with Special Language Needs.* Oceanside, CA: Academic Communication Associates.

Russell C. (1982) Coming alive down South. *American Demographics* 51, 14–25.

Sander E. (1972) When are speech sounds learned? *Journal of Speech and Hearing Disorders* 37, 55–63.

Schick FL, Schick R. (1991) *Statistical Handbook on U.S. Hispanics.* Phoenix: Oryx Press.

Seymour H, Ralabate P. (1985) The acquisition of a phonological features of black English. *Journal of Communication Disorders* 18, 139–148.

Seymour H, Seymour C. (1981) Black English and standard English contrasts in consonantal development of four- and five-year old children. *Journal of Speech and Hearing Disorders* 46, 274–280.

Shipley K, Maddox M, Driver K. (1991) Children's development of irregular past tense verb forms. *Language, Speech, and Hearing Services in Schools* 22, 115–122.

Stockman I, Vaughn-Cooke F, Wolfram W. (1982) *Developmental Study of Black English—Phase I.* Washington, DC: National Institute of Education. Publication NIE G-0135. Final Research Report (ERIC Clearinghouse on Language and Linguistics no. 245556).

Stockman I. (1986) Language Acquisition in Culturally Diverse Populations: The Black Child as a Case Study. In O Taylor (ed), *Nature of Communication Disorders in Culturally and Linguistically Diverse Populations* (pp. 117–155). San Diego: Singular Publishing Group.

Taylor O. (1986) *Nature of Communication Disorders in Culturally and Linguistically Diverse Populations.* San Diego: College-Hill Press.

Taylor O, Payne K, Anderson N. (1987) Distinguishing between communication disorders and communication differences. *Seminars in Speech and Language* 8, 415–427.

Terrell F, Terrell S. (1993) African-American Cultures. In DE Battle (ed), *Communication Disorders in Multicultural Populations* (pp. 3–37). Boston: Butterworth–Heinemann.

Terrell F, Terrell SL. (1983) The relationship between race of examiner, cultural mistrust, and the intelligence test performance of black children. *Journal of Consulting and Clinical Psychology* 31, 371–375.

Terrell SL, Terrell F. (1996) The Importance of Psychological and Sociocultural Factors in Providing Clinical Services to African-American Children. In AG Kamhi, KE Pollack, JL Harris (eds), *Communication Development and Disorders in African-American Children: Research, Assessment, and Intervention* (pp. 19–34). Baltimore: Paul Brookes.

United States Bureau of the Census. (1990) *Statistical Abstract of the United States: 1990* (110th ed). Washington, DC: U.S. Department of Commerce.

Valdes-Fallis G. (1978) *Language in Education: Theory and Practice: Code Switching and the Classroom Teacher.* Arlington, VA: Arlington Center for Applied Linguistics.

Vaughn-Cooke F. (1983) Improving language assessment in minority children. *Asha* 25, 29–34.

Wallace GL. (1993) Adult Neurological Disorders. In DE Battle (ed), *Communication Disorders in Multicultural Populations* (pp. 239–255). Boston: Butterworth–Heinemann.

Westby C. (1990) Ethnographic interviewing. Asking the right questions to the right people in the right way. *Journal of Childhood Communication Disorders* 13, 101–111.

Westby C. (1997) Multicultural Issues. In JB Tomblin, HL Morris, DC Spriesterbach (eds), *Multicultural Issues in Speech Language Pathology* (pp. 29–52). San Diego: Singular Publishing Group.

Wolfram W. (1983) Test interpretation and sociolinguistic differences. *Topics in Language Disorders* 3, 21–34.

Wolfram W, Fasold RW. (1974) *The Study of Social Dialects in American English.* Englewood Cliffs, NJ: Prentice-Hall.

Wyatt T. (1991) Linguistic constraints on copula production in black English child speech. Ph.D. diss., University of Massachusetts.

Wyatt T. (January 1995) Appropriate Speech and Language Assessment and Intervention of African-American Children. Presented at the American Speech-Language-Hearing Association Institute on Multicultural Literacy in Communication Sciences and Disorders, Sea Island, GA.

Wyatt T, Seymour H. (1990) The implications of code-switching in black English speakers. *Equity & Excellence: Special Issue: Language and Discrimination* 24, 17–18.

Zimmerman JR, Steiner VG, Pond RE. (1992) *Preschool Language Scale–3.* San Antonio: Psychological Corporation.

3

Differential Diagnosis for Young Children Presenting with Language Delay

Teris Kim Schery and Ashley S. Garber

Perhaps the most common referral complaint to any pediatric speech-language pathologist is that of delayed speech and language development. As federal legislation has lowered the age of mandatory special education to 3 years, with strong incentives to provide services to children in the birth to 2 years of age range (Amendment to the Education of the Handicapped Act [Public Law 99-457], reauthorized in 1986 as the Individuals with Disabilities Education Act), pediatricians, preschool educators, and parents have responded with increasing awareness of the importance of early intervention. Frequently, the symptom of earliest concern for young children is lack of "appropriate" speech and language development. Speech-language pathologists in medical facilities, school settings, and in private practice are being asked to answer questions and provide guidance concerning language development to families with children as young as 10 months of age (Bricker 1992). Often, these communication specialists serve as part of multidisciplinary teams, working to use and share information from medical specialists, as well as from psychologists, social workers, special educators, and others (Jones 1995; Richardson 1983).

Presented in this chapter are some of the most common issues in differential diagnosis encountered by the speech-language pathologist who works with children from birth to 5 years of age. This chapter focuses on very young children, because many practicing speech-language pathologists have not been trained to work with children under the age of 3 years, the age at which speech and language behaviors sufficient for evaluation were traditionally considered to be apparent (Siegel and Broen 1976). Psycholinguistic research since the 1980s has added much information to our knowledge of how language develops—from the earliest preintentional signals of the infant through preverbal and verbal intentional communication, the variable development of speech motor skills, and the sometimes asynchronous development of comprehension and production abilities (Chapman 1988; Miller 1988). More recently, the relationship of language development to early social skills and preliteracy development has been explored (Rice et al. 1993; van Kleeck and Schuele 1987). All of this information, as well as technological developments in brain imaging (Drayer 1993) and evaluation of the auditory system (Moller 1994), has meant that the speech-language pathologist who works with young children faces a complex differential diagnostic challenge. Ascertaining the underlying cause of a young child's language difficulty can lead to important treatment distinctions. However, even when this causal certainty cannot be achieved, a clinician's careful description of the nature of the language problem should facilitate appropriate referrals for further diagnostic evaluations, contribute meaningful recommendations to other professionals, allow delineation of a treatment plan that is appropriate for the child, and help guide parents and teachers in their understanding of the child and the child's needs. It is toward these goals that this chapter is dedicated.

RESEARCH ON LANGUAGE DELAY IN YOUNG CHILDREN

Late Talkers

Researchers have demonstrated substantial interest in the group of toddlers commonly referred to as *late talkers* (LTs). These are young children who present significantly restricted expressive language by 2 years of age. As the number of referrals of children of this age increase, research in this area becomes highly relevant to the clinical decision making of speech-language pathologists. Although definitions of an LT differ somewhat, most authors agree that children who use less than a 50-word productive vocabulary and are not producing any multiword utterances by 2 years of age should be considered in this group (Paul 1991; Rescorla 1989; Thal and Bates 1988). Paul also included children who do not have 10 intelligible words by 18 months. LTs are distinguished primarily on the basis of poor expressive skills and nonverbal cognitive skills that are thought to be within normal limits. However, studies have shown that, as a group, LTs also show significant deficits in receptive language, socialization, phonologic skills, articulatory skills, or any combination of these (Paul 1991; Paul and Smith 1993). Paul reported that findings from a longitudinal study of 30 LT children showed that 29% had deficits in receptive language and 62% had difficulties in socialization. The control group of toddlers developing language normally showed no deficits in these areas. LTs have also been found to show concomitant delays in grammar and phonology (Paul and Shiffer 1991; Paul et al. 1991). Stoel-Gammon (1987, 1991) suggested a phonetic inventory of four or five consonants with limited variety in vowel production by 24 months as indicative of LT phonology.

Follow-up studies have suggested that approximately one-half of the children identified as LTs by 2 years of age fail to catch up with their peers by 3 years of age (Paul 1993; Rescorla et al. 1997; Rescorla and Schwartz 1990; Thal et al. 1991). Rescorla and Schwartz (1990) reported that 4 year olds who were LTs obtained Developmental Sentence Scores (Lee 1974) below the tenth percentile. As preschoolers, LTs also performed significantly below age-matched controls on various measures of narrative ability and phonologic awareness, skills that have been shown to be related to academic success (Bishop and Edmunson 1987; Paul and Smith 1993). Substantial literature linking preschool speech and language impairments with difficulties in written language and academic achievement in the school-age years exists (Aram et al. 1984; Catts and Kahmi 1986). Therefore, to provide early intervention, it is important to use whatever information is available to determine which LT children are at risk for continuing language difficulty. On the other hand, it is helpful to know which characteristics of LTs predict that an individual child will be one of the almost 50% who are "late bloomers" and catch up with their peers by the school-age years. Such children should be exposed to more general language-stimulation programs and monitored in their development, while the labels and parental concerns that accompany a diagnosis of language impairment are avoided.

What predictors can help clinicians distinguish the "late bloomers" from those children who will continue to show language delay into the school years? Research evidence presents somewhat contradictory results, but the following factors have been implicated as risk factors (for long-range language delay) by at least one study:

- *Family history of language delay*. A positive history of language delay in the immediate or extended family increases the likelihood that the child will continue to have difficulties into the school years (Ellis-Weismer et al. 1993; Tallal et al. 1989; Tomblin 1989).
- *Socioeconomic status*. Lower socioeconomic status is associated with continuing language delay in some studies (Ellis-Weismer et al.

1993; Paul 1991; Rescorla 1989); however, the numbers of subjects in these studies have been small, and interpretation should be extremely cautious.

- *Gender.* LT girls, although fewer in number overall, are less likely to attain normal language and speech by kindergarten than boys (Paul 1993).
- *Ratio of consonants to total babble in prelinguistic vocalizations.* A lower proportion of consonants in the babbling of prelinguistic babies and toddlers was associated with poorer developmental language outcomes for children identified as LTs (Whitehurst et al. 1992).
- *Symbolic abilities, including use of symbolic play and symbolic gestures.* Lack of symbolic play and symbolic gestures for communication at 18–28 months of age was associated with poor receptive language as well as with expressive delays and with longer-range communication impairments (Rescorla and Goossens 1992; Thal and Bates 1988; Thal et al. 1991; Thal and Tobias 1992, 1994).

Additional proposed predictors, including size of initial vocabulary at 24 months of age (Fischel et al. 1989) and expressive language level relative to age at initial diagnosis (Rescorla and Schwartz 1990), have not distinguished "late bloomers" from LT children with continued problems. There is no known clear way of distinguishing the 50% of LT toddlers who "outgrow" their language delay from those who continue to have communication problems that adversely affect their social and academic performance during the school years. Clinicians must consider carefully the entire presenting case history and pattern of language performance to make informed clinical diagnostic decisions for such children. Because continuing research in this area should provide additional information in the future, speech-language clinicians need to remain current with emerging literature.

Neurologic Basis of Childhood Language Disability

Recent studies on the neurologic basis of developmental language disability in children offer important information for the clinician involved with differential diagnosis for young children with language delay. Traditionally, based on information from studies on adult aphasia, left-hemisphere damage was the explanatory model for the neurologic basis of specific language impairment in children (Benton 1964; Eisenson 1968; Kinsbourne and Hiscock 1977). However, recent research based on magnetic resonance imaging (MRI), a greatly improved technology for delineating damage to the brain, suggests that persistent and severe language disorders in young children are rarely a result of unilateral cortical lesions (Aram and Eisele 1994; Levin et al. 1987; Plante et al. 1991). Rather, such pervasive language disabilities seem to result when there is subcortical damage to anterior gray and white matter structures, regardless of the laterality of the lesion. Such lesions are associated with language and language-based learning disorders throughout the developmental period. Unilateral cortical lesions in young children most frequently result in language behaviors that parallel the developmental pattern of LT children, where onset and development of language are slow, but, by school age, abilities have normalized with minimal long-term language-learning deficits (Aram and Eisele 1992, 1994; Eisele and Aram 1993). Early unilateral cortical left-hemisphere damage is associated with delays in production of first words and with residual difficulty in processing and use of syntax. In contrast, there is some evidence that children with early right-hemisphere damage have more pronounced comprehension deficits in initial stages of language learning (Eisele and Aram 1993). Aram and Eisele (1994) speculated that delays in language development observed in these toddlers and preschoolers were a result of neural reorganization that, while imposing a delayed developmental schedule, ultimately resulted in normal or near-normal language abilities.

The speech-language clinician working on an interdisciplinary team is likely to have access to neurologic reports for some children with language delay. This information can be critically important in helping define the nature of the disorder. Although MRI scans are not routine, speech-language pathologists should be alert to the information they can contribute in conjunction with a neurologic evaluation, when available. It is important to check with parents to obtain any such reports from previous evaluations. There may be times when referral for a pediatric neurologic evaluation with consideration of an MRI scan is appropriate.

In summary, the most recent research on language delay in young children examines the nature of language and related social, symbolic, and academic abilities in LTs and attempts to distinguish those children who will "catch up" by school age from those who will continue to have pervasive difficulties. There is, as of yet, no definitive predictor(s) of the category into which any individual child will fall. However, some preliminary demographic variables and some increasingly documented neurologic variables are beginning to suggest to knowledgeable clinicians those children who are at greatest risk for long-term communication difficulties.

GATHERING PARENT INFORMATION

The parents of young children referred for delayed speech and language are a primary source for information that is critical to formulating a diagnosis and determining appropriate recommendations for treatment or referral. A parent or primary caregiver interview is of utmost importance in helping the clinician understand the nature of the problem and the family's concerns and viewpoints regarding intervention needs. It is imperative to consider young children first as part of a family system rather than in isolation (Bronfenbrenner 1977; Simeonsson 1989). The family's concerns, priorities, and resources are an important part of the ecology of the child's environment and must be taken into account in any evaluation effort (Crais 1995).

Obtaining a history of the child's problem and the history of language delays and difficulties in the rest of the family is an important goal of the parent information–gathering process. As discussed in the section *Late Talkers*, evidence for the predictive nature of familial language disorders in determining children who will not "outgrow" early language delays is increasing. Additionally, parents are generally the most informed source on the course of the child's language development, including age of first intentional communication, nature of babbling, and the course of preverbal and verbal communication (including any words that were used at one time and then disappeared). Such information, if available, can substantially assist the diagnostic process. Structured parental observations gathered in conjunction with an interview can be informative and assist in gathering specific data in a timely manner. In recent years, studies have shown a high correlation between parent and professional estimates of developmental behavior in young children, especially when the parent must indicate whether a specific behavior is currently exhibited by the child (Bloch and Seitz 1989; Bricker et al. 1995; Dale et al. 1989; Miller et al. 1995). This realization has led to the development of assessment tools that rely on parent reports and have acceptable properties of reliability and validity. One such instrument that is in common use is the MacArthur Communicative Development Inventory (Fenson et al. 1993). This parent report form has two separate versions: infants (ages 8–16 months) and toddlers (ages 16–30 months). Parents check off their child's comprehension and production vocabularies from among the 396 words that appear first in lexicons of young English-speaking children. It is appropriate for infants and toddlers using communicative gestures, first words, and two-word combinations. The available norms, gathered in three major U.S. cities, allow the child to be assigned to percentiles for age of language comprehension and production. Other parent report inventories (e.g., the Ages and Stages Questionnaires [Bricker et al. 1995] and the Parent/Professional Preschool Performance Profile [Bzoch 1987]) can also serve to enhance the role of parents or other caregivers in the assessment process. A more complete listing and discussion of these and other tools can be found in Crais and Roberts (1995).

DIFFERENTIATION OF DELAYED LANGUAGE DEVELOPMENT AND LINGUISTIC, DIALECTAL, AND CULTURAL DIFFERENCES IN LANGUAGE DEVELOPMENT

Family Evaluation

There is no better source than the immediate family members for exploring the sociocultural factors that can influence the course of the child's language development. The linguistic background of the family can affect the developmental course of language in young children, especially if all or some family members speak a language or dialect other than Standard American English (Battle 1993; Cheng 1991; Langdon 1994; Taylor 1986). The clinician must take special care to differentiate a delay in English based on a second-language developmental pattern from a true language disorder. In addition, it is important for clinicians to be sensitive to the family's cultural beliefs concerning the child's communication skills. Lynch and Hanson (1992) described some of the culturally specific differences in how families view children with any type of developmental disorder and variations in ways families are comfortable in discussing such problems. It is critical for the clinician who wants to communicate meaningfully with families to learn how the family views the child, any "differences" the child demonstrates, and the kinds of intervention options acceptable for the child and the family. For further information on linguistic, dialectal, and cultural factors in differential diagnosis of delayed language development see Chapter 2.

Evaluations from Other Agencies

Because the unfolding of language and speech is a sensitive developmental barometer that is implicated in a wide range of childhood disorders, the speech-language pathologist must be alert to information suggesting the entire range of possibilities. The differential diagnostic process for a young child with delayed speech and language can lead to a diagnosis of hearing loss, mental retardation, infantile autism, childhood schizophrenia, articulation disorders, reading disorders, specific language disorders, or a combination of these and other categories of disability (Richardson 1983). Evaluations of these children may have been made by other professionals before referral for speech and language assessment. Ideally, information should be gathered from all prior sources before undertaking the diagnostic process. This allows the speech-language pathologist to proceed with the most appropriate and efficient procedures, avoiding unnecessary duplication. Such information is also necessary to determine any further referrals that seem important following the communication assessment. Diagnostic procedures that systematically compile information on all prior professional and agency contacts before scheduling the diagnostic evaluation are well worth the effort involved.

Standardized Testing

Standardized testing is specifically designed to compare a child to a reference population to determine issues of relative delay and, thus, eligibility for services (Aiken 1988; Schery 1981). Standardized testing is therefore most useful for diagnostic purposes (as opposed to delineating a specific child's strengths and weaknesses to establish intervention goals, a task much better accomplished using other types of assessments, such as those that are criterion-referenced). Standardized measures are generally relatively easy to administer and score, because they have an established protocol and set of materials. This would seem to make them the ideal choice for purposes of establishing a differential diagnosis for a young child with language delay. However, the difficulty in relying on only standardized tests with very young children is that developmental skills, such as language, unfold in a highly variable sequence, and thus the predictive validity of standardized procedures can be poor, particularly for children younger than 3 years of age (Gibbs 1990; Maistro and German 1986). As stated previously, approximately 50% of the LTs in the studies reviewed in the section *Late Talkers* went on to develop normal language patterns, yet no test or procedure could reliably predict which half of the toddlers would be in that group and which half would continue to have significant language delays into the school years.

Particular dissatisfactions arise when clinicians try to find standardized tools that examine and profile early communication behaviors such as preverbal communication, play behaviors, and social-affective skills (Crais and Roberts 1995; Wetherby and Prizant 1992). Most speech-language pathologists conducting diagnostic evaluations of young children with language delay rely on some standardized measures to document the severity of the delay with normative data. (See Crais 1995 for a listing and description of standardized tests most commonly used with infants and toddlers.) However, especially with children younger than 3 years of age, standardized testing needs to be supplemented with less formal and more observational techniques to gain a representative overall picture of the child's communication abilities. Following is a discussion of some of these nonstandardized procedures.

Observational Assessments

Nonstandardized, observational assessments are particularly important in evaluating a young child for significance of language or speech delay. There are several areas essential for a complete picture of the child's abilities that have no formal standardized assessment available. In other cases, limited or suspect formal testing results can be validated with the more detailed, flexible, and naturalistic procedures found in observational assessments. This section briefly discusses several areas of evaluation for young children with suspected language delay that lend themselves to observational evaluation.

Play Behavior and Sensorimotor Cognitive Tasks

One of the basic determinations that the speech-language clinician must make regarding the significance of the communication delay in a young child is whether speech and language skills appear to reflect the child's overall developmental level. Although referral to a psychologist for a developmental evaluation is necessary to determine actual IQ (see Camarata and Swisher 1990; Reed 1994 for discussions of intelligence tests that are most valid for use with young children with language difficulties), general estimates of a young child's range of nonlinguistic developmental functioning can be obtained through observation of cognitive schema and motor skills during play behavior. This is particularly useful with children ages 3 years and younger who can be videotaped in play sessions with a parent, peer, or evaluator for later systematic observational scrutiny. Several schemes for evaluation of play behaviors are in general use, including the Symbolic Play Scale (Westby 1980, 1988); the Assessment, Evaluation and Programming System: AEPS (Bricker 1993); and the more extensive procedures described in Linder's (1993) play-based assessment. A related observational assessment for children functioning under 37 months developmental level is based on Piaget's stages of sensorimotor development. Miller and colleagues (1980) described a procedure to assess skills in Piagetian substages, such as object permanence and causality, through structured activities and evaluator observation. For children functioning at Piaget's preoperational level (generally 3–5 years of age), observational guidelines have been offered by Gill and Dihoff (1982) to assess skills such as sorting, haptic perception, and drawing. Table 3.1 lists cognitive observational protocols that can be used to screen these Piagetian stages. Such observations allow the speech-language clinician to estimate the child's level of functioning for developmental tasks that are not linguistic in nature. Comparison of these developmental estimates with the child's level of linguistic performance can suggest the need for further psychometric evaluation to rule out generalized delay.

Parental Language Input and Socioemotional Interaction

Family interactional variables associated with language learning, including quality of attention and language input, have been shown to influence differences in child language production (Hart and Risley 1992). The influence of maternal linguistic input on the development of productive language specifically in LT children has been examined by Paul and Elwood (1991), who found little difference among middle class families. However, Hoff-Ginsberg (1991) suggested that differences may be greater for children from other socioeconomic levels. The effects of environmental risk factors, including language opportunities and mother-child interaction, are reviewed in Brown and Edwards (1989), with the overall recommendation that the interactional dyad should become the focus of more attention in the identification of childhood language disorders. No specific criteria of appropriate parent-child linguistic input are in common use. Rather, only a global determination of the linguistic quality and contingent responsiveness of a caregiver's verbal input to young children (what has come to be called *motherese*) can be made. (See Snow 1972 and Hoff-Ginsberg 1986 for discussion of characteristics of motherese.)

Differentiation of Delayed Language Development and Socioemotional Disorders

Research has documented the probability that up to 50% of children with significant communication disorders have clinically identified socioemotional difficulties (Cantwell and Baker 1991; Prizant et al. 1990). In some cases, as in childhood autism, the socioemotional problem becomes the primary diagnosis, with language deficits seen as co-occurring symptoms (Baltaxe and Simmons 1990; Landry and Loveland 1988). (For more information on differential diagnosis of autism, see Chapter 9.) While diagnoses of emotional disorders must be made by a psychologist, psychiatrist, or neurologist familiar with *Diagnostic and Statistical Manual of Mental Disorders* (4th edition) (DSM-IV 1994), a speech-language pathologist must know when to refer a young child for such an evaluation. Prizant and Meyer (1993) developed a list of questions regarding socioemotional dimensions in the communication assessment of young children. Based on the parent interview and observation of the child's interactions with the caregiver and the examiner, judgments are made about the child's social relatedness, emotional expres-

Table 3.1
Assessment protocols used at the Bill Wilkerson Center for evaluation of children suspected of having language disorders

Test/Procedure (Standardized)	*Protocol**
Comprehension	
Sequenced Inventory of Communication Development (SICD)–Receptive (Hedrick et al. 1984)	A, B, C, D
Comprehension Checklist (Miller et al. 1980)	A, B, C
Peabody Picture Vocabulary Test (PPVT)–Revised (Dunn and Dunn 1981)	D, E
Clinical Evaluation of Language Fundamentals at Preschool (CELF-P) (Wiig et al. 1992)	E
Production	
SICD–Expressive	A, B, C, D
MacArthur Communicative Development Inventories (Fenson et al. 1993)	
Words and gestures	A, B
Words and sentences	B, C
Phonological Repertoire (Stark 1978)	B
Photo Articulation Test (Pendergast et al. 1984)	C
Arizona Articulation Proficiency Scale (2nd Edition) (Fedula 1986)	D
Goldman-Fristoe Test of Articulation (Goldman and Fristoe 1986)	E
Content/form analysis (Lahey 1988)	B, C, D
Renfrew Bus Story (Cowley and Glasgow 1994)	E
Language Assessment and Remediation Screening Procedure–Revised(LARSP) (Crystal et al. 1989)	C, D
Conversational sample	E
Systematic Analysis of Language Transcripts (SALT) (Miller and Chapman 1993)	E
Assigning structural stages (Miller 1981)	E
Pragmatic checklist (Bill Wilkerson Center) (Figure 3.1)	A, B, C, D
Pragmatic-idiosyncratic checklist (Bill Wilkerson Center) (Figure 3.2)	E

Table 3.1
Continued

Test/Procedure (Standardized)	*Protocol**
Cognition	
Sensorimotor tasks (Miller et al. 1980; Uzgiris and Hunt 1975)	A, B, C
Preoperational tasks (Gill and Dihoff 1982)	C
Oral Examination	
Oral Speech Mechanism Screening Examination–Revised (OSMSE–R) (St. Louis and Ruscello 1987)	B, C, D, E

*A = ages 1–12 months; B = ages 13–24 months; C = ages 25–30 months; D = ages 37–48 months; E = ages 49–60 months.

sion, sociability in communication, emotional regulation, communicative competence, and expression of emotion in language and play, as well as the clinician's subjective reaction to the child. Responses to this series of questions can help determine if a referral for further diagnostic work in the area of socioemotional functioning should be made.

Communicative Intentions and Pragmatic Skills

Pragmatics refers to the use of language for the purposes of social communication (Austin 1962; Bates 1976). There are different levels at which pragmatic communication skills can be examined. The first of these levels involves determination of the *communicative intentions* the young child is trying to convey through his or her gestural or verbal speech act (e.g., is the child commenting, requesting, greeting?) (Halliday 1975; Searle 1969). The clinical assessment of these communicative intentions involves observation to see if the child comprehends and expresses a range of intentions and notation of the linguistic forms or nonverbal ways in which such intentions are expressed. A second level of pragmatic assessment, *presupposition,* involves determining if the child is capable of taking the needs of the listener into consideration when formulating a message. Such knowledge is implicit when a child's message is formulated to assure shared contextual information, such as filling in background information that the listener would not already know. Aspects of informativeness include the topics a child chooses to

PRAGMATIC CHECKLIST

Bill Wilkerson Center

Name:______________________ DOB:_______ Date:_______

Communicative partner:_________ Communicative setting:_________

Performance rating scale: Behavior is (1) highly appropriate, (2) moderately appropriate, (3) borderline appropriate, (4) moderately inappropriate, (5) highly inappropriate

OBSERVATIONS

Performance rating **Examples and comments**

A. Speech act
__ Speech act pair analysis
__ Variety of speech acts

B. Topic
__ Selection
__ Introduction
__ Maintenance
__ Change

C. Turn taking
__ Initiation
__ Response
__ Insufficient information
__ Repair/revision
__ Informational redundancy
__ Interruption/overlap

D. Lexical selection
__ Specificity
__ Cohesion

E. Body language

Figure 3.1 Pragmatic checklist. The Bill Wilkerson Center, Nashville, TN. (Adapted from C Prutting, D Kirchner. [1987] A clinical appraisal of the pragmatic aspects of language. *Journal of Speech and Hearing Disorders* 12, 43–48.)

talk about, whether what is stated is new information, and the linguistic forms (e.g., deitic references, direct versus indirect pronouns, and cohesive devices). Furthermore, how a child changes such dimensions to accommodate listeners of varying ages and linguistic abilities is diagnostic. A third area of pragmatics focuses on *conversational discourse* skills that allow the child to maintain a dialogue with a conversational part-

PRAGMATIC-IDIOSYNCRATIC CHECKLIST
Bill Wilkerson Center

Name:____________________ DOB:_______ Date:_______

Communicative partner:_________ Communicative setting:_________

Check all that apply and give examples of client's speech-language patterns.

A. Undue hesitancy, dysfluency, garbling

_ Excessively prolonged pauses, searching, groping, delayed retrieval (e.g., "Bobby—went to—went home.")
Examples:

_ Overuse of meaningless starters to begin comments (e.g., and then, well)
Examples:

_ Overuse of stereotyped interjections and place holders (e.g., you know, um, er)
Examples:

_ Perseverative repetitions of words and phrases
Examples:

B. Overuse of word substitution patterns

_ Indefinites (e.g., somehow, something)
Examples:

_ General words lacking specificity (e.g., stuff, place, junk, man instead of proper name)
Examples:

_ Imprecise use of verbs (e.g., "He goes [says]....")
Examples:

_ Substitutions of phonetically similar words (e.g., saxophone, xylophone)
Examples:

Figure 3.2 Pragmatic-idiosyncratic checklist. The Bill Wilkerson Center, Nashville, TN. (Adapted from D German. [1979] Word-finding skills in children with learning disabilities. *Journal of Learning Disorders* 12, 43–48; E Schwartz, C Solot. [1980] Response patterns characteristic of verbal expressive disorders. *Language, Speech, and Hearing Services in Schools* 11, 139–144; and E Wigg, E Semel. [1986] *Language Disabilities in Children and Adolescents.* Columbus, OH: Charles Merrill.)

_ Synonym limitation substitutions (e.g., big for large, huge, wide)
Examples:

_ Circumlocution (e.g., "Those *things* you put on your feet." [galoshes])
Examples:

_ Within semantic class responses and imprecise word substitutions
Examples:

_ Borrowed terms or word formations (e.g., "The baby is *topsy turvey* [fell down].")
Examples:

_ Substitution of prefixes (e.g., "He is *ineducated* [uneducated].")
Examples:

_ Stereotyped phrases or terms (e.g., whatchamacallit, thingamajig)
Examples:

_ Excessive use of pronouns (e.g., "They chase him until he tells where she lives.")
Examples:

_ Inconsistencies (e.g., "I can't think of the word for that picture," "I always forget vase.")
Examples:

_ Paucity of expression (e.g., definitions or comparisons are inadequate, child relies on listener to prod and cue)
Examples:

Figure 3.2 *Continued*

ner over several turns. Specific behaviors to evaluate include the proportion of speech that is social (i.e., directed toward a listener) versus nonsocial and the child's abilities to initiate and maintain conversations, take turns effectively, and repair conversational breakdowns. While all of these aspects of pragmatic communication skill develop during the preschool period, the expression of a range of communicative intentions is the earliest, with some differentiation noted preverbally as early as 8–10 months of age (Bates et al. 1975).

Language Sample

Obtaining samples of a child's spontaneous language is an important nonstandardized assessment strategy, especially for children who are speaking with an average utterance length of more than two words (Klee 1985). Analyses of a language sample can delineate information about semantics, morphology, phonology, pragmatics, and syntax. Traditionally, syntax and morphology have been examined most widely, with measures of sentence complexity being tied to mean length of utterance (MLU) (Brown 1973) and via Developmental Sentence Scoring (DSS) (Lee 1974). These indices yield quantitative measures of the child's expressive language that can be used, together with norms, to evaluate the child's productive linguistic developmental status. There is a range of language sampling procedures that can be used by the clinician, each emphasizing a somewhat different aspect of the child's productions and each suggesting somewhat different ways to elicit the sample. (See Kemp and Klee [1997] or Reed [1994] for a discussion of the parameters involved in some of the most widely used procedures.) Several computer programs have been developed to assist in analyzing language samples, including Systematic Analysis of Language Transcripts (SALT Version 3.0) (Miller and Chapman 1993) and Computerized Profiling (Long and Fey 1993). The Language Assessment, Remediation and Screening Procedure (Crystal et al. 1989) can be helpful in assigning a developmental stage to syntactic and morphologic structures used in simple sentence productions (usually for children 25–48 months of age). SALT, used in conjunction with Miller's Assigning Structural Stages (1981), is helpful in analyzing MLU, syntax errors, and complex sentence development for more complicated samples (i.e., children at developmental ages 36 months and older). Videotaping a parent and child during unstructured play is a vehicle for collecting a language sample that later can be analyzed for semantic, morphologic, syntactic, and pragmatic information. It also provides information on parent-child interaction styles and language models.

Narrative Skills: Differentiation of Delayed Language Development and Language-Learning Disability

Recent research has documented a strong link between preschoolers' abilities to tell narratives and literacy acquisition in the school years (Dickinson and McCabe 1991; Feagans 1982; McCabe and Rollins 1994;

Michaels 1981). Results of a longitudinal study following 87 children with language delays (as well as children developing language normally) from the age of 4.0 to 5.6 years, found that the ability to recall a short story was the best predictor of subsequent language development (Bishop and Edmundson 1987). Beginning at about 22 months of age, children begin to refer to real past events, although by 2 years of age their narratives often concern negative events, such as injuries (Miller and Sperry 1988). Between the ages of 3 and 5 years, children tell each other longer and more complex narratives, progressing from single events to combining two or more events that occurred on one occasion. By 5 years of age, the typically developing child rarely has trouble sequencing events in oral narratives but often dwells on a climactic event at the end of the narration. Six-year-old children can usually use what is called a *classic narrative* (Johnston 1982; McCabe and Peterson 1991).

McCabe and Rollins (1994) developed a series of questions in flowchart format that assists a clinician in evaluating the structure and appropriateness of oral narratives for children between 2 and 7 years of age. Gillam and colleagues (1995) reviewed alternate approaches for assessing oral narratives for children in this developmental age range. Such an evaluation, in conjunction with in-depth language assessment, is particularly helpful for those older preschool children who present with mild to moderate communicative delays and for whom the question of a future language-based learning difficulty is a differential diagnostic issue. The Renfrew Bus Story is a procedure adapted by Cowley and Glasgow (1994) to screen narrative recall in the initial diagnostic evaluation. This standardized measure provides both quantitative (standard scores and percentile ranks for information and sentence length and scores for independence and complexity) and qualitative information (checklists for inferential skills and style) that can suggest areas for further evaluation when necessary.

Oral-Motor Skills: Differentiation of Delayed Language and Phonologic Disorders

Young children who present predominantly with language delay usually have some degree of delay in phonology and articulatory skills as well (Kent 1992). The differential diagnosis of children whose restricted expressive language is a result of motor constraints (i.e., dysarthria), difficulty with volitional sequential oral movements (i.e., apraxia), or both, as opposed to a primary language deficit, can be challenging even for the most experienced clinician (Shriberg et al. 1997). Kent and colleagues (1994) offered an extensive review of evaluation procedures to judge the intelligibility of children's speech and concluded that the primary factors that contribute to a child's intelligibility include relative accuracy of various phonetic contrasts, naturalness and appropriateness of prosodic variations, and use of conversational clarification and repair strategies. Rafaat and colleagues (1995) suggested, however, that speech-language clinicians' judgments of the severity of a child's phonologic impairment are notably unreliable for children under 3.5 years of age, perhaps because of the lack of contextual variables provided by the prosody and pragmatic components that are part of the speech of more fluent communicators. Marquardt and Sussman (1991) suggested some key speech characteristics of preschool children with developmental apraxia of speech, including a very limited phonemic repertoire, a high incidence of vowel errors, inconsistent articulation errors, altered prosody, and significant difficulty in imitating words and phrases. Nonspeech characteristics include impaired volitional oral movements (with better control for biologically based movements), decreased performance on sensory-oral tests, and the reliance on gestures in place of oral communication. Many of these are also characteristic of children with dysarthria, especially at young ages (Crary 1993). At any rate, it is important for the clinician to observe oral motor skills and make a preliminary judgment on the degree to which difficulties in this area contribute to the presenting delay or restriction of expressive language. Chapter 5 offers a more detailed discussion of differential diagnostic procedures for phonologic problems.

Sample Tests and Procedures

Table 3.1 lists tests and procedures for children from birth through 5 years of age as used by the diagnostic team at the Bill Wilkerson Center, Nashville, TN. Naturally, an individual assessment can vary from this suggested list of tests and procedures based on the child's interests, attitudes, and behaviors. The clinician must use information from the history and parent interview, as well as exercise clinical judgment, to determine what combination of standardized tests and informal observational techniques are useful in gathering the most informative data for a specific child.

RECOMMENDATIONS, REFERRALS, AND PARENT COUNSELING

Once the information has been assembled from medical and social histories, referral sources, and both formal and observational assessments, the speech-language pathologist must rely on clinical judgment to sift through and weigh the factors that are most salient in the overall picture. Parents or caregivers are entitled to the clinician's thinking at this point, even if unanswered questions remain. When a child is to be referred for additional evaluation by another professional, the family needs to be told where things stand, any impressions the clinician has formulated, and what additional information the new referral will provide.

If the amount and type of information the clinician or diagnostic team was able to gain from the evaluation is sufficient, a diagnosis can be communicated and treatment options can be discussed with the family. It is always a good idea to describe the child's behaviors and aptitudes (both strengths and weaknesses) to parents rather than just relying on a label (Crais 1993). The clinician should allow time for the parents to ask questions. If the clinician has used the parents during earlier stages of the evaluation to observe and validate the child's responses, the clinician should summarize and explain the child's performances in context so that family members feel overall coherence in the interpretation. Of course, different families have differing needs for detailed information and for direct involvement in the diagnostic process. The clinician must be sensitive to these variations, some of which may be culturally determined. Information should be provided in a way that will be most helpful to the family (Lynch and Hanson 1992). (See Chapter 2.) A number of different variables affect what kinds of intervention setting and schedule the family selects. Such things as family resources (e.g., time, money, transportation) play a part. It is important for the speech-language clinician to outline the variety of programs available in the family's community.

One of the most sensitive and difficult questions that a clinician must deal with when evaluating young children with language delay is a question that every parent has—whether spoken or not—"What will happen to my child? Will he [or she] be normal?" There is, of course, no definite answer that can be given, as much as the clinician would like to reassure the family. In the section *Late Talkers*, it was pointed out how variable the outcomes can be for children referred for delayed language when they are younger than 5 years of age (Paul and Smith 1993; Thal et al. 1991). In the same section, the risk factors that statistically indicate a greater likelihood of continuing communication difficulties into the school years (e.g., family history of delayed speech, low socioeconomic status, female gender, fewer consonants in prelingual babbling, less reliance on symbolic gesture) were reviewed. Indications of social-emotional difficulty, cognitive delays, or both are additional risk factors for development along a normal trajectory, as well as the severity of the initial delay. Yet each individual child is unique. Every experienced clinician knows several youngsters who, despite the presence of multiple risk factors, made remarkable progress. Perhaps the best response is the honest one: "We can't really tell how far he [or she] will go at this time, but help is available, and, together with your support, we can expect progress in the future. We are very hopeful, but we will have to take it one step at a time and reevaluate the program frequently to see if more can be done."

DECISION MATRIX AND CASE HISTORIES

The following nine cases have been selected to illustrate the range of diagnostic outcomes that can be seen among referrals of young children who present with language delay.

Figure 3.3 presents a decision matrix with nine possible outcomes illustrated by the clients. These children were selected to show contrasting differential diagnostic patterns. Clinicians will, of course, see children who present with some combination or variation of these patterns. The nine cases listed in Figure 3.3 are discussed in the following section. Key differential diagnostic points in the history and report of assessment results are indicated by double asterisks (**). The importance of these points is discussed in the final *Comments* section for each case.

Client 1: SG, Female, 2 Years, 1 Month, Hearing Loss

Birth history: Unremarkable

Medical history: Recurrent otitis media treated with antibiotics

Family history: **Recent Kurdish immigrants, have been learning English for 1.5 years; living with local sponsor family

Developmental history:

Motor milestones: Reportedly within normal limits (WNL)

Speech-language milestones: Mother is unsure of early vocalizations and the appearance of first word. SG reportedly put two words together at 2 years of age. About that time, parents started speaking English to SG: SG hears only English from sponsors and their children. SG reportedly says only a few "baby" words in Kurdish. At evaluation, SG spoke several single words and one two-word combination in English. The mother's primary concern was that words do "not come out clear[ly]." She stated that SG tries to talk in sentences but becomes very frustrated.

Behavior: Caregivers are concerned with "strong will" and aggressive behaviors. **Noncompliance and decreased attention to task were noted during evaluation.

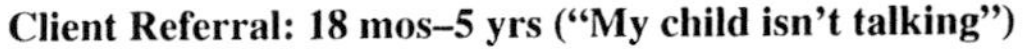

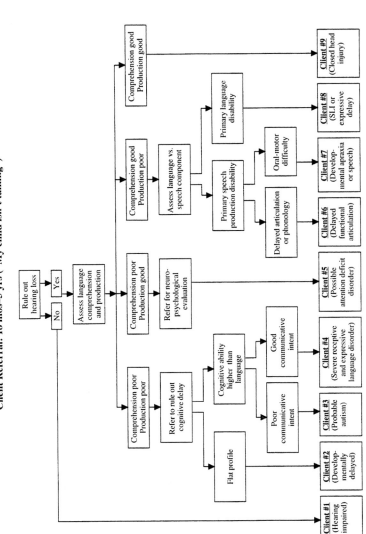

Figure 3.3 Through a series of decisions, the speech-language pathologist helps to answer a parent's concern, "Why isn't my child talking?" Nine cases illustrating differential diagnostic outcomes are discussed in this chapter. (SLI = speech and language impaired.)

Hearing: **Mother is concerned that SG "does not listen even if you stand before her." **Hearing evaluations attempted during and before the speech-language evaluation were inconclusive due to noncompliance and a refusal or inability to point to pictures.
Oral mechanism and fluency: WNL
Voice: **Distorted voice quality and nasal tone
Language testing:
**Sequenced Inventory of Communication Development (SICD)–Receptive: 18 months
**SICD–Expressive: 16 months
Diagnostic impressions: Receptive and expressive language skills were found to be severely delayed when compared to same-aged peers, even considering relatively recent exposure to English; questionable hearing.
Counseling and recommendations:

1. Follow-up audiologic evaluation to determine SG's hearing status.
2. Begin individual speech-language intervention on a weekly basis until conclusive results of hearing evaluation become available.
3. Supply information regarding suggested language stimulation techniques for use in the home environment and encourage consistent use of English for the time being.

Comments

A case such as SG's exemplifies the importance of ruling out hearing loss before making a final diagnosis of a child's speech and language performance. A sensory deficit makes language intervention critically important, but it should be undertaken with benefit of amplification. SG also illustrated the differential diagnostic complication presented when a child is from a bilingual family, and language performance might reflect limited exposure to English. In this case, SG was English-dominant, so testing was conducted in that language. SG received individual therapy for approximately 2 months before her hearing was successfully evaluated. In the interim, little progress was made with the language goals established, and behavioral issues interrupted therapy on a regular basis. Once mild to moderately severe bilateral sensorineural hearing loss was diagnosed, and binaural hearing aids were fitted, SG began to make more consistent progress, both with communication goals and with attention and behavior.

With the diagnosis of hearing impairment came the recommendation that SG's family participate in parent-infant therapy to address her speech-language-auditory skills, as well as to provide education on aspects of hearing loss. While this recommendation is a standard one for facilitating parental involvement, it needs to be made with the family's wishes in mind. For SG's parents, the demands of assimilating to a new culture made such involvement difficult and perhaps uncomfortable: They attended only twice. SG received intervention at the Wilkerson Center preschool for hearing-impaired children for a time. However, transportation became difficult after SG's parents moved into their own apartment almost 45 minutes away from the center. While SG's local public school system did not offer a specialized program for hearing-impaired children, it was decided that SG would have more consistent therapy seeing the speech-language clinician individually at the school near her home and attending a local integrated preschool.

Client 2: TG, Female, 3 Years, 1 Month
Developmental Delay

Birth history: **Genetic diagnosis with 17P+ chromosomal abnormality; supranumery digits removed at 8 months of age; **right anophthalmia (complete absence of eye tissue); fitted with a silicone implant at age 2 years, 11 months

Medical history: **Infantile spasms diagnosed in a hospital pediatric neurology department, treated with prescribed medication; hospitalization for dehydration and respiratory synticial virus at age 2 years, 6 months; recurrent otitis media treated with antibiotics

Developmental history:

Motor milestones: Sat alone at 9 months; crawled at 12 months; walked at 18 months of age

Speech and language milestones: Few early vocalizations; recent use of reduplicated babbling sounds and word approximations. **TG has a vocabulary of four words (i.e., *papa, mama, granny,* and *that*) used inconsistently. **Primary form of communication was through a combination of pointing, vocalizing, and making eye contact.

Behavior: **Eye contact was noted to be inconsistent. **TG engaged in some repetitive behaviors, such as staring at bright lights and vocalizing with whole body movements. She cried or screamed when tired or frustrated.

Play: **Observed play behaviors included rolling a ball, stacking blocks, and pushing buttons on a pop-up toy. TG mouthed most toys that were presented to her.

Other significant information: **A developmental evaluation at 2 years, 10 months, indicated that TG's cognitive, language, and gross and fine motor skills clustered at the 10- to 14-month level. As a result of that evaluation, TG attends a developmental preschool for approximately 24 hours per week. She is the only child of professional parents. Her mother now works part-time to devote attention to TG.

Hearing: WNL

Oral mechanism: WNL at time of evaluation. Earlier developmental evaluation indicated a delay in feeding skills. This issue has reportedly been addressed through her preschool program, and TG has recently begun self-feeding.

Language testing:

**SICD–Receptive: 12–16 months

**SICD–Expressive: 8–12 months

**Comprehension Checklist: 12–15 months

Phonology: Infrequent vocalizations consisting primarily of nonspecific reduplicated vowel and consonant-vowel syllables. These vocalizations were often accompanied by whole-body movements (e.g., rocking, bouncing). No word approximations were noted. **Her phonologic repertoire included consonants /b, d/ and a variety of vowels and diphthongs.

Semantics: **Parental report indicates an expressive vocabulary of approximately four words to code existence (e.g., *granny*). **TG reportedly does not code recurrence, rejection, or action. During the evaluation, TG did not produce any word approximations.

Pragmatics: **TG expressed a limited number of communicative intentions verbally and nonverbally, including requesting objects (e.g., reached for toy and made eye contact), protesting and rejecting (e.g., pushed objects away, cried), responding (e.g., turned to her name), and seeking attention (e.g., cried). She did not request actions or information, name, or comment.

Diagnostic impressions: TG demonstrated severely delayed receptive and expressive language skills when compared to children of her chronologic age. Receptive skills were judged to be at the 12- to 16-month level and therefore commensurate with cognitive levels reported on a developmental evaluation completed earlier in the year. Expressive language levels were mildly delayed when compared to cognitive and receptive skill levels. Specific concerns included limited communicative intentions, limited speech sound development, and lack of an expressive core vocabulary.

Counseling and recommendations:

1. Continue with developmental preschool program already in place.
2. Adjust the individualized family service plan to include individual speech-language therapy on a weekly basis in conjunction with her developmental programming. Goals should include the following:
   a. increasing imitation skills
   b. expanding communicative intentions expressed
   c. expanding comprehension of object labels and simple directions across settings
   d. building core vocabulary
3. Offer program of ongoing parent training to address areas of child development, appropriate expectations, and general speech-language stimulation techniques.

Comments

TG's chromosomal abnormality raised immediate concerns regarding her overall developmental prognosis. Although developmental evaluation and special preschool programming were pursued from an early age, slow speech and language development soon became an additional worry. Evaluation results indicating receptive language skills commensurate with cognitive ability suggested that TG's intensive developmental programming continued to be an appropriate service recommendation to address all areas of delay, including speech and language skills. The relative lag in expressive language, however, suggested that speech-language stimulation could complement the services already in place for TG. Recommendations also provide for involvement of the concerned parents to maximize the success of TG's intervention program.

Client 3: KK, Male, 2 Years, 6 Months, Autistic Characteristics

Pregnancy history: Remarkable for premature labor treated with prescribed medication from approximately 16–36 weeks gestation

Birth history: Nuchal cord × 2 (cord twice around neck); slight jaundice that resolved spontaneously

Medical history: Unremarkable

Developmental history:

Motor milestones: Reportedly WNL

Speech and language milestones: normal early vocalizations with early first meaningful word at 8 months of age. **KK reportedly used this word for several months and then stopped talking until approximately 1 month before the evaluation. **He now uses four words (*bite, drink, uhoh,* and *no*), as well as one learned phrase (*fee fi fo fum*). Parents have observed KK moving his mouth with speech on television and whispering words that his parents had used earlier. **KK communicates primarily by pulling his parents and pushing their hands toward desired objects.

Behavior: **Active with inconsistent attention to the examiner and to testing activities. Attention is limited to 1–2 minutes and only if interested in toys. KK did attend for several minutes to an activated music box. **Eye contact with the examiner and with his parents was limited and inconsistent.

Play: KK was observed to throw a ball, stack pegs repetitively, and climb on furniture to jump off. **Parents report that KK enjoys being with other children but does not play directly with them. **KK does not engage in pretend play and prefers household objects to toys. He enjoys spinning objects, banging on tables and objects, and making sounds with toys. **The parents described their son as "inquisitively different," in that he will look at objects (e.g., traffic signs) and patterns (e.g., his shadow) for extended periods of time and from all angles. **KK goes through stages of play interest: His current interest lies in collecting and holding sticks or other long objects.

Hearing, voice, and fluency: WNL

Oral mechanism: Not completed due to noncompliance. Parents reported no concerns with feeding; however, KK often does not chew his food and overfills his mouth.

Cognition: **Uzgiris-Hunt showed sensorimotor skills in Piagetian substages V (12–18 months of age) and VI (18–24 months of age)

Language testing:

**SICD–Receptive: 16 months

**SICD–Expressive: 12 months

**Comprehension Checklist: 15–17 months

Phonology: KK vocalized frequently, **primarily with repetitive vocalizations and unintelligible noises that were judged to be nonlinguistic and self-stimulatory in nature.

Semantics: Reported a total expressive vocabulary of four words used to code action (e.g., *drink, bite*) and mark rejection (e.g., *no*). No semantically meaningful utterances were used during the evaluation.

Pragmatics:

**Intentions: A limited number of communicative intentions were expressed nonverbally, including requesting objects (e.g., pulled parent by finger to object and pushed hand at object), requesting actions (e.g., pulled father to door and pushed hand in direction of door to have it opened), and protesting and rejecting (e.g., pulled away from examiner). **Responsiveness to verbal stimuli was observed to be inconsistent, as was eye contact. **No requesting of information nor commenting was observed or reported.

Diagnostic impressions: Severely disordered receptive and expressive language skills and questionable cognitive skills when compared to children of his chronological age. Specific concerns included markedly disordered pragmatic skills and limited play skills with stereotypical behaviors.

Counseling and recommendations:

1. Refer for a complete developmental evaluation to determine the relationship among speech-language skills, nonverbal cognitive skills, and overall development. This case was flagged for referral to a developmental psychologist with specific training in the differential diagnosis of children with pervasive developmental disorder and autism.
2. Individual or small group speech-language therapy to address the documented disorder of receptive and expressive language skills. A "transition class" has been established for children like KK (who await additional diagnosis through psychological evaluation) to ensure that individual goals are established in a structured group setting until appropriate placements can be made.

3. Developmental preschool programming for peer interaction and language stimulation.
4. Participation in a state-funded support program for ongoing coordination of services as necessary.

Comments

This case illustrates the importance of using detailed parental and clinical observations to provide a complete picture of a child's behavioral and social skills. Key diagnostic points (**) involving communication (i.e., disordered pragmatic skills, language regression) enabled a diagnosis of severe language disorder. However, for this child, developmental testing is crucial to the determination of any additional diagnosis. Because the term *autism* carries such emotional weight, the speech-language clinician is often restricted in counseling and making additional service recommendations until such a diagnosis is made. For KK, a diagnosis of autism was made, and speech-language therapy, as well as developmental programming, was planned to meet his specific needs. Key points reflecting poor social skills and atypical behavior patterns allowed appropriate service recommendations to be made initially and facilitated the later diagnosis.

Client 4: BC, Female, 2 Years, 9 Months, Severe Language Delay with Multiple Handicaps

Birth history: Slight jaundice; **respiratory difficulty requiring administration of oxygen; malformed right pinna

Medical history: **Agenesis of the corpus callosum and diffuse subcortical damage to frontal lobes diagnosed through MRI; **genetic work up indicated an uncharacterized syndrome of multifactorial inheritance; tenotomy at age 18 months to relieve tendons in ankles; recurrent otitis media resulting in placement of pressure equalization tubes at approximately 5 months of age; environmental allergies

Developmental history:

Motor milestones: Delayed; sat at 9 months; crawled at 11 months; began walking at approximately 20 months of age after surgery to lengthen the tendons in her legs and feet

Speech and language milestones: Few early vocalizations; **first word appeared at 22 months of age; current vocabulary of four words (i.e., *mama, uhoh, go,* and *dog*); **primary form of communication described as vowel-like babbling and pointing, paired with vocalizations. **BC's early intervention teacher has encouraged the use of sign language to supplement her communication skills.

Behavior: Pleasant; interacted well with the examiner; participated in a variety of activities, although she had to be redirected to on-task behavior on occasion. Reportedly, **BC often has tantrums when she becomes frustrated or does not "get her way." BC has pulled out some of her hair during these episodes. She protested during the evaluation by grabbing her head or hair.

Hearing: WNL

Oral mechanism: Exam could not be completed due to reticence. **BC has a history of feeding difficulties and oral sensitivity: She could not suck from a nipple at birth. No current concerns in this area. BC was noted to have a large oral cavity, widely spaced teeth, and **mild low tone in her cheeks.

Cognition: A developmental evaluation was completed 2 months before speech-language referral. Results of that assessment revealed **cognitive skills clustering at the 24-month level and **fine- and gross-motor skills at the 16-month level. Recommendations included participation in an early intervention program, continued physical and occupational therapy services, and a complete speech-language evaluation. **BC receives early intervention services in her home twice weekly for 1 hour and occupational therapy and physical therapy for 1 hour per week.

Language testing:

**SICD–Receptive: 20 months

**SICD–Expressive: 12 months

**Comprehension Checklist: 19–21 months

Phonology: **Vocalizations heard during the evaluation consisted primarily of prolonged consonant sounds (e.g., /mmmmm/). Reportedly, BC's phonologic repertoire includes the consonants /b, m, n, g/ and a variety of vowels and diphthongs.

Semantics: BC's expressive vocabulary reportedly includes a total of four words used to code existence (e.g., *mama, dog*) or action (e.g., *go*). During the evaluation, she did not produce any utterances with semantic meaning.

Pragmatics: **BC expressed a variety of communicative intentions nonverbally, including requesting objects (e.g., pointed to desired object), requesting actions (e.g., patted diaper and looked at mother), protesting and rejecting (e.g., shook head, pulled hair, threw toys), commenting (e.g., pointed to objects), responding (e.g., turned to name), greetings (e.g., waved), and seeking attention (e.g., gestured to her mother).

Diagnostic impressions: Severely delayed receptive and expressive language skills when compared to same-aged peers. Communication skills were judged to be below cognitive ability levels with more significantly depressed expressive language skills. Areas of concern included limited vocalizations, limited phoneme repertoire, and lack of a core receptive and expressive vocabulary; however, communicative intentions were observed to be good in relation to verbal skills.

Counseling and recommendations:

1. Individual speech-language therapy to address delays in receptive and expressive language skills with further assessment to determine the appropriateness of an alternative or augmentative communication system.

2. Expand BC's early intervention services to include an individualized education program with speech-language goals that can be implemented by transdisciplinary professionals (e.g., occupational therapists, physical therapists, speech-language pathologists).

Comments

When a child's cognitive levels have been established before a speech-language assessment, differential diagnosis attempts to determine to what extent communication skills are a relative weakness. For BC, the gap between receptive language skills and cognition was judged to be less significant than that between receptive and expressive communication abilities. BC's desire to communicate, along with her visible frustration in her inability to do so, were judged to be significant factors suggesting alternative or augmentative communication as a possible avenue for intervention. Transdisciplinary service delivery should involve all rehabilitation professionals in providing a common, coordinated set of objectives for BC.

Client 5: WT, Male, 4 Years, 7 Months, Attention Deficit Disorder

Birth and medical history: Unremarkable

Developmental history:

Motor milestones: WNL

Speech and language milestones: Normal early vocalizations, with first word and word combinations reportedly emerging "a little late." WT uses complete sentences; however, his mother reported him to have **"difficulty expressing himself" and **difficulty following directions. **Frustration with communication difficulties has been reported. WT attends preschool 2 days per week, and his teacher has expressed concern with his social skills and language abilities.

Behavior: **Active and eager to interact with the examiner. Attention to structured tasks was limited (i.e., 3–5 minutes). **WT demonstrated noncompliant behavior (e.g., spitting; pushing items away; using a deep, angry voice) when participating in expressive tasks in which verbal responses were required. **In general, attention decreased and noncompliance increased as the session progressed. These behaviors were judged to significantly affect WT's performance.

Hearing, oral mechanism, voice, and fluency: WNL

Language testing:

**Clinical Evaluation of Language Fundamentals Receptive Language: standard score: 50

**Clinical Evaluation of Language Fundamentals Expressive Language: standard score: 90

**Peabody Picture Vocabulary Test–Revised: standard score: 88

Phonology: WNL

Grammar:

Assigning Structural Stages: complex sentence skill development within Brown's Stage V++. (Stage V++ behaviors are most typical of children aged 48 months and older.)

Narrative:

Renfrew Bus Story:

Information: standard score, 81
Sentence length: standard score, 96
Complexity reference chart: average range
Independence score: below average score

Semantics: **Used indefinite statements, characterized by words lacking in specificity (e.g., "Let's talk about some more things right there") and **demonstrated word-finding difficulties (e.g., described objects ["That's what I brush my teeth with"] and demonstrated actions with his hands before naming them).

Pragmatics: WNL

Diagnostic impressions: Receptive language skills were found to be severely disordered when compared to chronologic-aged peers. General expressive language skills judged to be WNL, with a specific weakness noted in word-finding abilities. Results of the evaluation were interpreted with caution due to significant attentional difficulties and oppositional behaviors. Inappropriate behavior increased when verbal responses were required.

Counseling and recommendations:

1. Referral to a neuropsychologist for determination of the significance of attentional and behavioral characteristics
2. Individual therapy to address receptive language disorder and word-finding abilities. Because of noted parental frustration and their expressed desire to promote "appropriate conversation" with WT, a referral should be made to a speech-language pathologist experienced in family counseling and treatment of attention disorders.
3. Participation in a behavior-management program

Comments

WT's profile is a relatively unusual one for children referred for language delay, but it is seen occasionally with children who have attentional deficits or who demonstrate oppositional behaviors that interfere with comprehension testing. This case illustrates the need for close observation of a client's behavior as it affects standardized testing as well as communication skills in unstructured tasks. While WT's comprehension skills may not actually be "delayed," they are certainly impaired by his inability to attend consistently. On the other hand, difficulties in expressive language, which were more directly evidenced by observation than by standardized scores, appeared to have a direct effect on his confidence and therefore his behavior. A neuropsychological evaluation should aid in defining the parameters of the attentional and behavioral components of WT's communication difficulties. Medically supervised drug therapy may be indicated and should be closely coordinated with communication-skills training, as well as direct behavior management.

Client 6: VB, Male, 1 Year, 10 Months, Delayed Functional Articulation and Client 7: DL, Male, 1 Year 8 Months, Developmental Apraxia of Speech

VB

Birth history: Unremarkable

Medical history: Recurrent otitis media with pressure equalization tubes placed at 13 months of age; familial history of stuttering (father)

Speech and language milestones: Normal early vocalizations that decreased at the onset of bouts of otitis media. VB's first word appeared at 18–20 months of age; he currently has a vocabulary of eight to ten words. **Reportedly, VB has used several words on only one occasion. Elaborate gesture is VB's primary form of communication. He does not appear frustrated.

Hearing, voice, and fluency: WNL

Oral mechanism: Adequate structure. Functional assessment could not be completed due to reticence. Mild low tone in cheeks and open mouth breathing posture were observed. No history of drooling or mouthing toys.

Cognition: Uzgiris-Hunt showed sensorimotor skills in Piagetian substage VI (18–24 months).

Language testing:

  **SICD–Receptive: 24–28 months
  **SICD–Expressive: 12 months
  **Comprehension Checklist: 24 month range

Phonology: Vocalizations consisted primarily of **consonant-vowel (CV) single-syllable word approximations, symbolic noises (e.g., motor sound, *uhoh*), and CVCV reduplicated syllables. **His phonologic repertoire included the consonants /b, m, d, w/ and a variety of vowels and diphthongs. **Phoneme imitation was poor.

Semantics: **Used single-word utterances to code the semantic categories of existence (e.g., *ball*), rejection (e.g., *no*), and locative action (e.g., *up*). VB indicated no other categories coded verbally; however, he used **gesture to code attribution (e.g., stretched arms out to indicate *big*), action (e.g., put hand to mouth to indicate *eat*), and locative action (e.g., gestured *push*).

Pragmatics: Appropriate verbal and nonverbal intentions

DL

Birth and medical history: Unremarkable

Speech and language milestones: Limited early vocalizations. Parental report indicated that first word occurred at 13 months of age, with a current vocabulary of 10 words. No word combinations noted. **There is a history of one-time word use. **Majority of DL's words begin with the phoneme /d/; **other sounds are used infrequently. Primary form of communication described as grunt-like vocalization paired with gestures.

Hearing, voice, and fluency: WNL

Oral mechanism: Structure and function appeared to be adequate for speech production. Parental report indicated that DL avoids chewing "hard pieces of meat" because of their texture. No other feeding difficulties were reported. **DL was noted to mouth toys and chew on his fingers during the evaluation. **Inability to imitate phonemes, despite effort.

Language testing:

**SICD–Receptive: 28 months

**SICD–Expressive: 9–12 months

**Comprehension Checklist: 24 month range

Phonology: Vocalizations consisted primarily of consonants (C), vowels (V), CV syllables, and reduplicated CV syllables. **His phonologic repertoire included the consonants /w, m, d/ and a few vowels and diphthongs. **Inconsistent word productions with some vowel variation.

Semantics: Used word approximations to code existence (e.g., *dog*) and rejection (e.g., *no*).

Pragmatics: Appropriate verbal and nonverbal intentions

Diagnostic impressions of VB and DL: Both boys were found to demonstrate severely delayed expressive communication skills when compared to children of their chronologic ages. Specific concerns for each included performance suggestive of developmental apraxia of speech: limited phoneme repertoires, inconsistent articulatory productions, and histories of inconsistent word usage, along with poor ability to imitate phonemes.

Initial recommendations:

1. Individual diagnostic speech-language therapy with a clinician experienced in the diagnosis and treatment of oral-motor difficulties to determine the significance of oral-motor influences in the documented delays in speech and language
2. Provide information for suggested home language and speech stimulation techniques

Comments

These two cases are considered together to illustrate the importance and legitimacy of diagnostic therapy as a recommendation of initial speech-language evaluations. Key differential diagnostic points were originally similar for each child, yet final outcomes proved to be very different. DL was ultimately diagnosed with developmental apraxia of speech and required intensive individual speech therapy, in addition to small group speech-language therapy. After months of therapy, he continued to demonstrate difficulty sequencing sounds in words and words in phrases, along with an inability to gain stable articulatory patterns. VB, in contrast, was transitioned to small-group therapy after only 3 months of individual sessions and was terminated from the group 5 months later with speech and language skills within the broad limits of normal. Further complicating differential diagnosis in such cases is the overlying factor of depressed production. What looks like an expressive language delay may actually be avoidance of speech due to frustration or accommodation for listeners (i.e., limiting speech to what can be understood). Diagnostic therapy can be necessary to define such distinctions and to refine service recommendations.

Client 8: TD, **Female, 2 Years, 5 Months, Specific Language Impairment

Birth history: Delivery by emergency cesarean section secondary to fetal decelerations

Medical history: Occasional bouts of otitis media treated with antibiotics; familial history of Down syndrome (sister)

Family history: Middle class working parents; **father received "special help" with language and reading in school. TD attends day-care as a "peer model" at the developmental preschool where her sister receives services.

Developmental history:

Motor milestones: WNL

Speech and language milestones: Normal early vocalizations; **first word at 14 months (e.g., *bye bye*); recently combined words for the first time (i.e., *bye bye mama*); **current vocabulary of 40–50 words; communicates primarily through a combination of words and gestures; **observed frustration with communication.

Behavior: Active, eager to interact. Participated in structured and unstructured tasks with occasional verbal redirection required. Mother reported that TD does not play well with the children at her day-care.

Hearing and oral mechanism: WNL

Language testing:

**SICD–Receptive: 26 months, with scatter to 28 months

**SICD–Expressive: 20 months

**MacArthur Communicative Development Inventory (Words and Sentences):

Vocabulary: greater than the fifth percentile

Sentence complexity: fifth percentile

**Comprehension Checklist: 24 months

Phonology: Vocalizations consisted primarily of intelligible single-word utterances using the consonants /b, p, t, d, k, g, h, m/ along with a variety of vowels and diphthongs.

Semantics: Used single- and occasional two-word utterances to code a limited number of semantic categories, including existence (e.g., *cow, truck*), rejection or denial (e.g., *no*), and action (e.g., *look mama*). TD does not code attribution, possession, nonexistence, or recurrence.

Pragmatics:

Intentions: TD expressed a variety of communicative intentions verbally and nonverbally, including requesting objects (e.g., *cow* plus extended hand), requesting actions (e.g., *look*), naming (e.g., *truck*), and commenting (e.g., *oooh*).

Presupposition: not observed

Discourse: answered questions nonverbally; most speech directed socially

Diagnostic impressions: Moderate to severely delayed expressive language skills with borderline receptive skills. Specific concerns include limited expressive vocabulary and limited word combinations.

Counseling and recommendations:

1. Small group speech-language therapy on a weekly basis to address expressive language difficulties and monitor receptive language progress
2. Enrollment in a developmentally appropriate day-care or preschool with children with typically developing communication skills to serve as models
3. Supply the family with resources for home language-stimulation techniques

Comments

This case represents a common profile presented by toddler-age speech-language referrals—the LT whose parents seek reassurance that their child will "catch up on [his or] her own" or validation that their concerns have not been unfounded. While these questions cannot be answered definitively, key diagnostic points (**) do raise some red flags in this case that indicate the possibility of continued difficulties (e.g., gender, familial history of language and learning difficulties). Of equal importance in formulating service recommendations, however, may be issues such as frustration in communication, depressed peer interaction, and parental concern. Here, the recommendation for group speech-language therapy directly targets TD's language delay, as well as her social frustrations. Day-care services with more typical language models, as suggested, would complement efforts in both areas. The parents' desire for inclusion in the remediation process is met, for the short-term, with a supply of resources and ideas for home language-stimulation techniques. Later, counseling by the child's clinician will serve to maintain that parental involvement.

Client 9: JA, Female, 1 Year, 10 Months, Closed Head Injury

Birth history: Unremarkable

Medical history: **Skull fracture with loss of consciousness (15 minutes) sustained in motor vehicle accident at 11 months of age. Hospitalized for 3 days. **MRI indicated mild right frontal cortical damage. Hospitalized for pneumonia at 15 months of age; occasional bouts of otitis media

Family history: Single mother works at minimum wage job. JA and 3-year-old sister are cared for by a neighbor.

Developmental history:

Motor milestones: WNL, although JA stopped crawling for several months after accident. Currently, motor skills are age-appropriate.

Speech and language milestones: Normal early vocalization. **First word at 12 months. Current vocabulary of greater than 20 words and **has just begun to combine words. Uses some gestures.

Behavior: Shy, but warmed up and cooperated. Reportedly exhibits occasional head banging and wakes up with night terrors approximately once a month since the accident.

Hearing and oral mechanism: WNL

Cognition: Uzgiris-Hunt showed sensorimotor skills in Piagetian substage VI (18–24 months)

Language testing:

**SICD–Receptive: 24 months

**SICD–Expressive: 24 months

**MacArthur Communicative Development Inventory (Words and Sentences):

Vocabulary: sixtieth percentile

Sentence complexity: fiftieth percentile

Phonology: WNL. The consonants /w, b, p, m, n, t, d, g, f, k/ were heard during evaluation in generally intelligible word contexts along with a variety of vowels and diphthongs.

Semantics: Used single- and two-word utterances to code a variety of semantic categories, including nonexistence (e.g., *gone*), attribution (e.g., *blue*), and locative action (e.g., *here mommy*).

Grammar: **MLU of 1.8 morphemes. Language Assessment and Remediation Screening Procedure analysis (Crystal et al. 1989) indicates use of Stage II forms (1 year, 6 months, to 2 years), clause (e.g., verb plus object, *get ball*), and phrase (e.g., noun noun, *mommy baby*) structures. The language sample contained two examples of three-word utterances (e.g., *mommy baby bye*).

Pragmatics:

Intentions: JA expressed a variety of communicative intentions verbally, including requesting objects (e.g., *get ball*), requesting actions (e.g., *here mommy*), naming (e.g., *baby*), protesting (e.g., *no, no*), and commenting (e.g., *broken*).

Presupposition: not observed

Discourse: answered questions; most speech directed socially

Diagnostic impressions: Language and speech skills were found to be WNL for chronologic age and consistent with cognitive functioning. Good recovery from closed head injury.

Recommendations:

1. Reassure mother that early trauma has not affected JA's long-term development. Provide parent packet with suggested stimulation activities that mother or baby-sitter could incorporate into daily routine.
2. Refer 3-year-old sister to Head Start preschool in her area, with assumption that JA will benefit indirectly from some of Head Start's family services now and will benefit directly by enrolling when she is 3 years old.
3. Schedule re-evaluation in 6 months to monitor progress, in view of the history of head injury.

Comments

The history of closed-head injury and subsequent motor regression raises concerns, but JA appears to have made a very good developmental recovery. The MRI showing that damage was restricted to unilateral cortical involvement supports a positive prognosis for language outcomes. Key differential diagnostic points (**) included remarkably consistent age-appropriate receptive and expressive language abilities as reported by the mother (i.e., MacArthur), documented via formal tests (i.e., SICD), and substantiated by observational measures (i.e., MLU). Using words by 12 months of age and combining words into two- and three-word utterances before 24 months of age suggests that JA is not a LT, despite the potential setback from a brain trauma. Recommendations reflect the mother's need for reassurance and support and direct her to potential resources through Head Start that can benefit the children and the family without creating additional economic hardship.

REFERENCES

Aiken L. (1988) *Psychological Testing and Assessment* (6th ed). Boston: Allyn & Bacon.

Aram D, Eisele J. (1992) Plasticity and Recovery of Higher Cognitive Functions Following Early Brain Injury. In I Rapin, S Segalowitz (eds), *Handbook of Neuropsychology* (Vol. 6) (pp. 73–92). Amsterdam: Elsevier.

Aram D, Eisele J. (1994) Limits to a left hemisphere explanation for specific language impairment. *Journal of Speech and Hearing Research* 37, 824–830.

Aram D, Ekelman B, Nation J. (1984) Preschoolers with language disorders: 10 years later. *Journal of Speech and Hearing Research* 27, 232–244.

Austin J. (1962) *How To Do Things with Words*. New York: University Press.

Baltaxe C, Simmons J. (1990) The differential diagnosis of communication disorders in child and adolescent psychopathology. *Topics in Language Disorders* 10, 17–31.

Bates E. (1976) Pragmatics and Sociolinguistics in Child Language. In D Morehead, A Morehead (eds), *Normal and Deficient Child Language*. Baltimore: University Park Press.

Bates E, Camaioni L, Volterra V. (1975) The acquisition of performatives prior to speech. *Merrill-Palmer Quarterly* 21, 205–226.

Battle D. (1993) *Communication Disorders in Multicultural Populations*. Boston: Butterworth–Heinemann.

Benton A. (1964) Developmental aphasia and brain damage. *Cortex* 1, 614–617.

Bishop D, Edmundson A. (1987) Language-impaired 4-year-olds: distinguishing transient from persistent impairment. *Journal of Speech and Hearing Disorders* 52, 156–173.

Bloch J, Seitz M. (1989) Parents as assessors of children: a collaborative approach to helping. *Social Work in Education* 11, 226–244.

Bricker D. (1992) The Changing Nature of Communication and Language Intervention. In S Warren, J Reichle (eds), *Causes and Effects in Communication and Language Intervention* (pp. 361–375). Baltimore: Brookes Publishing Co.

Bricker D. (1993) *Assessment, Evaluation, and Programming System: AEPS Measurement for Birth to Three Years*. Baltimore: Brookes Publishing Co.

Bricker D, Squires J, Mounts L. (1995) *Ages and Stages Questionnaires: A Parent-Completed, Child-Monitoring System*. Baltimore: Brookes Publishing Co.

Bronfenbrenner U. (1977) Toward an experimental ecology of human development. *American Psychologist* 32, 513–531.

Brown B, Edwards M. (1989) *Developmental Disorders of Language*. London: Whurr Publishers.

Brown R. (1973) *A First Language: The Early Stages*. Cambridge, MA: Harvard University Press.

Bzoch K. (1987) *Parent/Professional Preschool Performance Profile*. Syosset, NY: Variety Pre-Schooler's Workshop.

Camarata S, Swisher L. (1990) A note on intelligence assessment within studies of specific language impairment. *Journal of Speech and Hearing Research* 33, 203–207.

Cantwell D, Baker L. (1991) *Psychiatric and Developmental Disorder in Children with Communication Disorder*. Washington, DC: American Psychiatric Press.

Catts H, Kamhi A. (1986) The linguistic bases of reading disorders: implications for the speech-language pathologist. *Language, Speech, and Hearing Services in the Schools* 17, 329–341.

Chapman RS. (1988) Language Comprehension in the Infant and Preschool Child. In D Yoder, R Kent (eds), *Decision-Making in Speech-Language Pathology*. Toronto: BC Decker, Inc.

Cheng L. (1991) *Assessing Asian Language Performance* (2nd ed). Oceanside, CA: Academic Communication Associates.

Cowley J, Glasgow C. (1994) *The Renfrew Bus Story*. Centreville, DE: The Centreville school.

Crais E. (1993) Families and professionals as collaborators in assessment. *Topics in Language Disorders* 14, 29–40.

Crais E. (1995) Expanding the repertoire of tools and techniques for assessing the communication skills of infants and toddlers. *American Journal of Speech-Language Pathology* 4, 47–59.

Crais E, Roberts J. (1995) Assessing Communication Skills in Infants and Preschoolers. In M McLean, D Bailey, M Wolery (eds), *Assessing Infants and Preschoolers with Special Needs* (2nd ed). Columbus, OH: Macmillan.

Crary M. (1993) *Developmental Motor Speech Disorders.* San Diego: Singular Publishing Group.

Crystal D, Fletcher P, Garman M. (1989) *The Grammatical Analysis of Language Disability* (2nd ed). London: Whurr Publishers.

Dale P, Bates E, Reznick S, Morisset C. (1989) The validity of a parent report instrument on child language at twenty months. *Journal of Child Language* 16, 239–249.

Diagnostic and Statistical Manual of Mental Disorders: DSM IV (4th ed). (1994) Washington, DC: American Psychiatric Press.

Dickinson D, McCabe A. (1991) A Social Interactionist Account of Language and Literacy Development. In J Kavanaugh (ed), *The Language Continuum* (pp. 1–40). Parkton, MD: York Press.

Drayer B. (1993) MR imaging advances in practice. *Journal of Computer Assisted Tomography* 17, 30–35.

Dunn LM, Dunn LM. (1981) *Peabody Picture Vocabulary Test-Revised.* Circle Pines, MI: American Guidance Services.

Eisele J, Aram D. (1993) Differential effects of early hemisphere damage on lexical comprehension and production. *Aphasiology* 5, 513–523.

Eisenson J. (1968) Developmental aphasia: a speculative view with therapeutic implications. *Journal of Speech and Hearing Disorders* 33, 3–13.

Ellis-Weismer S, Murray-Branch J, Miller J. (1993) Comparison of two methods for promoting productive vocabulary in late talkers. *Journal of Speech and Hearing Research* 36, 1037–1050.

Feagans L. (1982) The Development and Importance of Narratives for School Adaptation. In L Feagans, D Farran (eds), *The Language of Children Reared in Poverty* (pp. 95–116). New York: Academic Press.

Fenson L, Dale P, Reznick S, et al. (1993) *MacArthur Communicative Development Inventories.* San Diego: Singular Publishing Group.

Fischel J, Whitehurst G, Caulfield M, DeBarsyshe B. (1989) Language growth in children with expressive language delay. *Pediatrics* 82, 218–227.

Fudula J. (1986) *Arizona Articulation Proficiency Scale* (2nd ed). Los Angeles: Western Psychological Services.

Gibbs E. (1990) Assessment of Infant Mental Ability: Conventional Tests and Issues of Prediction. In E Gibbs, D Teti (eds), *Interdisciplinary Assessment of Infants: A Guide for Early Intervention Professionals* (pp. 77–90). Baltimore: Brookes Publishing Co.

Gill G, Dihoff R. (1982) Nonverbal Assessment of Cognitive Behavior. In B Campbell, V Baldwin (eds), *Severely Handicapped/Hearing Impaired Students* (pp. 77–113). Baltimore: Brookes Publishing Co.

Gillam R, McFadden T, van Kleeck A. (1995) Improving Narrative Abilities: Whole Language and Language Skills Approaches. In M Fey, J Windsor, S Warren (eds), *Language Intervention: Preschool Through the Elementary Years* (pp. 145–182). Baltimore: Brookes Publishing Co.

Goldman R, Fristoe M. (1986) *Goldman-Fristoe Test of Articulation.* Circle Pines, MN: American Guidance Services.

Halliday MAK. (1975) *Learning How to Mean: Explorations in the Development of Language.* London: Edward Arnold.

Hart B, Risley T. (1992) American parenting of language-learning children: persisting differences in family-child interactions observed in natural home environments. *Developmental Psychology* 28, 1096–1105.

Hedrick D, Prather E, Tobin A. (1984) *Sequenced Inventory of Communication Development–Revised*. Seattle: University of Washington Press.

Hoff-Ginsberg E. (1986) Function and structure in maternal speech: their relation to the child's development of syntax. *Developmental Psychology* 22, 155–163.

Hoff-Ginsberg E. (1991) Mother-child conversation in different social classes and communicative settings. *Child Development* 62, 782–796.

Johnston J. (1982) Narratives: a new look at communication problems in older language-disordered children. *Language, Speech, and Hearing Services in Schools* 13, 144–155.

Jones H. (1995) Issues in early childhood education: implications and directions for higher education. *Peabody Journal of Education* 70, 112–121.

Kemp K, Klee T. (1997) Clinical language sampling practices: results of a survey of speech-language pathologists in the United States. *Child Language Teaching and Therapy* 13, 161–176.

Kent R. (1992) Speech Intelligibility and Communicative Competence in Children. In A Kaiser, D Gray (eds), *Enhancing Children's Communication: Research Foundations for Intervention* (pp. 223–239). Baltimore: Brookes Publishing Co.

Kent R, Miolo G, Bloedel S. (1994) The intelligibility of children's speech: a review of evaluation procedures. *American Journal of Speech Language Pathology* 3, 81–95.

Klee T. (1985) Clinician language sampling: analysing the analyses. *Child Language Teaching and Therapy* 1, 182–198.

Kinsbourne M, Hiscock M. (1977) Does Cerebral Dominance Develop? In S Segalowitz, F Gruber (eds), *Language Development and Neurological Theory* (pp. 171–191). New York: Academic Press.

Lahey M. (1988) *Language Disorders and Language Development* (pp. 429–433). New York: Macmillan.

Landry S, Loveland K. (1988) Communication behaviors in autism and developmental language delay. *The Journal of Child Psychology and Psychiatry and Allied Disciplines* 28, 621–634.

Langdon H. (1994) Meeting the needs of the non-English speaking parents of a communicatively disabled child. *Clinics in Communication Disorders* 24, 227–236.

Lee L. (1974) *Developmental Sentence Analysis*. Evanston, IL: Northwestern University Press.

Levin S, Huttenlocher P, Banich M, Duda E. (1987). Factors affecting cognitive functioning of hemiplegic children. *Developmental Medicine and Child Neurology* 29, 27–35.

Linder T. (1993) *Transdisciplinary Play-Based Assessment: A Functional Approach to Working with Young Children* (rev ed). Baltimore: Brookes Publishing Co.

Long S, Fey M. (1993) *Computerized Profiling*. San Antonio, TX: Psychological Corporation.

Lynch E, Hanson M. (1992) *Developing Cross-Cultural Competence: A Guide for Working with Young Children and Their Families*. Baltimore: Brookes Publishing Co.

Mahoney G, Robinson C, Powell A. (1992) Focusing on parent-child interaction: The bridge to developmentally appropriate practices. *Topics in Early Childhood Special Education* 12, 105–120.

Maistro A, German M. (1986) Reliability, predictive validity, and interrelationships of early assessment indices used with developmentally delayed infants and children. *Journal of Clinical Child Psychology* 15, 327–332.

Marquardt T, Sussman H. (1991) Developmental Apraxia of Speech: Theory and Practice. In D Vogel, M Cannito (eds), *Treating Disordered Speech Motor Control.* Austin, TX: PRO-ED.

McCabe A, Peterson C. (1991) *Developing Narrative Structure.* Hillsdale, NJ: Erlbaum.

McCabe A, Rollins P. (1994). Assessment of preschool narrative skills. *American Journal of Speech Language Pathology* 3, 45–56.

Michaels S. (1981) "Sharing time": children's narrative styles and differential access to literacy. *Language in Society* 10, 423–442.

Miller J. (1981) *Assessing Language Production in Children.* Baltimore: University Park Press.

Miller J. (1988) Language Production in the Preschool Child. In D Yoder, R Kent (eds), *Decision-Making in Speech-Language Pathology.* Toronto: BC Decker, Inc.

Miller J, Chapman R. (1993) Systematic Analysis of Language Transcripts (SALT) (Version 3.0) [computer software]. Madison, WI: Language Analysis Laboratory, Waisman Center, University of Wisconsin.

Miller J, Chapman R, Branston M, Reichle J. (1980) Language comprehension in sensorimotor stages V and VI. *Journal of Speech and Hearing Research* 23, 284–311.

Miller J, Sedey A, Miolo G. (1995) Validity of parent report measures of vocabulary development for children with Down's syndrome. *Journal of Speech and Hearing Research* 38, 1037–1044.

Miller P, Sperry L. (1988) Early talk about the past: the origins of conversational stories of personal experience. *Journal of Child Language* 15, 293–315.

Moller M. (1994) Audiological evaluation. *Journal of Clinical Neurophysiology* 11, 309–318.

Paul R. (1991) Profiles of toddlers with slow expressive language development. *Topics in Language Disorders* 11, 1–13.

Paul R. (1993) Patterns of development in late talkers: preschool years. *Journal of Childhood Communication Disorders* 15, 7–14.

Paul R, Elwood T. (1991) Maternal linguistic input to toddlers with slow expressive language development. *Journal of Speech and Hearing Research* 34, 982–988.

Paul R, Shiffer M. (1991) Communicative initiations in normal and late-talking toddlers. *Applied Psycholinguistics* 12, 419–431.

Paul R, Smith R. (1993) Narrative skills in 4-year-olds with normal, impaired, and late-developing language. *Journal of Speech and Hearing Research* 36, 592–598.

Paul R, Spangle-Looney S, Dahm P. (1991) Communication and socialization skills at age two and three in "late-talking" young children. *Journal of Speech and Hearing Research* 34, 858–865.

Pendergast K, Dickey S, Selmar T, Soder A. (1984) *The Photo Articulation Test* (2nd ed). Austin, TX: PRO-ED.

Plante E, Swisher L, Vance R. (1991) MRI findings in boys with specific language impairment. *Brain and Language* 42, 52–66.

Prizant B, Meyer E. (1993) Socioemotional aspects of language and social-communication disorders in young children and their families. *American Journal of Speech Language Pathology* 2, 56–71.

Prizant B, Audet L, Burke G, et al. (1990) Communication disorders and emotional/behavioral disorders in children. *Journal of Speech and Hearing Disorders* 55, 179–192.

Rafaat S, Rvachew S, Russell R. (1995) Reliability of clinician judgments of severity of phonological impairment. *American Journal of Speech-Language Pathology* 4, 39–46.

Reed V. (1994) *An Introduction to Children with Language Disorders*. Columbus, OH: Merrill.

Rescorla L. (1989) The language development survey: a screening tool for delayed language in toddlers. *Journal of Speech and Hearing Disorders* 54, 587–599.

Rescorla L, Goossens M. (1992) Symbolic play development in toddlers with expressive specific language impairment. *Journal of Speech and Hearing Research* 6, 1290–1302.

Rescorla L, Roberts J, Dahlsgaard K. (1997) Late talkers at 2: outcome at age 3. *Journal of Speech, Language and Hearing Research* 40, 556–566.

Rescorla L, Schwartz E. (1990) Outcome of toddlers with specific expressive language delay. *Applied Psycholinguistics* 11, 393–408.

Rice M, Alexander A, Hadley P. (1993) Social biases toward children with speech and language impairments: a correlative causal model of language limitation. *Applied Psycholinguistics* 14, 473–488.

Richardson S. (1983) Differential diagnosis in delayed speech and language development. *Folia Phoniatrica* 35, 66–80.

Roth F, Spekman N. (1984) Assessing the pragmatic abilities of children: part 1 and part 2. *Journal of Speech and Hearing Disorders* 49, 2–53.

Schery T. (1981) Selecting assessment strategies for language disordered children. *Topics in Language Disorders* 1, 59–73.

Searle J. (1969) *Speech Acts: An Essay in the Philosophy of Language*. London: Cambridge University Press.

Shriberg L, Aram D, Kwiatkowski J. (1997) Developmental apraxia of speech: I. Descriptive and theoretical perspectives. *Journal of Speech and Hearing Research* 40, 273–285.

Siegel G, Broen P. (1976) Language Assessment. In L Lloyd (ed), *Communication Assessment and Intervention Strategies* (pp. 73–122). Baltimore: University Park Press.

Simeonsson R. (1989) Assessing Family Environments. In D Bailey, R Simeonsson (eds), *Family Assessment in Early Intervention* (pp. 167–184). Columbus, OH: Merrill.

Snow C. (1972) Mothers' speech to children learning language. *Child Development* 43, 549–565.

Stark R. (1978) Infant speech production and communication skills. *Allied Health and Behavioral Sciences* 1, 131–151.

St. Louis K, Ruscello D. (1987). *Oral Speech Mechanism Screening Examination–Revised*. Austin, TX: PRO-ED.

Stoel-Gammon C. (1987) Phonological skills of 2-year-olds. *Language, Speech, and Hearing Services in Schools* 18, 323–329.

Stoel-Gammon C. (1991) Normal and disordered phonology in two-year-olds. *Topics in Language Disorders* 11, 21–32.

Tallal P, Ross R, Curtiss S. (1989) Familial aggregation in specific language impairment. *Journal of Speech and Hearing Disorders* 54, 167–173.

Taylor O. (1986) *Nature of Communication Disorders in Culturally and Linguistically Diverse Populations*. San Diego: College-Hill Press.

Thal D, Bates E. (1988) Language and gesture in late talkers. *Journal of Speech and Hearing Research* 31, 115–123.

Thal D, Tobias S. (1992) Communicative gestures in children with delayed onset of expressive vocabulary. *Journal of Speech and Hearing Disorders* 35, 1281–1289.

Thal D, Tobias S. (1994) Relationships between language and gesture in normally developing and late-talking toddlers. *Journal of Speech and Hearing Research* 37, 157–170.

Thal D, Tobias S, Morrison D. (1991) Language and gesture in late talkers: a one year follow-up. *Journal of Speech and Hearing Disorders* 34, 604–612.

Tomblin B. (1989) Familial concentration of developmental language impairment. *Journal of Speech and Hearing Disorders* 54, 287–295.

Uzgiris I, Hunt J. (1975) *Assessment in Infancy: Ordinal Scales of Psychological Development*. Urbana, IL: University of Illinois Press.

van Kleeck A, Schuele C. (1987) Precursors to literacy: normal development. *Topics in Language Disorders* 7, 13–31.

Westby C. (1980) Assessment of cognitive and language abilities through play. *Language, Speech, and Hearing Services in the Schools* 11, 154–168.

Westby C. (1988) Children's play: reflections of social competence. *Seminars in Speech and Language* 9, 1–14.

Wetherby A, Prizant B. (1992) Profiling Young Children's Communicative Competence. In S Warren, J Reichle (eds), *Causes and Effects in Communication and Language Intervention* (pp. 217–253). Baltimore: Brookes Publishing Co.

Whitehurst G, Fischel J, Arnold D, Lonigan C. (1992) Evaluating Outcomes with Children with Expressive Language Delay. In S Warren, J Reichle (eds), *Causes and Effects in Communication and Language Intervention* (pp. 277–314). Baltimore: Brookes Publishing Co.

Wiig E, Semel E, Secord W. (1992) *Clinical Evaluation of Language Fundamentals–Preschool.* San Antonio, TX: Psychological Corporation.

4

Differential Diagnosis of Language Learning Disabilities

Alan G. Kamhi

Case 1

Adrian is a first grader who has not yet learned to read. He has been receiving speech-language therapy since he was 4 years old and still exhibits some speech and language delays. His receptive vocabulary is about a year and half below age level.

Case 2

Steve is a third grader reading at a first-grade level. He has difficulty remembering directions the teacher gives for completing assignments. He does not make any obvious errors in spoken language, though he does have difficulty telling a story or relating an event in front of the class.

Case 3

Michelle is a fifth grader. She had no problems in school until she got to the fourth grade, when she began to have difficulty completing her assignments in history and science. Although her handwriting and spelling are fine, she has difficulty organizing her thoughts on paper. Her mind often seems to wander in class.

Are these children language disordered, learning disabled, or reading disabled? Or are they more appropriately described as having dyslexia, language learning disabilities (LLDs), or attention deficit hyperactivity disorders (ADHDs)? The number of descriptors for students with developmental learning problems is not only confusing but in many cases detrimental to providing the best services for these students. The particular diagnostic category one would assign to the three sample cases depends more on professional territoriality and theoretical biases than on the specific behaviors exhibited by the students. Special educators are more likely to identify these children as *learning disabled*; speech-language pathologists prefer the terms *language disordered* or *language learning disabled*; physicians tend to prefer *ADHD* and *dyslexia*; and psychologists may use several of the terms.

The term *language learning disabled* is used by many speech-language pathologists to describe school-age children with language and learning problems. Use of this term has served to emphasize the language bases of the learning problems school-age children experience. As such, the term has played an important role in involving speech-language pathologists in serving children with reading and other academic problems. Although language learning disabled is a useful descriptor of school-age children who have difficulty with spoken language, written language, or more general learning problems, it has not received widespread use or acceptance outside of speech-language pathology.

The term *language learning disabled* will probably never be broadly used because the children it describes meet the criteria for a learning disability. In other words, the definition of LLD is essentially the same as the definition of a learning disability (LD). The National Joint Committee on Learning Disabilities, which includes the American Speech-Language-Hearing Association, has defined learning disabilities as follows:

> Learning disabilities is a general term that refers to a heterogeneous group of disorders manifested by significant difficulties in the acquisition and use of listening, speaking, reading, writing, reasoning, or mathematical abilities. These disorders are intrinsic to the individual, presumed to be due to central nervous system dysfunction, and may occur across the life span. Problems in self-regulatory behaviors, social perception, and social interaction may exist with learning disabilities but do not by themselves constitute a learning disability.
>
> Although learning disabilities may occur concomitantly with other handicapping conditions (for example, sensory impairment, mental retardation, serious emotional disturbance) or with extrinsic influences (such as cultural differences, insufficient or inappropriate instruction) they are not the result of those conditions or influences (National Joint Committee on Learning Disabilities 1988, p. 1).

In reading through the definition, the language bases of learning disabilities should be apparent. Listening, speaking, reading, writing, and reasoning all are language-based skills. The only exception is mathematics, and, in most cases, students who have problems in math also have problems in spoken or written language. It is extremely rare to find students who have problems solely with math. The term *dyscalculia* sometimes is used to describe the documented cases of students who have pure calculation or computation problems without associated language deficits.

A student with an LD or LLD can also have an ADHD. The *Diagnostic and Statistical Manual of Mental Disorders* (4th ed.) (1994) defines three subtypes of ADHD: (1) ADHD, combined type—individuals who have six or more symptoms of inattention and six or more symptoms of hyperactivity or impulsivity; (2) ADHD, predominantly inattentive type—six or more symptoms of inattentiveness but fewer than six symptoms of hyperactivity or impulsivity; and (3) ADHD, predominantly hyperactive-impulsive type—six or more symptoms of hyperactivity or impulsivity but fewer than six symptoms of inattentiveness. ADHD is a significant risk factor for learning problems, but not all children with ADHD are LD.

Because of the heterogeneous nature of LLDs, many attempts have been made to classify or identify subgroups of children with learning disabilities (Kamhi and Catts 1989; Lyon et al. 1993). For example, one can differentiate students according to the extent and nature of reading problems, the extent and nature of the spoken-language impairment, basic processing limitations, cognitive-intellectual abilities, environmental factors, and so forth. A framework for differentially diagnosing children with LLDs is presented in the section *Differential Diagnosis of Students with Language Learning Disabilities.* This framework reflects a broad-based approach to assessment, involving not only information about language abilities but also information about other organismic and environmental factors that can influence language and learning.

One of the primary purposes of differential diagnosis is to determine a particular student's strengths and weaknesses to develop appropriate intervention goals and strategies. Emphasis on individual differences needs to be balanced, however, by knowledge of the general patterns of language and language-related behavior that characterize children with LLDs. Differentiating language learning disabled students based on their history of spoken language impairment can also be useful. Subgroups and general characteristics of LLDs are discussed in the following sections *Subgroups of Children with Language Learning Disabilities* and *Characteristics of Children with Language Learning Disabilities.*

SUBGROUPS OF CHILDREN WITH LANGUAGE LEARNING DISABILITIES

The brief description of the three students that began this chapter is an example of three different subgroups of children with LLDs. The first child, Adrian, had been receiving speech-language therapy since he was 4 years old and still exhibited some speech and language delays. His receptive vocabulary was about a year and half below age level. He had not yet learned to read. Adrian is an example of a language learning disabled child with a history of a spoken language impairment. Many children who have a preschool language impairment have difficulty learning to read—the primary problem in children with LLDs (Bishop and Adams 1990; Catts 1993; Tallal et al. 1989). Children with preschool language impairments have deficiencies in many of the basic language abilities that are required for reading. Deficiencies have been found in lexical abilities (Catts 1993; Kail and Leonard 1986; Rice et al. 1990), syntactic production and comprehension (for reviews, see Johnston 1988; Kamhi 1996; Leonard 1989), narrative production and comprehension (Bishop and Adams 1992; Crais and Chapman 1987; Paul and Smith 1993), and phonologic awareness (Catts 1993; Kamhi and Catts 1986; Kamhi et al. 1988). Because of deficits in these areas, many children with preschool language impairments do not develop the necessary language foundation on which reading is based. Most important, language deficiencies during the preschool years are not limited to conversation but extend to narrative discourse and metalinguistic knowledge as well (Fey et al. 1995).

The second child, Steve, is a third grader reading at a first-grade level. Unlike Adrian, Steve had no history of a preschool language problem. He does not make any obvious errors in spoken language, though he does have difficulty telling a story or relating an event in front of the class. He has difficulty remembering directions the teacher gives for completing assignments. Many children with LLDs are like Steve. They have unremarkable preschool language histories but seem to "hit a wall" when they start school and have to make the formal transition from spoken to written language. Donahue (1986) suggested that some of these children may have spoken language problems that are too subtle to be detected during the preschool years. Another possibility is that the types of language problems these children have, such as in narrative discourse and the metalanguage area, are not typically noticed by parents, physicians, or even speech-language pathologists. Although these children probably have age-appropriate conversational skills when they enter school, spoken language deficiencies become more noticeable with the increased importance on other forms of discourse and metalinguistic abilities. It is important to note that children with very different language histories can resemble one another by the time they start school. In other words, by the time Adrian is in the third grade, his spoken and written language problems may be indistinguishable from those demonstrated by Steve.

The third child, Michelle, is in the fifth grade. Like Steve, Michelle had no history of spoken language problems, but, unlike Steve, she had no difficulty learning to read. In fact, she had no problems in school until she started the fourth grade, when she began to have difficulty talking about what she read and completing written work in class and at home. Although her word-recognition skills seemed fine, she had difficulty understanding what she was reading. She also had difficulty organizing her thoughts on paper, and her attention often seemed to wander in class. Michelle seems to have difficulty *reading to learn*. She did fine when the reading tests primarily measured her decoding and word-recognition skills; however, as reading tests became more heavily weighted toward comprehension, she did not do as well. It is unclear whether her current problems result from deficient comprehension skills or attentional, motivational, and instructional factors. Indeed, all of these factors may contribute in some way to her language learning problem.

Some scholars and educators (Taylor 1997; Harry 1992) would argue that there is a fourth subgroup of children with LLDs consisting of children from racial and ethnic minorities. Professionals across disciplines have become increasingly aware of the unique needs of children and youth with LLDs from racial and ethnic minority groups. A disproportionate number of these children have language learning problems and do not achieve the same levels of academic success as more advantaged peers. Children and youth from these diverse groups often are overrepresented or underrepresented in placements appropriate to their need. For example, many of these children do not receive any special services because they are performing comparably to their peers, many of whom perform below normative standards on measures of language and reading. Others, such as Glen in Case 4, typically the more disruptive students, may be misdiagnosed and inappropriately placed in classes for the behaviorally or emotionally disturbed (Harry 1992; Mercer 1973).

Children from low socioeconomic backgrounds are particularly at risk for language and literacy problems in school because they are raised in "low-print" environments that contain limited experiences with literacy artifacts and events. In many of these environments, children have limited exposure to adults who read and write a lot. As a result, they may not see the value in learning to read and write. When these children enter kindergarten, they are already behind middle class peers because of their limited literacy experiences. Many of these children never catch up to their middle class peers, either because they are seen as developing normally for their ethnic and socioeconomic background, or because they are placed in special education classes in which expectations often are low.

CHARACTERISTICS OF CHILDREN WITH LANGUAGE LEARNING DISABILITIES

Despite the different developmental histories children with LLDs can have, the kinds of language learning problems they experience are often similar. There is a vast body of literature that has attempted to characterize the language learning strengths and weaknesses of children with LLDs. There are also a number of comprehensive attempts to synthesize this literature (Gerber 1993; Kamhi and Catts 1989; Paul 1995; Wallach and Butler 1994). In this chapter, these sources are used in an attempt to provide a synopsis of the language and learning abilities of children with LLDs.

Phonologic Abilities

A large body of literature has found that there is a strong relationship between phonologic abilities and learning to read (Bryant 1991; Catts 1989a; Stanovich 1988; Wagner and Torgesen 1987). This body of research has approached phonologic abilities from a different perspective than speech-language pathologists have taken. Rather than focus on productive phonology, this research has examined individual differences in memory for phonologic information (Torgesen 1985), the retrieval of phonologic information from long-term memory (Wolf 1984), and phonologic awareness (Bradley and Bryant 1985). Some studies have also considered productive aspects of phonology (Catts 1986, 1989b; Kamhi et al. 1988). Children who perform well on measures of these phonologic abilities generally learn to read sooner than children who perform poorly on these tasks. Children with LLDs typically have deficiencies in these phonologic abilities. The extent of the deficiency is often related to the severity of the language learning problems the child demonstrates, particularly in the area of reading.

Phonologic Awareness

The phonologic awareness abilities of children with LLDs have received a lot of attention in the literature. *Phonologic awareness* is generally defined as awareness of, or sensitivity to, the speech sounds that comprise words (Stanovich 1988). In very young children (i.e., 2–3 years of age), phonologic awareness is frequently assessed by tasks that require sensitivity to rhyme or alliteration. At later ages, measures of phonologic awareness require children to identify, isolate, or in some way manipulate the sounds in words.

Children who are sensitive to the phonologic structure of words before receiving formal reading instruction have been found to read more easily than those who lack such sensitivity (Bradley and Bryant 1985; Felton and Wood 1989; Mann 1991; Torgesen et al. 1994; Wagner and Torgesen 1987). Torgesen and colleagues (1994), in reviewing the literature on phonologic awareness, found that the correlations between performance on phonologic awareness tasks in kindergarten and word-reading skills at the end of first grade fall within the range of 0.4–0.6. This strong relationship is consistent with the notion that some knowledge of the phonologic structure of words is needed to learn the alphabetic principle (i.e., that the letters in printed words correspond to the sounds in spoken language).

Consistent with this relationship, delayed development of phonologic awareness is commonly found in children who have difficulty learning to read (Bradley and Bryant 1985; Bruck 1992; Gough and Tunmer 1986; Juel 1988; Snowling 1981). Bradley and Bryant (1985), for example, found that children with reading disabilities were insensitive to rhyme and alliteration. Children were asked to choose the odd member from a list of spoken words, such as *lot, cot,* and *hat.* Even though the children with reading disabilities were 3.5 years older than the normal control subjects, they performed significantly worse on the task.

Importantly, the relationship between phonologic awareness and early reading performance is not unidirectional. A number of studies have found that reading instruction has a measurable impact on phonologic awareness skills (Bradley and Bryant 1985; Perfetti et al. 1987; Wimmer et al. 1991). This is not surprising given that learning the alphabetic principle focuses children's attention on the sounds in words. Because the relationship between phonologic awareness and reading is a reciprocal one, many questions remain concerning the timing and nature of the development of phonologic awareness and the extent to which particular measures of phonologic awareness predict reading performance.

Phonologic Memory

The ability to store information in long-term memory is crucial for normal language learning. To acquire language, children must match speech sound sequences to objects, actions, and events in the world. Learning the names of things requires perceptual analysis of the speech signal, constructing phonologic representations of the names, and storage of these representations in long-term or semantic memory. Memory limitations make it more difficult to perform tasks that require the simultaneous storage and processing of individual sounds in words

(Torgesen et al. 1994) or tasks that require the processing and analysis of long sequences of verbal information. Comprehension of spoken and written language requires this kind of processing.

Phonologic memory is typically assessed by memory-span tasks involving meaningful and nonmeaningful strings of verbal items. Difficulty with memory span tasks is a frequently reported characteristic of children with severe reading disabilities (Baddeley 1986; Torgesen 1985; Torgesen et al. 1994). A consistent finding in the literature is that there is a strong relationship between children's performance on phonologic memory tasks and early reading achievement. Children with spoken language impairments also do poorly on measures of phonologic memory (Kamhi and Catts 1986; Kamhi et al. 1988; Montgomery 1995). One would expect, therefore, that all children with LLDs will experience some difficulty with phonologic memory tasks.

Retrieving Phonologic Information

Word-finding problems have been documented in children with a wide range of language learning problems, including children with spoken language impairments (Catts 1993; Kail and Leonard 1986; Kamhi and Catts 1986), learning disabilities (German 1984), and dyslexia (Denckla and Rudel 1976; Wolf and Obregon 1992). Numerous studies have found a strong link between children's naming abilities and reading (Catts 1989a). Clinical observations have often revealed word-finding problems in the speech of children with reading disabilities (Johnson and Mykelbust 1967). Poor readers have also been shown to have difficulty recalling the names of common objects on tasks such as the Boston Naming Test (Wolf 1982). More recent studies have used "rapid automatic naming" tasks to evaluate naming abilities. These tasks require the rapid naming of a repeated series of five familiar letters, digits, colors, numbers, or objects. Individual differences in rapid naming in kindergarten have been found to be strongly predictive of later differences in reading in first grade and beyond (Felton and Wood 1989; Wolf 1986, 1991). The efficiency with which children can access phonologic codes thus provides some indication of children's general language learning abilities.

Speech Production Abilities

Children with LLDs also may have expressive phonologic delays. Speech delays often co-occur with developmental language problems during the preschool years. By the time these children enter school, the speech delay is often limited to late-emerging sounds (e.g., clusters and /l, r, s/). Even if a language learning disabled child does not have a history of speech delay, he or she may experience difficulty producing complex sound sequences. Clinical observations have indicated that poor readers often have difficulty producing complex sound sequences (Blalock 1982; Johnston and Mykelbust 1967). A number of studies have confirmed these clinical observations (Catts 1986, 1989b). For example, Catts (1986) found that adolescents with reading disabilities made significantly more speech-production errors than age-matched peers on tasks requiring naming pictured objects with complex names (e.g., *ambulance, thermometer*) and repeating phonologically complex words (e.g., *specific, aluminum*) and phrases (e.g., *brown and blue plaid pants*). The reading-disabled subjects generally made word-specific substitutions or omitted phonemes. In a follow-up study of college students with a history of reading disabilities, Catts (1989b) found that the students repeated complex phrases at a significantly slower rate and made more errors than nondisabled students. Other investigators have also found that children with reading disabilities have difficulty producing complex phonologic sequences (Apthorp 1995; Kamhi et al. 1988; Rapala and Brady 1990; Snowling 1980). One would expect, therefore, that most children with LLDs experience difficulty producing complex phonologic sequences.

Syntactic Abilities

The syntactic abilities of children with LLDs have been well documented in the literature (Doehring et al. 1981; Gerber 1993; Roth and Spekman 1989; Paul 1995). Research has shown that language learning disabled children between 7 years of age and adolescence show (1) reduced sentence length, (2) a higher incidence of syntactic and morphologic errors, and (3) a reduced ability to comprehend and produce complex sentences, particularly embedded sentences (Roth and Spekman 1989; Vogel 1977; Wiig and Semel 1975). Language learning disabled students also tend to show less elaboration of noun and verb phrases and use fewer adverbial modifiers and prepositional phrases than nondisabled peers. These children may also have difficulty expressing late-acquired grammatical morphemes, such as comparatives, superlatives, advanced prefixes, and suffixes.

Semantic Abilities

Students with LLDs often have vocabulary deficiencies. Some language learning disabled students have a history of receptive vocabulary delays; others develop vocabulary deficiencies because they do not read very well and typically read much less than average and good readers. Around third grade, reading becomes the major determinant of vocabulary growth (Nagy and Anderson 1984). Nagy and Anderson have estimated that average middle school children read million words a year, compared with only 100,000 words for the less motivated students and even fewer words for students with LLDs. The differences in reading volume between language learning disabled and nondisabled students leads to a "rich get richer and poor get poorer" phenomenon. As Stanovich (1986, p. 381) has noted, "the very children who are reading well and who have good vocabularies read more, learn more word meanings, and hence read even better. Children with inadequate vocabularies—who read slowly and without enjoyment—read less and, as a result, have slower development of vocabulary knowledge, which inhibits further growth in reading ability."

In addition to small vocabularies, children with LLDs typically have other semantic deficiencies. Nippold (1995), for example, discussed the restricted knowledge of word meanings these children have. Other investigators have documented difficulty with relational and abstract words (Wiig and Semel 1984), as well as problems understanding and using figurative language, such as metaphors, similes, and slang (Lee and Kamhi 1990; Paul 1995; Roth and Spekman 1989).

Pragmatic Abilities

Many children with LLDs have pragmatic difficulties. Paul (1995) noted that they typically do not talk much, and what they say is brief and unelaborated. Studies have shown that the language learning disabled student's language is often less assertive, tactful, and clear than their peers and more dysfluent and hostile (Brinton et al. 1988; Damico 1991; Donahue and Bryan 1983). Language learning disabled students have also been shown to have trouble making clarification requests and responses and are more likely to ignore the communicative bids of others and show poor topic maintenance (Paul 1995).

The pragmatic problems of language learning disabled students are not limited to conversational discourse. They also have difficulty with narrative, expository, and classroom discourse. Roth (1986), for example, found that story recall in language learning disabled children was characterized by (1) poor understanding of temporal and causal relations, (2) limited detail, (3) errors in information, and (4) decreased length of retelling. Many language learning disabled students also have difficulty answering inferential questions about stories (Gerber 1993).

The ability to generate stories is also impaired in many language learning disabled students (Liles 1987; Westby 1989).

Children with LLDs also have considerable difficulty with expository discourse (Westby 1989; Scott 1994). The expository discourse genre falls at the most literate end of the continuum of language styles (Paul 1995). Expository text provides the least contextual support and, as a result, places heavy demands on linguistic processes. Because even normally achieving students have difficulty with expository text, it is not surprising that children with LLDs have problems in this area. This difficulty is exhibited primarily in written, rather than spoken, language.

Reading and Writing Abilities

Although all children with LLDs have reading and writing difficulties, they do not necessarily show the same type of difficulty. Some children have particular problems with decoding and word-recognition processes, whereas others have particular difficulty with comprehension activities. Some students, of course, have both decoding and comprehension problems. Writing problems also can vary among students with LLDs. Some students have considerable difficulty learning the structural aspects of writing, such as grammar and punctuation, whereas others have problems generating, planning, and organizing texts. Most students with LLDs probably have problems with both the structural and the process components of writing.

Other Characteristics

There are other characteristics of students with LLDs that in many respects are just as important as their language learning abilities. These characteristics involve general knowledge, social-emotional abilities, problem-solving skills, attention abilities, and motivational states and attitudes. Students with LLDs may have deficiencies or problems in each of these areas. These problems can be the result of the LLD, or they may be associated with problems that co-occur with the LLD. In both cases, the behaviors that characterize the LLD and other abilities or attitudes are highly interactive. The causal connections that underlie language learning behaviors and related abilities and attitudes need to be considered in differentially diagnosing students with LLDs and designing effective remediation programs. In the next section, *Differential Diagnosis of Students with Language Learning Disabilities*, an assessment protocol that considers all of these factors is presented.

DIFFERENTIAL DIAGNOSIS OF STUDENTS WITH LANGUAGE LEARNING DISABILITIES

Much has been written about the assessment of children's language learning skills (Gerber 1993; James 1993; Lund and Duchan 1993; Paul 1995; Nelson 1993; Reed 1994). There is general agreement that the purposes of assessment are to (1) identify children with LLDs, (2) design appropriate intervention programs, and (3) monitor changes that result from intervention (James 1993). Lund and Duchan (1993) proposed five questions that should be answered in assessment.

1. Does the child have a language learning problem?
2. What is causing the problem?
3. What are the areas of deficit?
4. What are the regularities in the child's language learning abilities?
5. What is recommended for the child?

Nelson (1993) provided additional questions that are appropriate at different stages of the assessment and intervention process. Because assessment is an ongoing process, one must consider the types of assessments that occur during intervention. Some of Nelson's questions are:

1. Does the child qualify for services?
2. What kinds of services does the child need?
3. Which speech, language, and communication behaviors and strategies should be changed, and what kinds of procedures should be used to effect these changes?
4. Is progress occurring in therapy and are modifications in treatment objectives or procedures necessary?

James (1993, p. 186) wrote that "the task of assessing children's language would be relatively simple if language were easily quantified like height or weight." Language, however, is a multidimensional, complex, and dynamic entity involving many interrelated processes and abilities. Although it is possible to group students according to their overall pattern of language learning abilities, to a certain extent every student presents a unique pattern of language learning abilities. One of the major challenges in assessment is to describe the unique pattern language learning behaviors that each student with an LLD presents.

Some models of language assessment view language as a self-contained system that is independent from the social world in which people live. In recent years, there has been an increasing awareness that language use is a highly contextualized social activity that is influenced by participants, situations, language modes (i.e., speaking, writing, sign), and sociocultural factors (Damico 1992; Kovarsky 1992;

Nelson 1993). Assessments that are sensitive to this view of language attempt to describe language in as many different contexts as possible (e.g., home, classroom, playground). Such assessments clearly are more time-consuming than administering a few standardized tests or collecting a language sample in one setting; however, the benefits of such assessments should be obvious if one is interested in obtaining a true picture of a person's language abilities.

The components of a language learning assessment are described in the following outline. These components include instruments and procedures that provide information needed in determining the causal relationships that characterize language and learning disabilities.

I. *Language samples*
   - A. *Samples*. Obtain samples of the child's language in at least three different contexts (e.g., with friends, with an adult, and in the classroom). Also obtain at least two samples of the child's writing. One of the samples should be on a topic that the child has chosen.
   - B. *Transcription*. Follow procedures in Retherford (1993).
   - C. *Mean length of utterance*. Follow procedures in Retherford (1993).

II. *Story and event recall*
   - A. *Sample*. Have the child recall a short story and describe an event (e.g., a party, family trip, playing a game). For the recall story, read the child a brief story (150–200 words) and ask the child to recall the story in as much detail as possible.
   - B. *Transcription*. Transcribe stories into t-units (topic units). All conjoined sentences are treated as separate units. Do not forget to include the full version of the stories you ask the child to recall.

III. *The diagnostic report: Part 1*
   - A. *Developmental history*. Discuss pertinent medical and developmental information, particularly speech-language and academic development. Did the child have a preschool speech or language problem?
   - B. *Perceptual and memory processes*. Discuss the child's ability to detect, discriminate, and identify auditory input. Also, discuss the child's memory processes (e.g., short-term memory span for verbal and nonverbal information, encoding, storage, and retrieval processes). Is there a difference in the child's ability to process linguistic and nonlinguistic information?
   - C. *General knowledge and intelligence*. Measures of intelligence should be reported and discussed in this section. This section should also include information on academic strengths and weaknesses (e.g., geography, science, history, math).

D. *Social and emotional behaviors*. Include information about the child's emotional maturity, self-image, achievement motivation, peer relations, and so forth. Does the child have social-emotional problems beyond those caused by the LLD?

E. *Problem-solving and attentional behaviors*. Discuss the child's attentiveness, level of activity, and impulsivity and reflectivity. What is the child's general approach to solving problems and learning about the world? Does the child exhibit organizational problems?

F. *Instructional and environmental factors*. Provide information about the child's school and home environment. Are these environments conducive for language learning?

G. *Summary*. Briefly highlight some of the important findings from the first part of the evaluation.

IV. *The diagnostic report: Part 2: Language analyses*

A. *Phonology*. Phonology includes information about how the student processes phonologic information, particularly the ability to reflect on the phonologic properties of speech. Tasks should measure phonologic awareness, as well as the ability to produce complex phonologic sequences (Kamhi and Catts, in press).

B. *Semantics*. Include some measure of receptive vocabulary (e.g., Peabody Picture Vocabulary Test—Revised [Dunn and Dunn 1981]), as well as measures of instructional, textbook, and expressive vocabulary (Paul 1995). Definitional skills and knowledge of figurative language should also be examined.

C. *Syntax and morphology*. Assess receptive language in contextualized and decontextualized contexts (Paul 1995). Follow procedures in Retherford (1993) or similar descriptive analysis (Paul 1995). Analyses should consider grammatical morphology, word classes (e.g., pronouns, conjunctions), sentence type (e.g., negative, question), noun and verb phrase elaboration, and clause structure (i.e., simple versus complex).

D. *Conversational discourse*. Conversational discourse includes analysis of communicative intentions, topicalization, turn-taking skills, ability to make clarification requests and responses, ability to change registers, sensitivity to others (e.g., use of anaphora, politeness, rules), and nonverbal behaviors (e.g., proxemics, gestures, affective behaviors) (Brinton and Fujiki 1991; Paul 1995; Retherford 1993). Summaries should discuss the child's pragmatic abilities in relation to social and personal behaviors discussed in the previous section *Characteristics of Children with Language Learning Disabilities*. Is the child a good communicator and partner in discourse?

E. *Narrative discourse.* Determine the story and event structures and comment on the guiding scripts and use of various linguistic means to create narratives or events (Nelson 1993). Summaries should compare narrative and event recalls to conversational abilities.

F. *Reading and writing.* Include measures of decoding (word attack), comprehension, and writing skills, preferably using both norm-referenced tests and descriptive error analyses. Reading and writing abilities should be evaluated using different texts and topics. A portfolio type of assessment could be used for both reading and writing.

G. *Summary.* Compare and contrast the child's language abilities in the areas evaluated. This section should be more than just a summary of the previous sections.

V. *Diagnosis*

A. Generate some hypotheses about cause-and-effect relationships among physical structures, psychosocial behaviors, cognitive processes, instructional and environmental factors, language learning abilities, and academic performance.

B. Questions that should be addressed in this section include the following:

1. Are all language abilities equally delayed?
2. Are spoken and written language abilities equally delayed?
3. Which deficits seem to be primary and which secondary?
4. What kinds of interactions exist among the various structural, processing, psychosocial, language, and academic factors and abilities?

VI. *Recommendations and prognosis.* List some short- and long-term objectives for the child as well as other pertinent recommendations. Discuss some specific strategies to help the student function better in a regular classroom. Make some prognostic statements about the student's future academic performance and career choices.

The sections of the diagnostic process provide a framework for assessing language learning abilities and the processes and factors that can impact on these abilities. Detailed information about the assessment procedures and analyses have been provided by Paul (1995), Nelson (1993), and Retherford (1993). It is important to keep in mind that no assessment protocol is a substitute for an informed speech-language pathologist. As Siegel and Broen (1976, p. 75) wrote, "the most useful and dependable 'language assessment device' is an informed clinician who feels compelled to keep up with developments in psycholinguistics, speech pathology, and related fields, and who is not slavishly attached to a particular model of language or of assessment."

LEARNING DIFFERENTIAL DIAGNOSIS: A COMMITMENT TO CAUSAL QUESTIONS

Comprehensive differential diagnosis is not easy. There are no shortcuts in learning how to assess the many factors that can impact language. Computer analyses can save time, but clinicians first need to learn how to analyze language and language-related behaviors.

Although a good differential diagnosis can take time, it does not typically involve all of the components described in the previous section. As clinicians become more experienced, they gradually internalize the framework of an assessment protocol and become proficient in analyzing and interpreting test information and observational data. Although the "time factor" is often given as the reason that comprehensive assessment protocols cannot be performed, clinicians would make the time if they were convinced of the value of such assessments. Because differential diagnosis is closely linked to causal questions, clinicians must recognize that addressing causal questions and identifying students' strengths and weaknesses have significant and beneficial implications for treatment.

Much has been written about the importance of causal questions (e.g., see the clinical forum in the April 1991, issue of *Language, Speech, and Hearing Services in Schools*). Robert Hubbell (1981, p. 105) began his chapter on causation in child language disorders as follows:

> If something goes wrong, it's natural to ask why. If the car won't start, you start looking for causes. Out of gas? Battery dead? If a child develops red blotches and a high fever, the physician likewise looks for causes. Similarly, if a child demonstrates impairments in the use of language, we wonder why.

Hubbell went on to note that the search for causal factors in LLDs has been frustratingly difficult. A primary reason for this difficulty is that many individuals have assumed that one causal factor could explain the LLD. Causation, however, is a complex process. This complexity is best seen by contrasting three different views of the process of causation: (1) the linear cause-and-effect model, (2) the interactional model, and (3) the transactional model. These models are discussed briefly in the following sections. For a more detailed discussion, see Hubbell (1981) or Sameroff (1975).

Linear Cause-and-Effect Model

In the linear cause-and-effect model, often referred to as the *medical model*, there is a direct, one-to-one relationship between cause and effect. The physician, for example, diagnoses the cause of a disease by considering its symptoms or effects. The logic of this model is that for each effect there is a cause and for each cause there is a resulting effect. The term *linear* refers to the direct connection between cause and effect. There are two contrasting applications of the linear cause-and-effect model, one that emphasizes the child's constitution, and the other that emphasizes the child's environment. The term *constitution* refers to the child's neurophysical makeup and genetic endowment. As Hubbell (1981) notes, both views of the linear cause-and-effect model have a severe shortcoming. A language disorder does not depend solely on constitutional factors or solely on environmental factors. Both constitutional and environmental factors influence language development and thus contribute to LLDs.

Interactional Model

The interactional model acknowledges that a child's development results from the interaction between constitutional and environmental factors. The example Hubbell (1981) provided is of a child who is born premature and then does not receive adequate medical care. Such a child is at a higher risk than one who suffers from only one of these conditions. The interactional view, however, is still an oversimplification of the process of causation. First, it assumes that constitution and environment do not change over time. Second, it assumes that constitutional and environmental factors do not influence one another. The transactional model addresses both of these concerns.

Transactional Model

Unlike the previous two models, the transactional model includes change over time and acknowledges the reciprocal influences of constitutional and environmental factors (Hubbell 1981; Sameroff 1975). Consider, for example, two children from different families who are diagnosed as having a severe developmental language disorder because they are using less than 10 words at 2 years of age. Assume that the intelligence level and other constitutional factors are similar in the two children. In one family, there are two older normal siblings. The family is resentful that they now have a child with a language disorder. They specifically resent the stigma of having such a child and the trouble he will cause them throughout his development. By 5 years of age, this child is not only severely language delayed but also has significant behavior problems. He is a very aggressive child and, as a result, has no close friends and is generally not liked by other children his age. His teachers find him noncompliant, and he shows little motivation to improve his language abilities or engage in other school-oriented activities.

In contrast, the parents of the other child with a developmental language disorder have no other children. Although they are disappointed that their child has a language disorder, they try to provide the best possible learning environment for him. By 5 years of age, his language is still delayed but only by a year or so. He is able to enter a normal kindergarten classroom. Although he is at risk for reading problems, his parents, clinicians, and teachers have exposed him to literacy activities for the last 3 years. He is already able to recognize many words by sight. He is well liked by other children and teachers because of his caring and empathetic nature.

The example of these two children illustrates the difficulty in identifying etiology and causal factors. Neither environmental nor constitutional factors alone can explain the language and language-related behaviors of children when they are 5 years old. The diagnostic process should include clinical hypotheses about the cause-and-effect relationships that affect children's language learning (Kamhi 1984). The hypotheses should consider the relationship between the structures and mechanisms, processes, and behaviors that impact language learning. Although it can be difficult to formulate such hypotheses, treatment that is based on these hypotheses can be better tailored to students' strengths and weaknesses than treatment that is not based on such hypotheses.

IMPLICATIONS OF DIFFERENTIAL DIAGNOSIS FOR IDENTIFICATION AND TREATMENT

In addition to questions about the child's language learning and related behaviors, the assessment and diagnostic process must also determine whether the student qualifies for services. Questions about possible goals and intervention procedures and treatment progress are also part of the assessment and diagnostic process (Lund and Duchan 1993; Nelson 1993). The following are the pertinent questions:

1. Does the student qualify for services?
2. What kinds of services does the student need?
3. What are the areas of deficit?

4. What are the regularities in the student's language learning abilities?
5. Which behaviors (e.g., language, cognitive, social) and strategies should be changed, and what kinds of procedures should be used to effect these changes?
6. Is progress occurring in therapy and are modifications in treatment objectives or procedures necessary?

The first question a clinician or team of educators must answer is whether the student qualifies for services. For many clinicians, determining whether the student qualifies for services and under what label or category represents the extent of the diagnostic process. In most cases, clinicians have to determine whether the student meets eligibility criteria established by each state's department of education. Some large cities have their own eligibility criteria. Eligibility decisions often involve proving that the student's language learning abilities are significantly below age level or significantly discrepant from IQ. Norm-referenced tests, rather than descriptive analytic procedures, are almost always used to qualify a student for services, although many states now allow clinicians to use both procedures to qualify children for services.

To determine which kinds of services students need, clinicians need to answer questions about areas of deficit and the regularities in the student's language learning abilities (i.e., questions 3 and 4 above). Answering these questions requires the kind of comprehensive assessment described in this chapter.

Recall that Adrian, in one of the three examples that began this chapter, was a first grader who had not yet learned to read. He had been receiving speech-language therapy since he was 4 years of age and still exhibited some speech and language delays. A comprehensive evaluation indicated that he still had some cluster reduction and gliding (i.e., w/r). Although his language sample contained some complex sentences, the majority of his utterances (90%) were simple sentences. He still showed some inconsistent use of auxiliary *be*. Pragmatically, he had excellent social skills and was a good communicator despite his speech and language delay. He had lots of friends and was one of the more popular students in the class. He sometimes acted out in class; his teachers complained that he played the "class clown" too much. He expressed a variety of communicative intentions, showed age-appropriate turn-taking and topicalization skills, and showed sensitivity to the listener's communicative needs. Adrian's parents were both college educated and would be considered upper middle class. His paternal grandfather and uncle both remembered having some difficulty learning to read. Cognitively, Adrian performed within normal age limits on a measure of nonverbal intelligence. He had difficulty, however, learning things like numbers, the alphabet, and other information that appears best learned by rote memory. His attentional and motivational skills were good, if he was interested in the activity. Although his parents provided a rich literacy environment, filled with books and magazines, Adrian showed little interest in being read to and did not like reading or writing.

Adrian is a classic example of a child with a developmental language impairment. He already has experienced difficulty learning to talk and is now experiencing difficulty learning to read. The speech-language pathologist, classroom teacher, and special educator need to recognize Adrian's social, pragmatic, and cognitive strengths. The difficulty he has with learning information by rote memory explains, in part, some of his language learning problems. Learning for Adrian and students like him should occur in a meaningful, contextually rich, nurturing environment. Because Adrian is a motivated learner, he should be involved in figuring out which strategies help him learn. His parents also should be involved in planning and implementing his education program.

Another example provides a contrast with Adrian.

Case 4

Glen is an African American first grader who goes to a large urban school and is being raised by his maternal grandmother with seven other siblings and cousins. Glen, like a lot of his classmates, reads below grade level. He was also disruptive in class, always jumping out of his seat and getting into fights with other students. He made it very difficult for the classroom teacher to maintain order and discipline. Because of his disruptiveness, the classroom teacher referred him to special education with the hope that his reading delay was severe enough to qualify him for placement in a resource room. The speech-language pathologist was involved in the evaluation and found that his receptive language abilities were more than one standard deviation below the mean. He was not easy to test because of attentional and behavior problems. As a result, he performed within the mild retarded range on the Stanford-Binet test. He did not do much better on a nonverbal measure of intelligence. Eliciting a language sample was difficult, but, in conversation with peers, he appeared to have no difficulty communicating. His language contained a number of dialectal forms.

A differential diagnosis of Glen's language learning strengths and weaknesses was particularly important, because many children from ethnic and racial minorities are classified as emotionally disturbed or mentally retarded because they do not perform well on standardized tests (Harry 1992). It was not easy to classify Glen, even if he met the discrepancy criteria to qualify as learning disabled, because the disability did not appear to have a constitutional origin. In reality, he did not meet the criteria for learning disabilities because he did not perform within the normal range on the measure of intelligence. Despite Glen's low performance profile, his cognitive and language learning abilities were comparable to his peers. The reason Glen was singled out for referral was not because of his language or reading abilities but because of his disruptive behavior in class.

The problems Glen, and children like him, have in learning to read and in other academic areas require solutions that go beyond differential diagnosis. Differential diagnosis can identify the problem, its potential causes, and characterize students' language learning strengths and weaknesses. It cannot, however, change the circumstances that cause and perpetuate the problem for Glen and his classmates. This does not mean that a differential diagnosis has no value for students like Glen; it can have considerable value for those educators and professionals who plan to help such students. By identifying the environmental and instructional factors that play a significant causal role in the language learning problem, differential diagnosis forces educators to think about ways to improve the educational outcome for students like Glen. Glen and his classmates need resourceful and creative teachers who work together to improve the learning environment and show these students the value of language and literacy. These teachers need to figure out ways to channel Glen's energy into productive activities in the classroom.

This brief discussion of Adrian and Glen illustrates the importance of differentiating language learning differences and delays stemming from sociocultural and environmental factors from developmental LLDs that are constitutionally based. It would be a mistake to provide services only to a disruptive student like Glen, when his classmates have language learning problems that would be viewed as disabilities if they occurred in middle-class students. It is not possible, however, for speech-language pathologists to provide direct services to large numbers of students with language learning delays. The solution is for the clinician to develop a collaborative model of service delivery. Rather than having to provide direct services to all the students with language and literacy needs, consultation and collaboration with regular and special education teachers and other school personnel can be helpful. These collaborative efforts get speech-language pathologists into the classroom where their differential diagnostic skills can be employed to identify the particular language learning strengths and weakness of the students. The clinician may not only spend more time with the students with LLDs, but also may become involved in improving the language and literacy skills of other students who are not reading at grade level.

CONCLUSION

The major benefit of differential diagnosis is that it keeps clinicians from accepting simple solutions to complex problems. Determining why students have language learning problems and how best to treat these difficulties is a complex problem. It is a natural tendency to attempt to simplify this problem by looking for commonalities that link students with LLDs. Clinicians who focus too much on commonalities run the risk, however, of treating all the students the same. These clinicians have the same objectives for students depending on their developmental level and use the same strategies and procedures to target particular objectives. At the other extreme are clinicians who focus too much on individual differences. These clinicians run the risk of becoming too focused on what makes students different and fostering these differences rather than teaching the skills and strategies needed to function at the same levels as other students. Focusing too much on individual differences can be just as much an oversimplification as focusing too much on commonalities. The view of differential diagnosis presented in this chapter encourages clinicians to notice both the similar patterns of performance and the individual differences in students with LLDs. Although this chapter has discussed some of the treatment implications of this kind of differential diagnosis, I am sure that a few skeptics remain. It is not sufficient just to give differential diagnosis "a try." However, if a clinician thinks it is not worth the effort, it probably will not be. Clinicians need to recognize the importance and value of addressing the assessment and diagnostic questions discussed in this chapter. If clinicians are convinced of the value of the questions, they will spend whatever time is needed to seek the answers.

REFERENCES

Apthorp H. (1995) Phonetic coding and reading in college students with and without learning disabilities. *Journal of Learning Disabilities* 28, 342–353.

Baddeley A. (1986) *Working Memory*. New York: Oxford University Press.

Bishop D, Adams C. (1990) A prospective study of the relationship between specific language impairment, phonological disorders, and reading retardation. *Journal of Child Psychology and Psychiatry* 31, 1027–1050.

Bishop D, Adams C. (1992) Comprehension problems in children with specific language impairment: literal and inferential meaning. *Journal of Speech and Hearing Research* 35, 119–129.

Blalock J. (1982) Persistent auditory language deficits in adults with learning disabilities. *Journal of Learning Disabilities* 15, 604–609.

Bradley L, Bryant P. (1985) *Rhyme and Reason in Reading and Spelling*. Ann Arbor: University of Michigan Press.

Brinton B, Fujiki M. (1991) *Conversational Management with Language-Impaired Children*. Rockville, MD: Aspen.

Brinton B, Fujiki M, Sonnenberg E. (1988) Responses to requests for clarification by linguistically normal and language-impaired children in conversation. *Journal of Speech and Hearing Research* 53, 383–391.

Bruck M. (1992) Persistence of dyslexics' phonological deficits. *Developmental Psychology* 28, 874–886.

Bryant P. (1991) Phonological awareness is a pre-cursor, not a pre-requisite of reading. *Mind and Language* 6, 102–106.

Catts H. (1986) Speech production/phonological deficits in reading disordered children. *Journal of Learning Disabilities* 19, 504–508.

Catts H. (1989a) Phonological Processing Deficits and Reading Disabilities. In A Kamhi, H Catts (eds), *Reading Disabilities: A Developmental Language Perspective* (pp. 101–132). Boston: Allyn & Bacon.

Catts H. (1989b) Speech production deficits in developmental dyslexia. *Journal of Speech and Hearing Research* 54, 422–428.

Catts H. (1993) The relationship between speech-language impairments and reading disabilities. *Journal of Speech and Hearing Research* 36, 948–958.

Crais E, Chapman R. (1987) Story recall and inferencing skills in language/learning-disabled and nondisabled children. *Journal of Speech and Hearing Disorders* 52, 50–55.

Damico J. (1991) Descriptive Assessment of Communicative Ability in Limited English Proficient Students. In E Hamayan, J Damico (eds), *Limiting Bias in the Assessment of Bilingual Students* (pp. 157–217). Austin, TX: PRO-ED.

Damico J. (1992) Language assessment in adolescents: addressing critical issues. *Language, Speech, and Hearing Services in Schools* 24, 29–35.

Denckla M, Rudel R. (1976) Rapid automatized naming (R.A.N.): dyslexia differentiated from other learning disabilities. *Neuropsychologia* 14, 471–479.

Diagnostic and Statistical Manual of Mental Disorders: DSM IV (4th ed). (1994) Washington, DC: American Psychiatric Press.

Doehring D, Trites R, Patel P, Fiedorowicz C. (1981) *Reading Disabilities: The Interaction of Reading, Language, and Neuropsychological Deficits*. New York: Academic Press.

Donahue M. (1986) Linguistic and Communicative Development in Learning Disabled Children. In S Ceci (ed), *Handbook of Cognitive, Social, and Neuropsychological Aspects of Learning Disabilities* (Vol 1) (pp. 263–291). Hillsdale, NJ: Erlbaum.

Donahue M, Bryan T. (1983) Conversational skills and modeling in learning disabled boys. *Applied Psycholinguistics* 4, 251–278.

Dunn LM, Dunn LM. (1981) *Peabody Picture Vocabulary Test —Revised*. Circle Pines, MI: American Guidance Service.

Felton R, Wood R. (1989) Cognitive deficits in reading disability and attention deficit disorder. *Journal of Learning Disabilities* 22, 3–13.

Fey M, Catts H, Larrivee L. (1995) Preparing Preschoolers for the Academic and Social Challenges of School. In M Fey, J Windsor, S Warren (eds), *Language Intervention: Preschool Through the Elementary Years* (pp. 3–38). Baltimore: Brookes Publishing Co.

Gerber A. (1993) *Language-Related Learning Disabilities: Their Nature and Treatment*. Baltimore: Brookes Publishing Co.

German D. (1984) Diagnosis of word-finding disorders in children with learning disabilities. *Journal of Learning Disabilities* 17, 353–358.

Gough P, Tunmer W. (1986) Decoding, reading, and reading disability. *Remedial and Special Education* 7, 6–10.

Harry B. (1992) *Cultural Diversity, Families, and the Special Education System*. New York: Teachers College Press.

Hubbell R. (1981) *Children's Language Disorders: An Integrated Approach*. Englewood Cliffs, NJ: Prentice-Hall.

James S. (1993) Assessing Children with Language Disorders. In D Bernstein, E Tiegerman (eds), *Language and Communication Disorders in Children* (3rd ed). Columbus, OH: Merrill.

Johnson D, Myklebust H. (1967) *Learning Disabilities: Educational Principles and Practices*. New York: Grune & Stratton.

Johnston J. (1988) Specific Language Disorders in the Child. In N Lass, L McReynolds, J Northern, D Yoder (eds), *Handbook of Speech-Language Pathology and Audiology* (pp. 685–715). Philadelphia: BC Decker, Inc.

Juel C. (1988) Learning to read and write: a longitudinal study of 54 children from first through fourth grades. *Journal of Educational Psychology* 80, 437–447.

Kail R, Leonard L. (1986). Word-finding abilities in language-impaired children. *ASHA Monographs 25*.

Kamhi A. (1984) Problem solving in child language disorders: the clinician as clinical scientist. *Language, Speech, and Hearing Services in Schools* 15, 226–234.

Kamhi A. (1996) Linguistic and Cognitive Aspects of Specific Language Impairment. In M Smith, J Damico (eds), *Childhood Language Disorders* (pp. 97–118). New York: Thieme.

Kamhi A, Catts H. (1986) Toward an understanding of developmental language and reading disorders. *Journal of Speech and Hearing Disorders* 51, 337–347.

Kamhi A, Catts H. (1989) *Reading Disabilities: A Developmental Language Perspective*. Boston: Allyn & Bacon.

Kamhi A, Catts H (in press). Phonological Abilities in Reading. In N Creaghead, P Newman, W Secord (eds), *Assessment and Remediation of Articulatory and Phonological Disorders* (3rd ed). Columbus, OH: Merrill.

Kamhi A, Catts H, Mauer D, et al. (1988) Phonological and spatial processing abilities in language and reading impaired children. *Journal of Hearing and Speech Disorders* 53, 316–327.

Kovarsky D. (1992) Ethnography and Language Assessment: Toward the Contextualized Description and Interpretation of Communicative Behavior. In W Secord (ed), *Best Practices in School Speech-Language Pathology* (pp. 115–123). New York: Harcourt Brace Jovanovich.

Lee R, Kamhi A. (1990) Metaphoric competence in learning disabled children. *Journal of Learning Disabilities* 23, 478–483.

Leonard L. (1989) Language learnability and specific language impairment in children. *Applied Psycholinguistics* 10, 179–202.

Liles B. (1987) Episode organization and cohesive conjunctions in narratives of children with and without language disorders. *Journal of Speech and Hearing Research* 30, 185–196.

Lund N, Duchan J. (1993) *Assessing Children's Language in Naturalistic Contexts* (3rd ed). Englewood Cliffs, NJ: Prentice-Hall.

Lyon G, Gray D, Kavanagh J, Krasnegor N. (1993) *Better Understanding Learning Disabilities: New Views from Research and Their Implications for Education and Public Policies*. Baltimore: Brookes Publishing Co.

Mann V. (1991) Phonological Abilities: Effective Predictors of Future Reading Ability. In L Rieben, CA Perfetti (eds), *Learning to Read: Basic Research and Its Implications* (pp. 121–133). Hillsdale, NJ: Erlbaum.

Mercer J. (1973) *Labeling the Mentally Retarded.* Berkeley: University of California Press.

Montgomery J. (1995) Sentence comprehension in children with specific language impairment: the role of phonological working memory. *Journal of Speech and Hearing Research* 38, 187–199.

Nagy W, Anderson R. (1984) How many words are there in printed school English? *Reading Research Quarterly* 19, 304–330.

Naremore R. (1980) Language Disorders in Children. In T Hixon, L Shriberg, J Saxman (eds), *Introduction to Communication Disorders* (pp. 177–217). Englewood Cliffs, NJ: Prentice-Hall.

Nelson N. (1993) *Childhood Language Disorders in Context: Infancy Through Adolescence.* Columbus, OH: Merrill.

Nippold M. (1995) Language norms in school-age children and adolescents: an introduction. *Language, Speech, and Hearing Services in Schools* 26, 307–308

Paul R. (1995) *Language Disorders from Infancy Through Adolescence.* St. Louis: Mosby.

Paul R, Smith R. (1993) Narrative skills in 4 year olds with normal, impaired, and late-developing language. *Journal of Speech and Hearing Research* 36, 592–598.

Perfetti C, Beck I, Bell L, Hughes C. (1987) Phonemic knowledge and learning to read are reciprocal: a longitudinal study of first grade children. *Merrill-Palmer Quarterly* 33, 283–319.

Rapala M, Brady S. (1990) Reading ability and short-term memory: the role of phonological processing. *Reading and Writing* 2, 1–25.

Reed V. (1994) *An Introduction to Children with Language Disorders* (2nd ed). New York: Macmillan.

Retherford K. (1993) *Assessing Children's Language in Natural Contexts* (3rd ed). Englewood Cliffs, NJ: Prentice-Hall.

Rice M, Buhr J, Nemeth M. (1990) Fast mapping word-learning abilities of language-delayed preschoolers. *Journal of Speech and Hearing Disorders* 55, 347–359.

Roth F. (1986) Oral narrative abilities of learning-disabled students. *Topics in Language Disorders* 7, 21–30.

Roth F, Spekman N. (1989) Higher-Order Language Processes and Reading Disabilities. In A Kamhi, H Catts (eds), *Reading Disabilities: A Developmental Language Perspective* (pp. 159–197). Boston: Allyn & Bacon.

Sameroff A. (1975) Early influences on development: fact or fancy? *Merrill-Palmer Quarterly* 2l, 267-294.

Scott C. (1994) A Discourse Continuum for School-Age Students: Impact of Modality and Genre. In G Wallach, K Butler (eds), *Language-Learning Disabilities in School-Age Children and Adolescents: Some Underlying Principles and Applications* (pp. 219–252). Columbus, OH: Merrill-Macmillan.

Siegel G, Broen P. (1976) Language Assessment. In L Lloyd (ed), *Communication, Assessment and Intervention Strategies.* Baltimore: University Park Press.

Snowling M. (1980) The development of grapheme-phoneme correspondence in normal and dyslexic readers. *Journal of Experimental Child Psychology* 29, 294–305.

Snowling M. (1981) Phonemic deficits in developmental dyslexia. *Psychological Research* 43, 219–234.

Stanovich K. (1986) Toward an interactive compensatory model of individual differences in the development of reading fluency. *Reading Research Quarterly* 16, 32–71.

Stanovich K. (1988) Explaining the differences between the dyslexic and the garden-variety poor reader: the phonological-core variable-difference model. *Journal of Learning Disabilities* 21, 590–604.

Tallal P, Curtiss S, Kaplan R. (1989) *The San Diego Longitudinal Study: Evaluating the Outcomes of Preschool Impairment in Language Development*. Washington, DC: NINCDS.

Taylor O. (1997) Foreword. In A Kamhi, K Pollock, J Harris (eds), *Communication Development and Disorders in African Children: Research, Assessment, and Intervention* (pp. ix–xi). Baltimore: Brookes Publishing Co.

Torgesen J. (1985) Memory processes in reading disordered children. *Journal of Learning Disabilities* 18, 350–357.

Torgesen J, Wagner R, Rashotte C. (1994) Longitudinal studies of phonological processing and reading. *Journal of Learning Disabilities* 27, 276–286.

Vogel S. (1977) Morphological ability in normal and dyslexic children. *Journal of Learning Disabilities* 10, 292–299.

Wagner R, Torgesen J. (1987) The nature of phonological processing and its causal role in the acquisition of reading skills. *Psychological Bulletin* 101, 192–212.

Wallach G, Butler K. (1994) *Language-Learning Disabilities in School-Age Children and Adolescents*. New York: Merrill.

Westby C. (1989) Assessing and Remediating Text Comprehension Problems. In AG Kamhi, HW Catts (eds), *Reading Disabilities: A Developmental Language Perspective* (pp. 299–360). Boston: Allyn & Bacon.

Wiig E, Semel E. (1975) Productive language abilities in learning disabled adolescents. *Journal of Learning Disabilities* 8, 578–586.

Wiig E, Semel E. (1984) *Language Assessment and Intervention for the Learning Disabled*. Columbus, OH: Merrill.

Wimmer H, Landerl K, Linortner R, Hummer P. (1991) The relationship of phonemic awareness to reading acquisition: more consequence than precondition but still important. *Cognition* 40, 219–249.

Wolf M. (1982) The Word-Retrieval Process and Reading in Children and Aphasics. In K Nelson, (ed), *Children's Language* (Vol 3) (pp. 437–493). New York: Gardner Press.

Wolf M. (1984) Naming, reading, and the dyslexias: a longitudinal overview. *Annals of Dyslexia* 34, 87–136.

Wolf M. (1986) Rapid alternating stimulus naming in developmental dyslexias. *Brain and Language* 27, 360–379.

Wolf M. (1991) Naming speed and reading: the contribution of the cognitive neurosciences. *Reading Research Quarterly* 26, 123–141.

Wolf M, Obregon M. (1992) Early naming deficits, developmental dyslexia, and a specific deficit hypothesis. *Brain and Language* 42, 219–247.

5

A Framework for Differential Diagnosis of Developmental Phonologic Disorders

Paul N. Deputy and Audrey D. Weston

A developmental phonologic disorder is a speech disorder of known or unknown origin that has an onset during the developmental period (Shriberg et al. 1994a). Children with developmental phonologic disorders are heterogeneous with respect to etiology and severity and include preschool children with intelligibility deficits and school-age children with /s/ or /r/ distortions. Shriberg and Kwiatkowski (1994) identified two major disorder subtypes. The first group consists of children who make excessive speech-sound substitutions and omissions that persist past the age of 4 years. These children are described as having speech delay. Children in the second group have residual errors, the maintenance of distorted production of one or more speech sounds beyond the expected age of normalization. These children may or may not have had prior speech delay. Both the speech delay and residual error subgroups are also heterogeneous, each subgroup presenting disorder characteristics as diverse as any other single communication disorder category.

Clinical identification of a developmental phonologic disorder frequently occurs within the first few minutes of an initial assessment. For example, immediate diagnosis of speech delay can occur when a clinician must rely on a parent to interpret a preschooler's communication attempts. Likewise, a clinician may quickly determine that a referred school-age child's lateral lisp represents a socially significant residual articulation error. However, even when clinicians make relatively immediate disorder identification that is further verified by normative data, the clinical work of differential diagnosis has only just begun.

Differential diagnosis of children with suspected developmental phonologic disorders requires comprehensive consideration of many variables related to the communication process (Meitus and Weinberg 1983) to clarify the presence and nature of a disorder and any associated secondary problems (Lynch 1978). The diagnostic process should enable a clinician to estimate the severity of involvement, state a prognosis for normalization of communication ability, and make specific treatment recommendations. The literature devoted to developmental phonologic disorders includes limited discussion of differential diagnosis (Dodd 1995; Richardson 1983). However, differential diagnosis is necessary because of the numerous variables related to speech production. Deputy (1984) expressed the need for a descriptive framework that can differentiate among subgroups and individuals. Approaches to subgroup classification of individuals with developmental phonologic disorders also reflect ongoing attempts to identify both causal and maintenance factors. Diverse variables have been explored, including associated behavioral phenomena (Arndt et al. 1977), cognitive-linguistic and educational performance factors of older children (McNutt and Hamayan 1984), treatment outcomes (Bishop and Edmondson 1987), normalization profiles (Shriberg et al. 1994a, b; Whitehurst and Fischel 1994), etiologies (Shriberg and Kwiatkowski 1994; Shriberg 1994, 1997), linguistic typologies (Ingram 1997), and speech subgroups (Dodd 1995). On several bases, empirically verified subgroups have been identified and have added to professional understanding of children who fail to develop articulate speech at expected ages.

Subgroups identified in research have provided sharper investigative focus and thus have increased the validity of inferential statistical findings. However, as of this writing no classification system provides sufficient understanding of individuals for detailed clinical decisions. The order a classification system imposes on a diverse population occurs by ignoring many individual differences. On the other hand, a differential diagnosis embraces individual differences, facilitates clinical hypotheses about causal and contributing factors and expected speech normalization, and suggests individualized intervention strategies. Although classification systems can provide clinical direction in assessment, only differential diagnosis is uniquely dedicated to tailor-made service delivery, because it allows a clinician to move beyond diagnosis and subgroup classification and provide a thorough description of the child's presenting symptoms. Thus, differential diagnosis can facilitate critical thinking about accumulated quantitative and qualitative data and motivate data-based intervention decisions.

The purpose of this chapter is to present evaluative tasks that form a clinically useful framework for differential diagnosis of children with suspected developmental phonologic disorders. A framework is a prerequisite for accurate diagnosis and effective, efficient treatment, because of the disorder complexities and variability found in children whose speech development is delayed. Misarticulating children typically present overlapping symptoms (e.g., both phonologic and articulatory problems), with a variety of possible etiologies and contributing factors and numerous viable intervention choices. The framework suggested in this chapter for differential diagnosis divides the collection and organization of descriptive data used for assessment into two categories suggested by Shriberg and Kwiatkowski (1982a) and reflected in Bernthal and Bankson's (1993) characterization of phonologic assessment and related factors. These major categories, speech production characteristics and causal correlates, have guided data collection and helped to organize profiles of children with developmental phonologic disorders in the ongoing programmatic research of Shriberg and colleagues. This research, spanning more than two decades, has yielded much descriptive data in these categories, as reviewed in a report by Shriberg and Kwiatkowski (1994).

Within this framework, an eclectic perspective is adopted to summarize the types of data that facilitate describing and understanding a child's developmental phonologic disorder. Clinicians can select from many alternative procedures related to evaluation, assessment, and diagnosis in the area of phonology that have evolved based on reported research and collective clinical experience. The proposed framework accommodates alternative procedures. Rather than list or describe specific procedures that can be found elsewhere in the literature (Bernthal and Bankson 1993; Creaghead et al. 1989; Elbert and Gierut 1986; Hodson and Paden 1991; Ingram 1989; Lowe 1994), this chapter identifies the types of speech production and causal correlates information that an assessment protocol should yield. It also underscores how the proposed framework provides for integration and interpretation of clinical observations to differentiate a child from other subgroups and individuals and to facilitate intervention decisions. Two case studies illustrate the application of the framework through realistic scenarios confronting clinicians in public school, clinic, and hospital settings. This chapter identifies implications for intervention consistent with the assessment of the descriptive data. Although there are still no definitive diagnostic paradigms that are universally accepted and used, this chapter is based on the belief that clinical application of an organizational and conceptual framework facilitates the delivery of more effective service to clients. It is with this idea in mind that the framework for differential diagnosis of developmental phonologic disorders is presented.

DESCRIPTION AND ASSESSMENT OF DEVELOPMENTAL PHONOLOGIC DISORDERS

To assess children with developmental phonologic disorders, a typical protocol derived from the literature would likely include some or all of the following components: (1) case history and parent interview; (2) hearing screening; (3) sampling and analysis of two types of speech production, including single-word citation forms and connected speech; (4) stimulability testing of erred sounds; (5) oral peripheral examination; (6) speech motor ability assessment; (7) receptive and expressive language screening; (8) intelligibility and severity estimate; (9) observation of other aspects of communication, such as voice, prosody, fluency, and pragmatics; and (10) informal description or classification (e.g., speech delay versus residual errors). As warranted by individual characteristics, the protocol can also include additional assessments, such as receptive and expressive language, auditory skills, or other skill areas and modalities. Referral to coprofessionals (e.g., educational psychologists, audiologists, physicians) or collection of existing assessment results is also a common feature of a typical protocol. If a clinician sees such a protocol as a checklist, data can be compartmentalized, which can prevent a conceptual understanding of the disorder in terms of speech production characteristics and causal correlates. If this process took place, data collection and organization for purposes of clinical integration and interpretation could be limited, interfering with assessment and differentiation of a child's individual disorder characteristics.

In this chapter, elements of the above protocol are organized into the two basic descriptive categories—speech production characteristics and causal correlates. With the culminating section, *Integration and Interpretation: Data Assessment,* this three-part framework provides an effective plan for the description of an individual child and a strategy for integration and interpretation of the data. Using the proposed framework can help clinicians first to categorize children into subgroups and second to recognize each child's unique, individual speech production and speech-learning characteristics. The many individual differences seen clinically involving speech production characteristics and causal correlates require a clinician to have a data management framework that facilitates comparison and differentiation of observations. Appropriate intervention strategies have much greater potential to emerge from a comprehensive differential diagnosis plan than from less-structured or incomplete data collection efforts.

Speech Production Characteristics

Children with developmental phonologic disorders exhibit much variability in their speech production characteristics. Speech production characteristics are considered in this section to subsume two broad areas: segmental phonology (e.g., consonant production) and nonsegmental phonology (e.g., speech rate). Three common aspects of a phonologic assessment—intelligibility estimation, dynamic assessment, and severity estimation—are typically included under the topic of speech production characteristics. *Intelligibility* is generally conceptualized as the extent to which a speaker's intended words are understood by a listener (Kent 1992). *Dynamic assessment* is a reconceptualization of stimulability based on an expanded view of exploring the phonologic "learning potential" of children with developmental phonologic disorders (Bain 1994). *Severity* is a term that encompasses a broad conceptualization of the degree to which a disorder impedes effective communication functioning (Shriberg and Kwiatkowski 1982b). All three aspects form less circumscribed areas than either segmental or nonsegmental parameters. Although highly related to speech production, clinical measurement, estimation, and description, these three aspects often encompass more than segmental and nonsegmental characteristics. All three aspects are potentially impacted by causal correlate characteristics that should be considered for a more comprehensive understanding of the factors involved. For these reasons, intelligibility, learning potential, and severity, although highly related to segmental and nonsegmental parameters, are discussed in the section *Integration and Interpretation: Data Assessment*, which considers broader-based integrated data assessment. These three areas are considered to be critical components of assessment for children with developmental phonologic disorders.

A deficit in segmental phonology constitutes an essential disorder characteristic; thus, a child's speech-sound realizations, based on single-word speech samples, continuous speech samples, or both, require analysis. Generally, a clinician completes both independent and relational analyses (Stoel-Gammon and Dunn 1985), although the relative emphasis given the two types of analysis can vary depending on client characteristics. An independent segmental analysis yields an inventory of the phonetic features, phonemes, or phoneme classes that a child uses without regard to his or her articulatory accuracy in comparison with an adult model. A relational analysis requires comparison of a child's realization of consonants and vowels with conventional adult speech production, using various approaches to estimate error rates and describe observed error sounds, types, patterns, or any combination.

In addition to articulation deficits, a child with a developmental phonologic disorder may also exhibit nonsegmental deviations. Included in this category is an aspect of speech production involving larger analysis units than individual segments. This involves the ability to combine and coarticulate individual consonants and vowels to form various syllable shapes and syllable combinations. Thus syllable production is included as an aspect of nonsegmental phonology. Typical nonsegmental, or prosodic, parameters include pitch contours, stress, and rate. Overall precision is included as a prosodic parameter, because, perceptually at least, imprecision transcends individual segment production. Phrasing (e.g., repetitions and revisions) is also included among prosodic parameters. Table 5.1 is an outline of a structure for collecting and organizing single-word and continuous speech data to describe a child's phonologic domain characteristics. It represents the speech production component of the three-part framework used for differential diagnosis of developmental phonologic disorders. Combined with two other components (Tables 5.2 and 5.3), it can be used to describe thoroughly the relevant speech production features of a child with a developmental phonologic disorder.

Segmental Phonologic Data

Children with speech delay produce multiple speech-sound substitution and omission errors. Their error patterns are often described in terms of phonologic processes (Hodson 1986; Ingram 1981; Shriberg and Kwiatkowski 1980) or feature deficiencies (Bernhardt and Stoel-Gammon 1994; Blache 1989; Costello and Onstine 1976; Elbert and Gierut 1986; McReynolds and Engmann 1975). Many children with speech delay also have limited phonetic inventories that constrain both segmental and syllable shape output. Their speech output may or may not reveal prosodic deviations, but intelligibility is generally reduced. Other children, considered to have residual articulation errors, produce age-inappropriate distortions (i.e., phonetic-level deviations) of one or more sounds. Some of these children have had previous speech delay and some have not. As with children with speech delay, nonsegmental symptoms vary; however, intelligibility may or may not be compromised by the speech production errors. Identification of children with either speech delay or residual articulation errors requires consideration of a child's segmental errors in relation to the child's chronological age. The speech delay category is generally relevant through the ages of 6–7 years, while the residual category is considered after the

Table 5.1
Collection of speech production data

- A. Segmental data
  - 1. Independent analysis
    - a. Consonant inventory
    - b. Cluster inventory
    - c. Place, manner, and voicing contrasts
    - d. Vowel and diphthong inventory
  - 2. Relational analysis
    - a. Error summary
      - (1) Consistent misarticulations
      - (2) Inconsistent misarticulations
      - (3) Accuracy summary (PCC)
    - b. Error pattern summary
      - (1) Prevalent feature deficiencies
      - (2) Syllable structure processes
      - (3) Substitution processes
      - (4) Assimilation (harmony) processes
      - (5) Phonetic level errors
    - c. Disparity among levels of linguistic complexity
- B. Nonsegmental data
  - 1. Syllabic level observations
    - a. Syllable and word-shape inventory
    - b. Syllable and segment interactions
  - 2. Global features
    - a. Pitch contours
    - b. Stress
    - c. Rate
    - d. Precision
    - e. Phrasing

PCC = percentage of consonants correct.

age of 7–8 years, whenever specific sound distortions persist beyond the age of expected normalization.

Collection of Data

Any protocol used to assess a child for a suspected developmental phonologic disorder, speech delay, or residual articulation error includes the collection and analysis of segmental speech production data. Many factors, however, influence individual clinician preferences for specific types of speech samples and approaches to data analysis, including client characteristics, procedural efficiency, clinician knowledge and skill, and theoretical views. The most common types of speech samples include citation forms generated from word lists (e.g.,

Table 5.2
Collection of causal correlates data

A. Mechanism data
    1. Speech
    2. Voice
    3. Hearing
    4. Speech motor
    5. Neurologic observations
B. Cognitive-linguistic data
    1. Cognitive
    2. Receptive language
    3. Expressive language
    4. Academic achievement
C. Psychosocial data
    1. Age
    2. Gender
    3. Family dynamics
    4. Individual behavioral characteristics

Table 5.3
Three critical assessment areas

A. Intelligibility assessment
    1. Quantitative
    2. Qualitative
    3. Related causal correlates factors
B. Dynamic assessment
    1. Capability
        a. Error stimulability
        b. Discrimination of erred sounds
    2. Focus
        a. Attention
        b. Motivation and effort
        c. Self-monitoring
C. Severity assessment
    1. Quantitative
    2. Qualitative
    3. Related causal correlates factors

published articulation tests) or informal clinician protocols, imitated or elicited sentences, and continuous speech-language samples. The latter sample type requires the most time for collection, transcription, and analysis, even when a clinician uses a speech-analysis software package such as Programs to Examine Phonetic and Phonologic Evaluation Records (PEPPER) (Shriberg 1986) or Macintosh–Interactive System for Phonological Analysis (Mac-ISPA) (Masterson and Pagan 1993).

Attention to several procedural details can enhance the quality of audiotaped samples and transcription and analysis efficiency. A basic goal is obtaining samples of sufficient quality to facilitate whatever level of transcription (Shriberg and Kent 1995) a clinician decides to complete, ranging from an orthographic gloss of a child's intended words to narrow phonetic transcription of a child's realized phones. Quality recording equipment and careful procedures can help clinicians avoid poor quality, noisy audiotapes that provide little use. A good, reliable desktop audiocassette recorder and accompanying external microphone are essential pieces of clinical equipment that can be obtained for about the same cost as many published tests. Both Shriberg and Kent (1995) and Shriberg (1986) suggest several practical recording procedures to help both beginning and experienced clinicians improve the listening quality of audiotaped samples. Suggestions address helping children feel comfortable with recording equipment and monitoring mouth-to-microphone distance. When collecting a sample from a child whose speech intelligibility is poor, a clinician should routinely gloss the child's utterances on the audiotape to facilitate later recognition of the child's words. Clinicians may find it helpful to have a child's parent or caretaker present during collection of a sample. Without embarrassing the child, this person may be able to identify words that are problematic, particularly if the clinician has told the parent beforehand that he or she may occasionally ask the child, "if Dad or Mom knows about that?"

Word inventories, or articulation tests, whether published or informally produced, are the quickest way to obtain segmental data. Although the literature is equivocal about how accurately citation form data represent an individuals' conversational speech, word lists are considered a valued tool (Bernthal and Bankson 1993) and are widely used by clinicians. They provide at least an approximate inventory of the main errors exhibited by a child and an estimate of the number of sounds misarticulated. They allow preliminary description of error types, phonologic processes, or phonetic feature deficiencies. One advantage is that they can also be used when a child's intelligibility is so poor that a clinician cannot adequately transcribe a continuous speech sample (Schmitt et al. 1983). However, many word inventories do not provide representative data on syllable and word shapes, and all provide limited information for intelligibility estimation.

Despite many arguments in support of continuous speech as one source of data (Morrison and Shriberg 1992), our past and present dialog with clinicians indicates that phonetic transcription and phonologic analysis of continuous speech-language samples is often not formally completed as part of the assessment process. In spite of the constraints of large caseloads, selective inclusion of continuous speech in assessment protocols is encouraged, given certain client characteristics. First, whenever a child also has suspected language involvement, a clinician can increase clinical efficiency by using the same sample for multiple purposes (Weston et al. 1989). This allows for analysis of morphophonemic interactions between speech production competence and grammatical forms that involve increased phonologic complexity (Paul and Shriberg 1982). Another use for continuous speech includes observation of noteworthy discrepancies, or disparity, between a child's errors in single words and in dialog. In particular, some children's omission and assimilation errors occur primarily in continuous speech (DuBois and Bernthal 1978; Johnson et al. 1980). Continuous speech samples also provide a better basis for intelligibility estimates. Continuous speech analysis is important when a child displays many or unusual error patterns that cannot be identified through citation forms alone. Finally, as delineated in the next two paragraphs, continuous speech data facilitates more complete independent and relational analyses that are presumably more representative of the typical output of the child.

Analysis

Analysis of children's segmental speech output, based on word citations, continuous speech, or both, generally assumes both independent and relational perspectives (Stoel-Gammon and Dunn 1985). Independent analyses of segmental speech output yield several types of data that provide a picture of a child's phonetic abilities without consideration of correspondences between child and representative adult surface forms. This type of analysis can be especially important in the evaluation of a child with an expressive vocabulary of less than 50 words, because rule-based phonetic output is not expected of children in the first 50-word stage (Stoel-Gammon and Stone 1991). However, clinical consideration of phonetic inventory is important for most children with suspected speech delay. Incomplete phonetic inventories are common, especially among children with more severe delays, and a speech evaluation should reveal any inventory deficiencies. Most clinical protocols yield relative frequency tallies of the consonant segments that appear in a child's speech output, including data on realized consonant clusters and singletons. Segment data reflect the place, manner, and voicing features included in a child's inventory. In addition, vowel and diphthong inventories are important for children producing vowel distortions (Pollock 1991). Furthermore, information, such as a child's preferred or "default" articulations, can be suggested by sounds that appear frequently (Bernhardt and Stoel-Gammon 1994). Detailed inventories can summarize the segments and phonemic features that a child realizes in different word positions (i.e., initial, medial, or final), revealing any specific word-position constraints on output. Also inventories can be examined in terms of the syllable releasing or arresting function of erred segments (Deputy and Shine 1994; Shine 1989). An additional concern of independent analysis, an inventory of realized syllable shapes, is addressed in the next section along with other nonsegmental aspects of phonology.

Many approaches to relational analysis, comparison of the child speech forms with adult phonology, have appeared in the literature (e.g., Ingram 1989; Stoel-Gammon and Dunn 1985), beginning with traditional error-type description of children's sound changes as segmental omissions, substitutions, distortions, and additions. For continuous speech samples, error-type description yields phoneme-by-phoneme accuracy and error-type rates, as well as an overall measure of percentage of consonants correct (PCC), which provides a severity-of-involvement index (Shriberg 1986; Shriberg and Kwiatkowski 1982b). The PCC has relevance especially for preschool children with speech delay (i.e., those who make many consonant substitutions and deletion errors). Shriberg et al. (1997a) describe six alternative measures of conversational speech proficiency that may be more appropriate for some clients (e.g., the Percentage of Consonants in the Inventory for toddlers). A traditional approach makes few theoretical assumptions about potential cognitive-linguistic bases of children's speech production errors. Most articulation tests, such as the Photo Articulation Test (Pendergast et al. 1984) and Bankson-Bernthal Test of Phonology (BBTOP) (Bankson and Bernthal 1990), suggest error-type scoring of test phonemes. Most speech analysis software provides for traditional description of the error topography reflected in a transcribed speech sample (Shriberg 1986).

In contrast, later sound-change analyses have emphasized children's error patterns, with specific approaches emerging from alternative theoretical perspectives on the acquisition of speech, such as children's acquisition of distinctive features (Blache 1982; Costello 1975; Singh and Polen 1972) or hierarchical feature systems as reviewed in Bernhardt and Stoel-Gammon (1994) and children's use of phonologic processes as speech output simplification strategies (Stampe 1969, 1973). Theoretically based analysis procedures can facilitate subsequent interpretation and treatment decisions. Often, specific approaches include strategies for organizing data with guidelines for selecting treatment targets. For example, Hodson and Paden (1991) suggested determining phonologic process percentage occurrence scores and further ranking processes according to their presumed costliness to intelligibility. A clinician can then use these data to determine what processes should be treated and which should receive treatment priority. Elbert and Gierut (1986) provided a set of guidelines using production data to determine a child's level of underlying knowledge of each phoneme. To encourage generalization, they suggested that initial intervention objectives address a child's "least knowledge" phonemes.

Nonsegmental Phonologic Data

Nonsegmental phonologic data are also important in describing a particular child's speech production, whether or not clinically significant deviations appear. Thus, a data-collection protocol should include prosodic domain observations of a child's speech output on at least two levels. The first prosodic level involves the process of coarticulating segments to form syllables and syllable combinations. In much of the previous literature, analysis of this function was often included in sections on segmental assessment due to the logic that segments were combined to form syllables. However, this is a broader speech production function, because, as expressed by earlier researchers (Kelso and Munhal 1988; McDonald 1964), segments in syllables are overlapping, and producing syllables is a process that both depends on and spans segments. On a word level, a child's syllable and word-shape realizations reflect the child's ability (1) to use phonetic segments for particular syllabic functions (e.g., releasing and arresting); (2) to combine different phonetic segments within one syllabic unit (e.g., to cluster consonants and to mark different places of articulation); and (3) to combine syllables to form more complex canonical word shapes (e.g., consonant vowel consonant vowel [CVCV] and CVCCVC), while still maintaining phonetic accuracy across syllable and lexical boundaries.

Perspectives on syllable-segment interactions presently stem from nonlinear phonologic theories discussed by Bernhardt and Stoel-Gammon (1994) in their tutorial on assessment and treatment applications. They reviewed evidence that the development of syllable shapes (e.g., CV, CVC, and CCVC) and phonetic features (e.g., continuance or velar place of articulation) proceeds both independently and interdependently. Thus, a clinician may most efficiently bring about improved speech production by using the child's current inventory of phonetic features to expand syllable-shape inventory. Similarly, a child may most quickly expand his or her phonetic feature inventory when new features are introduced into strengthened syllable positions. The interaction between segmental and nonsegmental syllable data illustrates why this information should be considered in an assessment framework intended to facilitate effective treatment decisions. This is further clarified in the examples in the next paragraph.

Collection of Data

Syllable and word-shape data can be tallied along with segmental data using either a child's citation forms or words from continuous speech-language samples. Both independent and relational analyses can reveal deficiencies in syllable realizations. For example, a syllable shape inventory that includes a preponderance of CV syllables but few CVC syllables suggests problems in using syllable-arresting consonants. As an interpretive aid, Shriberg (1986) provided reference data on expected syllable-shape distributions in children's continuous speech-language samples. Mismatched proportions of intended versus realized syllable shapes can also signal deficiencies. For example, a ratio of only two realized initial-consonant-cluster monosyllables to 20 such intended syllables suggests limited ability to produce consonant sequences. Many clinicians have learned to view children's syllable-shape deficiencies from the perspective of phonologic processes, invoking the concept of whole-word versus segment-change processes (Bernthal and Bankson 1993). However, specific consideration of a child's apparent deficiencies in the realization of particular syllable shapes and positions can lead to differences in treatment in comparison to a phonologic process approach (Bernhardt and Stoel-Gammon 1994). Clinicians may find that close inspection of a child's syllable realizations yields potentially valuable clinical insight.

The second prosodic level includes more global surface features of a child's typical utterances, including use of pitch contours, stress, rate, and phrasing (e.g., repetitions and revisions). Unlike word-level data, which can be tallied from either word inventories or discourse samples, most of these prosodic evaluations call for continuous speech sampling. Shriberg et al. (1990) suggested that a clinician use only conversational samples as opposed to story-based original or retold narratives that may not reflect a child's typical prosody. Their Prosody-Voice Screening Profile is a procedure to code utterance-level observations. Guidelines for interpreting obtained prosody data, as well as voice data, are available in Shriberg et al. (1992). Whether a clinician chooses to use the screening procedure, he or she will find that the Prosody-Voice Screening Profile content broadens critical thinking about developmental phonologic disorders as well as many other communicative disorders. Clinicians can find an additional helpful resource in the work of Hargrove and McGarr (1994), which focuses more on prosody remediation and prosody use in treatment.

Although precision can also be viewed as a segmental phenomenon, particularly when attempting to transcribe segments judged distorted or perceptually in between some phonetic category (e.g., voiced and voiceless), it is included in the area of prosody in this chapter because it also can be a more global process that transcends segments. Usually imprecision, even though transcription decisions often involve a segment, involves syllable formation and can affect vowels as well as consonants. Children are usually imprecise across syllables affecting the general production of the segments as opposed to specific distortions on a particular segment. Clinicians are familiar with children who have minimal identified segmental deviations but have reduced intelligibility due to general imprecision. Intervention techniques other than those commonly used in segmental deviations may be more appropriate. Although a procedure for measuring general imprecision has not yet been devised, a subjective impression of this phenomenon can be helpful to interpretation.

Analysis

Even without additional causal correlates evidence, descriptive prosodic data can suggest much about the nature of a child's speech production disorder. For example, the excessive occurrence of whole-word and part-word repetitions, revisions, and pauses may signal that a phonologic disorder is a component of a more comprehensive language problem (Deputy et al. 1982). Given the complexity involved in the cognitive organization and linguistic expression of experiences (Weiss 1995), many children with language disorders have phrasing problems. Similarly, observed sound repetitions and prolongations, perhaps accompanied by unusual stress patterns, can suggest coexisting speech delay and stuttering. Finally, rate deviations (e.g., excessive slowness) and perhaps lack of contrastive stress or a monotonic pitch contour suggest a need to investigate for corroborating evidence of speech motor involvement. These three examples illustrate the importance of prosodic description, with each example suggesting different diagnoses and different treatment implications.

Causal Correlate Characteristics

In addition to variability in speech production characteristics, children with developmental phonologic disorders can also present a wide variety of symptoms and behaviors subsumed under the umbrella term *causal correlates*. As reviewed by Bernthal and Bankson (1993), many factors in this category can be associated with speech development problems, even though research has demonstrated true causal relationships with relatively few variables (Shriberg et al. 1994a). Causal correlates evaluation can contribute important information to the differential diagnosis process, such as indicating appropriate referrals and determining factors that influence intelligibility, severity, and prognosis. Causal correlates observations can also help a clinician select appropriate treatment approaches.

Three subcategories provide a comprehensive classification system for causal correlates: (1) mechanism factors, (2) cognitive-linguistic factors, and (3) psychosocial factors. Collecting data to identify and describe these factors can involve (1) informal or structured observation; (2) formal or standard procedures; (3) review of case histories, previous diagnostic reports, and treatment records; and (4) interviews with caregivers and other professionals (e.g., teachers). Table 5.2 outlines the basic structure of the causal correlates component of the framework leading to differential diagnosis of developmental phonologic disorders.

Mechanism Data

Mechanism factors potentially related to developmental phonologic disorders include deviations of the structure and function of the speech, voice, and hearing mechanisms. These also include positive histories of conditions associated with any one mechanism (e.g., many episodes of otitis media with effusion). Shriberg and Kwiatkowski (1994) listed 86 possible mechanism factors, such as neurologic integrity and neurologic differences (e.g., neurologic "soft signs"). They also included consideration of genetic factors (e.g., close relatives who have or have had speech-language disorders) as a possible mechanism causal correlate. Although Shriberg and Kwiatkowski's (1994) research indicated that mechanism factors are relatively infrequent among the developmental phonologic-disordered population, there is potential involvement in any individual case that could have an impact on the nature and treatment of the disorder.

Prominent deficits of the speech and hearing mechanism form traditional diagnostic groupings, consisting of etiologic disorder categories such as cleft palate, hearing impairment, and neurologically based speech disorders (e.g., dysarthria, apraxia) (Smit 1994). Most of the research regarding developmental phonologic disorders excludes disorders of known origin and considers children with speech delay or residual errors as generally a separate population. Child phonology issues also pertain to "special populations" that overlap with "mechanism" disorders and include cultural factors such as American English dialects of sociocultural groups and first language–influenced English (Bernthal and Bankson 1994). The specific problems of special populations may differ, yet there is often a phonologic component that includes segmental and nonsegmental deviations that can be analyzed similarly.

Individuals with structural deficits, sensory deficits, neuromotor deficits, or any combination of these can show widely differing segmental and nonsegmental patterns and other causal correlates deficits that must be considered. To address the phonologic component of special populations, specific assessment procedures may be needed (e.g., Trost-Cardamone and Bernthal 1993; Locke 1980a, b). Differential diagnosis procedures often indicate a need for a particular treatment focus depending on special population characteristics. For example, in the speech of a client who has a cleft palate, the phonologic process of backing may have unique diagnostic significance and treatment implications. Similarly, an increased emphasis on auditory identification and discrimination of sounds related to final-consonant deletion may hold special relevance when working with phonology disorders related to persons with hearing impairment.

Several published protocols facilitate a direct examination of the speech mechanism (e.g., Dworkin and Culatta 1980; Robbins and Klee 1987; St. Louis and Ruscello 1987), and typical evaluation parameters have been summarized by Hall (1994). These procedures include systematic observations of the structure and function of all aspects of the oral mechanism and related structures (e.g., face, jaw, lips, tongue, velum, teeth, palate, pharynx). Typically, protocols help the clinician make judgments about structure and function across three levels: normal, questionable, and deviant. Included in an examination of the speech mechanism is an evaluation of vocal mechanism integrity, including a perceptual judgment of voice quality, as this has been found to be a coexisting factor in some cases of developmental phonologic disorders (Shriberg and Kwiatkowski 1994).

An additional standard procedure is screening the hearing of each child with a developmental phonologic disorder to examine hearing acuity. Although hearing acuity most frequently is not a primary factor, frequent middle-ear infections can contribute to a developmental phonologic disorder (Roberts and Clark-Klein 1994; Shriberg and Kwiatkowski 1994; Shriberg and Smith 1983). For example, clinicians may observe factors, such as a history of middle-ear infections or tympanometry results, that indicate the need for appropriate referrals. Another aspect of the hearing process commonly addressed in the phonology literature is speech-sound discrimination. Although the research findings are equivocal regarding the association between misarticulation and poor discrimination (Bernthal and Bankson 1993), some children may have difficulty discriminating specific target sounds. Clinicians may wish to assess a child's ability to discriminate error sounds using procedures suggested by Locke (1980a, b).

Most protocols for examination of the speech mechanism contain nonspeech oral-motor and speech-motor tasks. Many clinicians include observation of speech-motor skills either through informal or more formal (Riley and Riley 1985) means. This includes (1) diadochokinetic tasks, which are repeated syllable strings with alternating place, manner, or voice features (Riley and Riley 1985); (2) syllable-sequencing tasks with shifting vowels and consonants (McDonald 1964); and (3) production of syllables with increasingly complex syllabic structures (Shine 1989). Each task represents a skill prerequisite to development and maintenance of articulate speech. The first requires maintaining ongoing syllable production in a smooth and appropriately rapid manner, termed here *horizontal speech motor skill* because of the ongoing, repetitive nature of the task. The second requires motor vigilance in maintaining accurate productions, termed *vertical speech motor skill* because of the depth of phonetic context constant consonant and vowel shifting requires. This relates to McDonald's deep-testing concept. The third requires maintaining horizontal and vertical motor integrity during increasing syllabic complexity, which could be termed *integral motor skill*. Crary (1993), Hall et al. (1993), Hayden (1994), and Velleman and Strand (1994) discussed the use of similar procedures with children exhibiting observed or suspected speech motor control problems. Many clinicians consider persistent forms of speech motor control difficulty to be an etiologic condition known as *developmental apraxia of speech* (Hall et al. 1993). It should be noted that there is controversy about the nature and existence of developmental apraxia of speech (Crary 1983; Guyette and Diedrich 1981; Parsons and Crary 1984; Shriberg et al. 1997b; Velleman and Strand 1994). Consistent with and related to a speech motor evaluation is a screening for neurologic "soft signs," or indications of difficulty involving strength and range of movement. Referral to a pediatric neurologist is often also indicated. For cases involving traumatic brain injury or cerebral palsy, clinicians can generally obtain neurologic data from the examining physician.

The literature suggests several possible indicators of speech motor-control problems (Crary 1993; Deputy 1984; Hall et al. 1993; Velleman and Strand 1994): (1) inability to sequence syllables; (2) disparity in accuracy among levels of linguistic complexity; (3) a prevalence of phonologic processes involving syllable structure, assimilation, and voicing; (4) reduction of complex morphophonemic productions; (5) slow, weak, inaccurate nonspeech oral motor movements, possibly including limited range of motion; and (6) difficulty in integrating newly learned sounds into more complex linguistic levels. The last indicator has received a great deal of attention in the literature. Identified problems include difficulty with the production of syllable-structure hierarchies, inability to efficiently respond to contrasting or highly motivating activities, and a tendency to retain reduced productions in spite of maturity and extensive treatment (Crary 1993; Hall et al. 1993; Velleman and Strand 1994). A framework for differential diagnosis that facilitates integration and interpretation of speech production data with mechanism data can be helpful in sorting out and confirming the presence of these indicators for individuals or groups.

Cognitive-Linguistic Data

Professionals have investigated potential relationships between the development of articulation proficiency and intelligence, language ability, and academic achievement. As summarized by Bernthal and Bankson (1993), articulation proficiency is related to standardized intelligence test scores, primarily when they fall below the normal range. Although individuals with mental retardation have a high incidence of articulation impairment, IQ scores are poor predictors of articulatory proficiency among individuals with normal intelligence.

Researchers, however, have observed positive relationships between articulation development and language development. Disorders of phonology and language co-occur in 60–80% of children identified with either type of disorder (Tyler and Watterson 1991). Yet, individual clinical profiles reveal that misarticulating children have highly variable language abilities, ranging from using complex syntactic structures to a restricted mean length of utterance that constrains social interaction and expression of basic needs. Among children identified with speech delay, 50–75% exhibit some clinically significant delay in language production, especially affecting morphology and syntax (Hodsen and Paden 1981; Shriberg 1994; Shriberg et al. 1994a). Children in this subgroup make many errors involving past tense, plurals, possessives, and pronouns. Morphophonemic complexity may increase the frequency of language form errors, but many errors also occur even when obligatory forms are phonemically simple. In comparison, the child whose grammatical errors result from impaired phonology should have normal expressive language form in contexts unaffected by the child's error pattern (Paul and Shriberg 1982).

In addition to expressive language delay, 10–40% of children with speech delay have language-comprehension delay (Shriberg and Kwiatkowski 1994). Children with isolated delays in articulation have the most favorable prognosis for development of normal speech and little risk of later reading or other academic problems (Bishop and Adams 1990; Bishop and Edmondson 1987). However, children with early syntactic restrictions, especially reduced mean length of utterance, are at risk for poor academic achievement (Bishop and Adams 1990), even though many will develop correct production of speech sounds. Children with concomitant language comprehension delay have the least favorable prognosis, both for the development of normal speech and for academic achievement (Whitehurst and Fischel 1994). This is especially true for children whose speech-language delay is secondary to general cognitive delay or another developmental disorder.

Assessment considerations for school-age children with residual articulation errors differ somewhat in comparison to those for a child with speech delay. Among the former group, a clinician can expect to encounter variability with regard to cognitive-linguistic performance. School clinicians have remediated such problems as lateral lisps and derhotacized /r/ sounds in children who excel academically, as well as in children with severe learning disabilities. However, academic achievement can be difficult for the child with abnormal distortion errors who also has a history of speech-language delay (Shriberg and Kwiatkowski 1988). When assessing a child in this category, the assessment protocol generally calls for collaboration with other school personnel, such as classroom teachers, reading specialists, and educational psychologists, to collect and interpret data.

The co-occurrence of either expressive language or language comprehension delay influences the focus and context of intervention. Appropriate treatment decisions for individual children depend on thorough consideration of a child's speech-language strengths and deficits. For example, clinicians need sufficient data to decide the relative amount of direct treatment each deficit area will receive. This is not a question to be taken lightly, given that the literature reports conflicting results regarding treatment effects on phonology when language is treated and vice versa (Fey et al. 1994; Hoffman et al. 1990). Regardless of co-occurring language problems, when phonologic deficits are severe, considerable direct treatment of phonology appears to be warranted (Tyler and Sandoval 1994).

The frequent co-occurrence of speech and language disorders, together with related prognosis and treatment issues, suggests that clinicians should question the language abilities of all children seen for possible speech delay. As a profession, speech-language pathology has advanced beyond the time when a clinician could focus on remediating articulation errors without consideration of potential relationships between speech-language characteristics and reading and writing development (see Chapter 4). Recognizing relationships can lead to the development of more integrated and effective intervention approaches in school settings. For an individual child, a combination of case history, referral information, and direct, informal observation can indicate the need for comprehensive language evaluation.

Discussion of a language evaluation falls outside the scope of this chapter (see Chapter 3). However, a typical phonologic disorders assessment protocol readily facilitates expressive language screening through procedures for sampling a child's connected speech. A continuous speech-language sample can serve as a potential source of assessment data for both speech and language. In addition, the collection of several continuous samples over time (e.g., before the intervention begins and as treatment progresses) facilitates a clinician's monitoring of treatment efficacy. Aspects of the sampling process also can contribute to psychosocial observations and to intelligibility and dynamic assessments.

Psychosocial Data

Important psychosocial data for clinical consideration include (1) age, (2) gender, (3) family dynamics, and (4) individual behavioral characteristics. Age is a critical variable in differential diagnosis. Many of the speech patterns clinicians evaluate are consistent with normal speech development. When that is the case, the clinician's role is to provide developmental information that allays the concerns of caregivers. Children younger than 3 years old who have limited phonetic inventories are likely to be referred for evaluation because of language development concerns rather than speech. Although professionals have increasingly considered relationships between phonetic constraints and delayed language development (e.g., Stoel-Gammon and Stone 1991), the diagnosis for very young preschoolers in this category is more likely to be language delay or late talking than speech delay. Most commonly, children are referred because of speech production concerns during their fourth year. Diagnoses of speech delay occur primarily between the ages of 4 and 7 years, although developmental status can be a concern before 4 years of age. Diagnoses of residual errors primarily apply to children beyond the age of 7–8 years or whenever retained distortion errors are no longer age appropriate. Recall that children diagnosed with residual articulation errors may or may not have histories of previous speech delay, so that clinicians in public-school settings assess many children who have never received prior, early-intervention services.

Two facts related to gender are clinically important. First, at certain ages and for certain sounds, females tend to be somewhat ahead of males in phonologic acquisition (Smit et al. 1990), and clinicians may need to consider these gender differences. Second, gender ratios among children diagnosed with speech delay favor males by nearly 3 to 1, especially when children have coexisting speech and language delays (Shriberg 1994). This gender discrepancy, in combination with a high incidence of familial speech-language involvement, supports the idea that heredity plays a major role in children's abnormal speech development (Felsenfeld et al. 1995; Shriberg 1994).

Beyond age, gender, and familial transmission, research has identified few relationships between developmental phonologic disorders and psychosocial variables such as socioeconomic status and personality traits. For most psychosocial variables, clinicians can expect to encounter as much variability among clients as the general population. However, clinicians should attempt to identify any factors that can have implications for intervention, such as a child's apparent communicative frustration or a factor that may contribute to the maintenance of a child's speech errors (e.g., a child's reluctance to attempt specific speech tasks). For diagnostic consideration, potentially noteworthy factors pertain to the client's family dynamics and behavioral characteristics, concepts that others have variously described as environmental influences (Nation and Aram 1984) and psychosocial inputs and behaviors (Shriberg and Kwiatkowski 1994) are included in the psychosocial category. Our approach to describing a child from a psychosocial perspective addresses several questions relevant to these concepts and are exemplified in the next two paragraphs.

Family dynamics can be considered from the perspective of interactions among family members. What is the level of family concern over a child's speech errors? Do caregivers attempt to correct the child's speech or talk for the child? Do they compare the child unfavorably to siblings and other children? Do parental expectations for behavior seem consistent with the child's developmental level? Does parental management of the child's behavior seem effective? Does the child receive positive feedback for desirable behavior? Variables in this category can influence a child's self-perceptions as a talker and a learner, which can in turn influence a child's response to treatment. Clinicians treating young children have unique opportunities to serve as teaching models for caregivers, as well as for children.

The practitioner should also note possible signs of communicative anxiety or frustration that may be revealed as reticence to talk or as "giving up" when a listener fails to understand. Childhood aggression, as reported during a parent interview, can also be related to a child's intelligibility problem. Observations in this category can influence treatment decisions such as whether to begin treatment versus scheduling the child for a later re-evaluation and whether to target goals aimed at providing a child with early success. In addition, it is also important to observe how a child responds to specific types of speech and language tasks (e.g., clinician-structured training or play-oriented formats). To what types of stimuli does a child attend? What types of activities seem to motivate a child's best speech efforts? What types of reinforcement seem effective with a child? Does the child seem able to monitor errors and make changes when listener feedback indicates uncertainty about an intended word? These types of variables provide intervention direction, such as indicating the types of therapy activities most likely to elicit desired speech responses.

Clinician opportunities to observe family dynamics and a child's behavior occur throughout the assessment process, beginning with review of referral information, case history, and caregiver interview and continuing in combination with all formal and informal evaluation procedures. Appropriate assessment procedures, to be discussed under *Dynamic Assessment*, can especially reveal an individual child's response to alternative teaching approaches.

Integration and Interpretation: Data Assessment

When assessment activities have been carried out that provide comprehensive data about the speech production and causal correlates characteristics of a child with a developmental phonologic disorder, the descriptive phase of the differential diagnostic process has been completed. The clinician then must integrate and interpret the obtained descriptive data, as well as conduct a dynamic assessment of the child's ability to respond to antecedent or consequential events structured by the clinician. This data assessment phase incorporates three additional assessment areas: intelligibility, stimulability, and severity of involvement. These three areas help a clinician to further define the nature of the disorder and make treatment decisions, such as formulating treatment objectives and delineating specific treatment strategies. Table 5.3 illustrates the basic structure of the data assessment component of the framework. It is the third component in a three-part framework (see Tables 5.1 and 5.2). The first two components are primarily descriptive, whereas the third component, involving three critical assessment areas, emphasizes integration of various aspects of the descriptive data, as well as observation of the child's learning potential. Further elaboration of these concepts follows in the sections on the three aforementioned assessments: *Intelligibility Assessment, Dynamic Assessment,* and *Severity Assessment.*

Intelligibility Assessment

Although many professionals define *speech intelligibility* as involving recognition of a speaker's intended words, viewpoints differ regarding the role of many variables that can influence word recognition. Some recommend that *intelligibility* be narrowly defined as word recognition based primarily on information present in the acoustic signal itself (e.g., Yorkston et al. 1996). Others take a view that incorporates a range of potential influences, including listener variables (e.g., experience with deviant speech patterns) and communicative-context variables (e.g., topic knowledge shared by interactants), in addition to speech production variables (Shriberg and Kwiatkowski 1982b). Yorkston and colleagues (1996) used the term *comprehensibility* to distinguish the latter view from the former, more narrow, view. Their perspective considers many variables, such as a speaker's pragmatic ability to monitor communication breakdowns and other variables that contribute to a person's overall communicative competence. As Kent (1992) emphasized, speech intelligibility influences many aspects of a child's social use of language. Kent advocated that assessment of intelligibility should incorporate both perspectives (i.e., acoustic cue clarity and communicative competence issues). Thus, intelligibility assessment challenges the clinician to "explain" a child's intelligibility deficit by considering a number of potentially interacting factors, many of which may fall outside the domain of speech production.

Several authors have reviewed or suggested approaches to the unique clinical challenge of measuring, estimating, or describing intelligibility (e.g., Gordon-Brannan 1994; Hodge 1996; Kent et al. 1994; Morris et al. 1995). Approaches tend to reflect either a narrow or broad consideration of intelligibility influences. Scores based on listener recognition of single-word recitations presumably reflect the primary influence of acoustic information. Examples of instruments that provide such scores include (1) Test of Children's Speech (Hodge 1996), (2) CID Picture SPINE (Monsen et al. 1988); and (3) the Preschool Speech Intelligibility Measure (Morris et al. 1995). In contrast, a measure such as the Intelligibility Index (Shriberg and Kwiatkowski 1982b), which is the percentage of nonquestionable glossed words in a transcript of continuous speech-language, reflects the influence of many variables (e.g., a child's clarification skills and whether a parent was present, as an informant, during the sample collection).

Concerning the relative clinical value of such extremes, Kent (1992) believed that single-word intelligibility tests are especially useful because controlled, closed-set word lists systematically sample a range of phonetic contrasts and can reveal the linguistic contrasts that a child does not mark. Thus, such a test can provide clinical insight as to the intelligibility effects of particular error patterns. However, Kent suggested that a clinician also use a sample of continuous speech to make judgments about factors other than segmental variables that affect a child's overall communicative competence (e.g., prosody and voice characteristics or language-domain variables). Rate and stress patterns can logically affect intelligibility. For example, consonant deletion errors in combination with reduced or deviant stress marking can substantially reduce a listener's ability to segment and identify a child's intended words. This broader focus on intelligibility involves more qualitative clinical judgments. For example, a clinician should consider his or her experience with child speech forms and time spent in transcription among factors that represent a best-case scenario in word recognition. Care must be taken to avoid underestimating a child's intelligibility problems outside the clinic, especially when communication involves nonfamily members.

Because a child's intelligibility varies from context to context, attempts to quantify this aspect of speech fall short of precision. No doubt, this has prompted many clinicians to use subjective ratings to reflect qualitative judgments about a child's level of intelligibility. In this approach, clinical estimation of intelligibility commonly relies on scales, some with anchors such as "highly unintelligible," "cannot be understood," or "completely intelligible" (Gordon-Brannan 1994). Often clinicians consider the impressions of caregivers or teachers in making qualitative judgments about intelligibility. Hodge and Hancock (1994) suggested a form that is useful for obtaining others' estimates of a child's speech handicap. Although the reliability of such qualitative estimates may be questionable, judgments have some ecological validity and may have considerable use in the differential diagnosis process, in view of the complexity involved in trying to understand a child's overall communicative competence.

To understand a child's intelligibility deficit requires that the clinician examine other variables in addition to speech production. Many causal correlate variables can influence a child's intelligibility. For example, among mechanism factors, a clinician may determine that a deviation in structural integrity of the speech mechanism underlies a child's resonance problems, a parameter known to detract from speaker intelligibility (Curtis 1970). Similarly, within the cognitive-linguistic area, a child's expressive language abilities have implications for how well listeners can understand the child. Some language factors in this category bear little relationship to a child's speech patterns. For example, the length of an utterance can influence intelligibility (Weston and Shriberg 1992), perhaps by increasing or decreasing the demands on the listener. Thus, the loquacious child who freely initiates topics may especially challenge a listener. On the other hand, the two- or three-word utterances of a child with limited language ability may be mostly intelligible, especially when the child tends to talk mostly about stimuli present in the environment.

Similarly, psychosocial variables can either mitigate or exacerbate a child's intelligibility problems. A child's sensitivity to communication breakdowns can sometimes bring about articulation improvement or lead to vocabulary modifications. Consequently, the talkative child may not fair too poorly if language skills are sufficient to allow a child to select alternative ways to say the same thing or to define problem words. On the other hand, more reticent children may try to decrease intelligibility problems by avoiding communication. Some children may use a quiet voice, poor eye contact, and other avoidance tactics that detract from their communication attempts. Social-context variables also fall into this category and include such factors as the degree of knowledge shared by speaker and listener and the listener's experience with child speech (Kent 1992). Factors in this category can make a child more or less intelligible depending on who the listener is.

For these and many other factors, a child's speech error rates and types do not have a direct relationship with his or her intelligibility, particularly when conceptualized broadly. In view of the many factors influencing intelligibility estimates, we believe that both quantitative and qualitative observations have considerable clinical use for diagnosis and treatment. Quantitative measures, such as those obtained from single-word closed-set tests, can provide useful pre-and post-treatment comparisons (Morris et al. 1995), in addition to aiding the identification of a child's most detrimental speech errors (Hodge 1996). However, from the perspective of estimating the degree of social handicap and determining overall severity of involvement, qualitative judgments of intelligibility deficit also play an important role. Furthermore, qualitative judgments can lead to the identification of factors other than speech errors that underlie or contribute to a speaker's intelligibility deficit.

Dynamic Assessment

Dynamic assessment procedures allow a clinician to estimate a child's potential to learn specific aspects of phonology and language and also to identify the conditions that can foster skill acquisition (Minick 1987). This can contribute highly useful information to help a clinician make optimal treatment recommendations, since treatment involves learning and change. These activities differ from the majority of assessment protocol activities that help a clinician determine if a disorder is present through comparison of observed and expected speech production proficiency and identify any causal or maintaining factors (e.g., prior episodes of otitis media, expressive language delay, cognitive delay, orofacial anomaly). The above can be considered measures and observations of existing conditions and constitute "static" assessment.

In the context of developmental phonologic disorders "dynamic" assessment can help to identify antecedent stimuli (e.g., auditory model or phonetic placement cues), linguistic complexity levels (e.g., isolation, words, and phrases), and communication consequences (e.g., situations in which improved articulation receives reinforcement) that can facilitate change in speech production (Bain 1994). Encompassing the traditional concept of stimulability testing (Carter and Buck 1958; Deidrich 1983; Madison 1979; Milisen 1954), dynamic assessment allows for manipulation of factors that may foster phonologic learning. Speech-language pathologists determine a child's ability to modify erred production of speech sounds and apply this information in several ways, such as selecting sounds for treatment (Hodson and Paden 1991; Bain 1994), determining productive phonologic knowledge (Dinnsen and Elbert 1984; Elbert and Gierut 1986), or deciding the appropriate linguistic complexity level of intervention stimuli (Bernthal and Bankson 1993; Creaghead et al. 1989; Elbert and Gierut 1986). In addition, data support the idea that high stimulability is a favorable prognostic indicator (Powell et al. 1991).

Bain (1994) proposed that clinicians use the concept of dynamic assessment to increase the number of variables typically considered in conjunction with traditional stimulability. By making systematic observations of the conditions associated with a child's success or failure on a specific speech-sound target, a clinician can determine (1) a child's readiness to learn a new phonetic skill (e.g., to produce /ʃ/) at a particular point in development, (2) the factors that influence a child's improved production of a specific sound (e.g., placement cues, linguistic contrasts, or extrinsic rewards), and (3) environmental changes that can facilitate the child's speech development or functioning (e.g., a specific type of therapy approach or increasing parental information about speech development).

Dynamic assessment can be viewed as encompassing two concepts identified by Kwiatkowski and Shriberg (1993): *capability* and *focus*. Speech production capability relates directly to the maturity and integrity of the physiologic, neurologic, perceptual, and cognitive-linguistic foundations, prerequisites for realizing phonetic targets. However, for a child to accomplish phonetic expression, particularly involving emerging skill, some level of attention, self-monitoring, and motivation are also presumed prerequisites: Focus includes these and similar cognitive states. In sum, knowing a child's capability helps to determine what new articulation skills can be taught; understanding focus helps to determine the most effective elicitation and teaching approaches. Thus, dynamic assessment includes determining capability for phonologic growth, as well as how a child's level of focus can affect changes in habituated speech-sound production.

Based on dynamic assessment procedures, Deputy (1992) and Deputy and Shine (1994) suggested a straightforward categorization of phonemes according to a child's level of production of each, drawing on both independent and relational analysis data and dynamic assessment data (Table 5.4). First-level sounds (Level I) include those that appear regularly in a child's output or are within his or her capability. These sounds further separate into IA- and IB-level sounds, with IA including sounds the child uses in all contexts with accuracy at the mastery level. These are considered sounds included in a child's phonemic inventory because he or she uses them contrastively. The IB category includes sounds with lower accuracy rates and perhaps some distributional error patterns. These are considered sounds that appear in a child's phonetic inventory, because they can be produced but are not used in the sense of the adult model. Second-level sounds are considered error sounds and also include two subgroups: IIA sounds are sounds a child can produce with auditory or visual modeling but that are seldom or never used correctly in spontaneous speech, and IIB sounds are sounds that can be produced through more extensive demonstration and phonetic teaching methods. A third level includes sounds that do not appear in the phonetic inventory and that a child cannot produce even after considerable phonetic teaching and trial. The resulting level of production organization facilitates a clinician's selection of specific sounds for use in treatment.

Severity Assessment

Severity assessment enables a clinician to further qualify the nature of a child's developmental phonologic disorder. Commonly, clinicians use an interval scale of severity with corresponding descriptors, such as "mild," "moderate," or "severe," to reflect their clinical judgment or estimate of a child's severity of involvement. This estimate serves several purposes. First, it provides a statement of the extent of a child's

Table 5.4
Level of speech sound production

Level I	Sounds that the client can produce	
	IA	Sounds that can be produced easily and used contrastively in speech (phonemic inventory)
	IB	Sounds that can be produced easily on request and are not used contrastively or even used in speech (phonetic inventory)
Level II	Stimulable sounds	
	IIA	Sounds that are stimulable with salient auditory or visual models
	IIB	Sounds that are stimulable with a moderate amount of demonstration and probing
Level III	Sounds that the client cannot produce	
	IIIA	One example was produced either with considerable demonstration and teaching or spontaneously, but it cannot be produced voluntarily
	IIIB	No production or approximation of the phone observed

Source: Adapted from PN Deputy, RE Shine. (1994, November) Integrating Treatment Approaches for Phonologic/Articulatory Problems and Disorders. Short course presented at the meeting of the American Speech-Language-Hearing Association, New Orleans.

speech delay to parents and other professionals who may have involvement with the child and family. Second, severity estimation can serve to identify children who meet treatment eligibility criteria, either through state or federally funded programs or services reimbursable through a third-party payer. Third, severity judgments relate to many treatment decisions, such as the nature of therapy (e.g., direct versus indirect, group versus individual) and how much therapy time per week a child will receive. Finally, severity can relate to a child's prognosis for normalized speech and the projected normalization time span. However, prognosis must be approached cautiously, because, as of this writing, the factors that predict normalization within a certain period of time remain largely unknown (Shriberg et al. 1994a). Thus, the clinical significance of estimated severity may relate most closely to intervention decisions.

Estimating a child's severity of involvement requires primary consideration of a child's speech production characteristics relative to chronological age, although professional opinion differs about the critical variables and whether quantitative or qualitative indices should be used. Many clinicians think that speech-error variables, such as rate, consistency, and uniqueness, should all be considered. For example, the uniqueness of speech errors can provide information about the nature of a disorder and can conceivably influence severity impressions. A 4-year-old child who is retaining natural processes (Shriberg and Kwiatkowski 1980), such as stopping or cluster reduction, may simply sound like a younger child. In contrast, a child with uncommon patterns, such as initial consonant deletion, apicalization (Ingram 1981), or extensive substitution of initial /h/ or /j/ as a "favorite sound" (Ferguson and Macken 1983), may sound qualitatively "unusual" and, thus, more severe. However, relationships between clinician ratings and such qualitative differences have received limited research attention. The role played by variables associated with erred sounds, including frequency, age of acquisition, syllable and word positions, consistency, and error type, has not yet been determined. Still, a clinician has available several alternative observations for severity assessment. Although causal correlates and intelligibility variables possibly warrant consideration for individual children, a clinician may first obtain a quantitative index of severity based on speech measurement and then decide if other types of information indicate adjustment of a rating based on quantitative data.

Several published articulation test protocols yield data that can lead to assignment of a severity adjective. These estimates are especially relevant for children with speech delay and may often be necessary to document service eligibility. One quantitative approach involves comparing an individual child's articulation abilities to a normative sample. The use of percentile ranks and standard scores for this purpose is exemplified by the BBTOP (Bankson and Bernthal 1990). With these data, a clinician can apply criteria such as 1.0–1.5 standard deviations (SDs) below the mean indicating mild-to-moderate disability, 1.5–2.0 SDs below the mean indicating moderate disability, and more than 2.0 SDs below the mean indicating severe disability. The BBTOP includes a developmental scale score that adds to the validity of obtained results. This score provides for comparison of an individual child's performance on each consonant with a representative group score. Thus, a clinician can evaluate a child's BBTOP performance with considerable specificity.

A second quantitative approach is based on speech production accuracy data yielded by phonetic transcription of 5-minute continuous speech samples. The PCC (Shriberg and Kwiatkowski 1982b) provides an objective severity metric for children who make high numbers of omission and substitution errors (i.e., children with speech delay). For this population, the measure correlates positively with clinician judgments of relative severity, so that a clinician can feel confident that PCC provides a valid severity index when Shriberg and Kwiatkowski's scoring and computational guidelines have been followed. PCC scores divide into four ordinal categories: (1) ≥ 85% = mild; (2) 65–85% = mild-moderate; (3) 50–65% = moderate-severe; and (4) ≤ 50% = severe. Clinician adjustments to this scale can be suggested when a child (1) is older than approximately 8 years or primarily exhibits distortion errors (i.e., has residual errors), (2) exhibits deviant nonsegmental phonologic characteristics, or (3) has involvement in causal correlate areas (e.g., concomitant language delay). Although the validity of PCC as a severity index has received empirical support, many clinicians simply do not have the time required to transcribe and analyze a continuous speech sample, especially when intelligibility is a concern.

An alternative approach takes a child's error patterns and their presumed effect on intelligibility into consideration. Hodson (1986) and Hodson and Paden (1991) ranked a child's severity of involvement using a four-level continuum from mild to profound. A clinician determines a phonologic deviancy score that accounts for error patterns and their relative frequency of occurrence. Error patterns associated with the greatest cost to intelligibility contribute the most to obtained scores, increasing estimated severity.

In general, however, professionals differ in their views of whether a child's speech intelligibility should influence clinical estimation of severity of involvement. For example, Shriberg and Kwiatkowski (1982b) advocated that the accuracy of a child's continuous speech should be the primary consideration for describing the severity of a child's speech disability. These researchers prefer the relative objectivity of articulatory accuracy rates over the greater subjectivity reflected in intelligibility estimates. However, others (e.g., Smit 1994) view the clinical concepts of severity and intelligibility more synonymously. This latter perspective may reflect the majority of clinicians. As reviewed by Gordon-Brannan (1994), intelligibility is the most frequently cited factor in deciding the extent of a child's phonologic disorder.

Separation of intelligibility and severity is difficult in clinical practice, because the concepts overlap in how they influence intervention decisions. The concerns of family members or teachers for a child's intelligibility problems frequently lead to referral in the first place, and such concerns have considerable face validity as estimates of the extent of a child's speech handicap. Thus, the opinions of lay persons deserve clinical consideration in determining whether intervention is indicated, and few clinicians would overlook family concerns and base severity assessment entirely on a quantitative index such as articulatory accuracy rates. Similarly, few would base a severity estimate solely on the degree of expressed concern for intelligibility.

One way to ascertain the degree of concern held by significant persons in a child's life is through the use of rating scales. Hodge and Hancock (1994) suggested a possible format that asks a respondent to rate the negative effect that a child's speech disability has on a number of communication aspects, including, for example, the frequency and quality of communication interactions. Their five-point scale ranges from "no effect" to "profound." Such ratings can provide real-life documentation of a child's progress through comparison of pre- and postintervention perceptions. When clinical efficiency is particularly important, a rating scale approach can provide key information for severity assessment.

DIFFERENTIAL DIAGNOSIS: DATA-BASED CLINICAL DECISIONS

The following two conceptual case studies illustrate varying, but real, possibilities confronting clinicians in public school, clinic, and hospital settings, urban or rural. Both cases fall into the category of speech delay but display differing speech production and causal correlate characteristics that suggest different intervention approaches. Each illustrates application of various assessment, evaluation, and diagnosis approaches that have evolved from research findings and clinical experiences reported since the 1920s. We invite readers to foster their own critical thinking and consider how their current clinical procedures could contribute to the description and decisions for each case. The cases are reported in a format consistent with the three-part diagnostic framework. A block-reporting form, including a place for summarizing observed speech production data, causal correlate data, and information from the critical data assessment areas, can be created for clinical use (Deputy et al. 1997). Not all categories pertain to a particular case and only germane aspects need to be reported for an individual client. In addition to the summarized assessment data, the reporting form should include space to summarize diagnostic conclusions and treatment implications, listed as a fourth concluding item in the data-assessment section.

The case studies illustrate the many general clinical decisions that emerge from the differential diagnosis process. Some of these decisions include: (1) whether a developmental phonologic disorder is present, (2) the etiologic and associated factors that may be involved with the disorder, (3) whether treatment is indicated, (4) the prognosis for normalization, and (5) what the general nature of treatment should be (e.g., motor, cognitive-linguistic, pragmatic). Given decisions that a developmental phonologic disorder exists and that treatment is warranted, the clinician can make related intervention decisions such as (1) referral recommendations, (2) treatment setting (e.g., clinic, home stimulation, developmental preschool), (3) whether intervention should be direct or indirect, (4) who should be involved, and (5) who should monitor objectives.

There are three major treatment focuses represented in the literature (Deputy and Shine 1994) that illustrate how differential diagnosis and related decisions lead to differences in clinical direction. The three focuses can be identified as production, meaning, and intelligibility. Issues related to production emphasize phonetic-level skills (i.e., learning how to produce segments); integrating new production skills in various syllable and word shapes; and sequencing syllable trains smoothly, accurately, and rapidly (Riley and Riley 1985). A meaning focus relates to using production skills and cognitive-linguistic competence to express meaning through phonemic contrasts. An intelligibility focus emphasizes maintenance of production skills and cognitive-linguistic competence in the context of functional speech acts (i.e., communicative effectiveness). These alternative treatment focuses show how differential diagnosis helps match individual characteristics with specific treatment issues and needs, thus creating efficacious treatment consistent with the current knowledge base. This framework can also accommodate decisions about established approaches, such as cycles (Hodsen and Paden 1991), production training (Crary 1993; Shine 1989) and a phonologic-process approach (Ingram 1989), as well as recent approaches such as nonlinear phonology (Bernhardt and Stoel-Gammon 1994) and metaphonology (Howell and Dean 1995). However, no matter how sophisticated the treatment procedure or approach, psychosocial factors, such as the attitude and behavior of the child, must also be considered (Deputy 1992; Deputy and Shine 1994). No approach is effective when the child is hiding under the table. This framework is comprehensive, facilitating consideration of all child issues, including critical psychosocial observations.

CASE STUDY 1

Sherry is a preschool child who is 4 years and 10 months old. Family, friends, and relatives often have difficulty understanding her. Her oral language reveals multiple articulation and grammatical errors. Other aspects of her oral language also appear delayed. Neurologic soft signs have been observed.

I. Speech production characteristics

A. Segmental data
  1. Independent analysis
    a. *Consonant inventory:* Nearly complete. Missing sounds include palatal fricatives, affricates, and the voiced interdental fricative; few syllable-final fricatives; and no syllable-final liquid /l/.
    b. *Cluster inventory:* Syllable-initial stop + glide and syllable-final nasal + stop.
    c. *Place, manner, and voicing contrasts:* All contrasts present except palatal place for fricatives.
    d. *Vowel and diphthong inventory:* Complete.
  2. Relational analysis
    a. Error summary
      (1) *Consistent misarticulations:* /ʃ, ʒ, ʧ, ʤ, r, ð/
      (2) *Inconsistent misarticulations:* /l, k, t, s, z, v, θ/
      (3) *Accuracy summary* (PCC): PCC = 52%; PCC initial = 74%; PCC final = 47%; PCC singletons = 65%; and PCC clusters = 31%.
    b. Error pattern summary
      (1) *Prevalent feature deficiencies:* Not summarized.
      (2) *Syllable structure processes:* Final consonant deletion (FCD), especially fricatives, and cluster reduction (CR).
      (3) *Substitution processes:* Liquid simplification (LS), stopping of fricatives (S), palatal fronting (PF), backing (B).
      (4) *Assimilation (harmony) processes:* Assimilation (A), especially affecting words with both velar and alveolar targets with inconsistent fronting and backing patterns.
      (5) *Phonetic level errors:* Voicing errors, especially prevocalic voicing. Vowel distortions, particularly neutralization and dipthong reduction.
    c. *Disparity between levels of linguistic complexity:* FCD and phonetic changes occur primarily in continuous speech. Other error patterns occur in both citation forms and continuous speech.

B. Nonsegmental data
  1. Syllabic level observations
    a. *Syllable and word-shape inventory:* Sherry uses a variety of monosyllabic shapes and combines basic syllable shapes to produce both disyllables and multisyllables with expected frequency. Syllable shapes affected primarily by CR and FCD processes.
    b. *Syllable and segment interactions:* Many more errors occur for postvocalic consonants than for prevocalic consonants. Velar and alveolar place features are vulnerable to assimilation when occurring within the same syllable.

2. Global features
    a. *Pitch contours:* Normal.
    b. *Stress:* Normal.
    c. *Rate:* Normal.
    d. *Precision:* No general imprecision.
    e. *Phrasing:* Part- and whole-word repetitions are frequent, appearing in more than half of utterances exceeding five words.

II. Causal correlate characteristics

A. Mechanism data
1. *Speech:* Normal structures and nonspeech functions.
2. *Voice:* Normal.
3. *Hearing:* Two documented instances of transient, mild conductive loss within last 12 months. Two ventilating tube placements, first at age 2 years, 10 months, and again at 4 years, 4 months. Hearing acuity for pure tones is currently within normal limits.
4. *Speech motor:* Difficulty with both horizontal and vertical syllable sequencing tasks.
5. *Neurologic observations:* Gross motor clumsiness; poor balance; toe-walking. Questions about attention-deficit disorder from both neurologic and psychological reports. Father had "speech problems." Fourteen-year-old brother diagnosed with attention deficit–hyperactivity disorder.

B. Cognitive-linguistic data
1. *Cognitive:* A standard IQ score, Kaufman Brief Intelligence Test (K-BIT) = 109 (Kaufman and Kaufman 1990).
2. *Receptive language:* Standard scores. Test of Auditory Comprehension of Language-Revised (TACL-R) = 93 (Carrow-Woolfolk 1985); Preschool Language Scale-3 (PLS-3) Auditory Comprehension = 89 (Zimmerman et al. 1992); Peabody Picture Vocabulary Test–Revised (PPVT-R) = 97 (Dunn and Dunn 1981). Parents are not concerned about Sherry's ability to understand oral language. She follows the teacher's directions in her preschool setting.
3. *Expressive language:* PLS-3 Expressive Communication = 67. Mean length of utterance = 3.8. A speech-language sample analysis indicates many morphology errors. Poor discourse ability suggested by very low rate of contingent responses and topic maintenance, limited narration of personal events, and poor story retelling.
4. *Academic achievement:* Preschool teacher observations indicate normal interest in play objects and activities. No other educational testing has been completed.

C. Psychosocial data

1. *Age:* 4 years, 10 months.
2. *Gender:* Female.
3. *Family dynamics:* Lots of parental attention. Parental concern seems commensurate with child's communication difficulty. Behavior management is positive. Parents encourage talking and provide translation.
4. *Individual behavioral characteristics:* Child seems immature. Outgoing and pleasant; short attention span; impulsive responder; task avoider.

III. Data assessments

A. Intelligibility assessment

1. *Quantitative:* 22% of words in transcribed sample unintelligible or questionable.
2. *Qualitative:* Speech production errors of segment deletions, assimilations, and phonetic-level changes seem especially costly. Parents estimate friends and relatives understand only about half of what Sherry says.
3. *Related causal correlates factors:* Lack of shared conversational focus with a listener. Sherry is frequently "silly" in her interactions, which may be an avoidance behavior.

B. Dynamic assessment

1. Capability
   a. *Error stimulability:* Can correctly produce most erred sounds in imitated citation forms (level IIA–syllables and words). Cannot produce palatal fricatives or affricates (level III).
   b. *Discrimination of erred sounds:* Frequent perceptual confusions between /t/ and /k/ and between /s/ and /ʃ/.
2. Focus
   a. *Attention:* Avoids speech tasks. Often responds by "singing" requested words, wiggling, avoiding eye contact. Likes pretend play that emphasizes meaningful language.
   b. *Motivation and effort:* Does not like to try new speech sounds.
   c. *Self-monitoring:* Rarely self-corrects, even when listener does not understand. Does not modify phonetically given clarification requests.

C. Severity assessment

1. *Quantitative:* PCC of 52% falls at the lower boundary of the moderate-severe range (50–65%).
2. *Qualitative:* Considering causal correlates factors below, her involvement is considered severe.
3. *Related causal correlates factors:* Questionable speech motor skill status and concomitant expressive language delay.

D. Clinical decisions

1. *Diagnostic conclusions:* Sherry has a severe delay in the development of speech with a concomitant delay in expressive language morphology and syntax. Her family history suggests a possible genetic etiology. Her middle-ear history suggests fluctuating hearing levels as a contributing factor. Other causal correlates factors potentially contributing to her speech-language delay include (a) problems with speech-motor coordination, as suggested by evidence such as the persistence of assimilation processes and voicing changes and poor performance on nonmeaningful syllable sequencing tasks; and (b) behavioral characteristics, such as poor attention and avoidance of communication, which may help to maintain her disorder.
2. *Treatment implications:* Sherry should receive direct intervention to decrease her use of error patterns and improve expressive language form. To improve speech-motor ability, nonmeaningful syllable-sequencing tasks are recommended, possibly approached through short intervals of drill interspersed between higher-interest activities. An auditory trainer can be used to increase perception of her error sounds. Given her preference for meaningful speech "play" and her high stimulability for many error sounds, intervention should emphasize contrasting activities to address error patterns most costly to intelligibility (e.g., cluster reduction and assimilation). When accurate production of target words is established, it should be integrated into language context, such as simple stories that emphasize topics of interest to Sherry. Parents should be encouraged to provide frequent auditory models for error sounds during reading activities. In addition, Sherry's "silly" behaviors should be discussed with parents, and they should be encouraged to decrease their communication attempts with Sherry until she is more responsive to them.

CASE STUDY 2

Sam is an elementary-school student who is 6 years and 4 months old. His parents report that he used to be harder to understand than he is presently. He has been in treatment since the middle of his kindergarten year and is now entering the first grade. He is average or above in his academic endeavors. He is beginning to withdraw in new social situations and complains of being teased. His parents have enrolled him in a university speech-language hearing clinic as a supplement to his public school treatment.

I. Speech production characteristics
   A. Segmental data
      1. Independent analysis
         a. *Consonant inventory:* Complete, except for misarticulations of /l/ and /r/.
         b. *Cluster inventory:* Limited to a few productions of specific *s*-clusters.
         c. *Place, manner, and voicing contrasts*: All contrasts present.
         d. *Vowel and diphthong inventory*: Complete except for consistent distortion of rhotic vowel and rhotic (*r*-colored) diphthongs.
      2. Relational analysis
         a. Error summary
            (1) *Consistent misarticulations:* /k, g, n, l, r/ and clusters /st, sk, sw, sl/.
            (2) *Inconsistent misarticulations:* Production of /sp/, /sm/, and /sn/ are inconsistent in continuous speech. Error type inconsistency of /l/ due to occasional j/l substitution, rather than the typical w/l substitution.
            (3) *Accuracy summary* (PCC): PCC 82%.
         b. Error pattern summary
            (1) *Prevalent feature patterns:* Not summarized.
            (2) *Syllable structure processes:* CR.
         c. *Substitution processes:* Fronting (F), LS.
            (1) *Assimilation (harmony) processes*: Not observed.
            (2) *Phonetic level errors:* Not observed unless /r/ and final /l/ distortions are considered phonetic changes.
         d. *Disparity between levels of linguistic complexity:* Misarticulations and error patterns are fairly consistent between linguistic levels ranging from words to continuous speech. There is higher accuracy on /sp/, /sm/, and /sn/ at the word level.
   B. Nonsegmental data
      1. Syllabic integration features
         a. *Syllable and word-shape inventory:* Expected variety of mono- and multisyllabic productions.
         b. *Syllable and segment interactions:* Vowelization of final /l/.
      2. Global features
         a. *Pitch contours:* Normal, except rising affect when frustrated.
         b. *Stress:* Normal.
         c. *Rate:* Normal.
         d. *Precision:* No observed general imprecisions.
         e. *Phrasing:* Normal.
II. Causal correlate characteristics
   A. Mechanism data

1. *Speech:* No structural, functional, or speech motor problems identified.
2. *Voice:* Normal.
3. *Hearing:* Normal.
4. *Speech motor:* No difficulty observed, some trouble integrating level IIA sounds into more complex syllable shapes and new multisyllabic words.
5. *Neurologic observations:* Normal.

B. Cognitive-linguistic data

1. *Cognitive:* Wechsler Intelligence Scale for Children–Revised (WISC-R) (Wechsler 1991) indicates an overall IQ of 120, with verbal IQ of 110.
2. *Receptive language:* Previous screenings have been passed. No observed or reported reason to suspect difficulty in this area.
3. *Expressive language:* Long elaborated sentences in connected speech. Existence of specific language form errors: (a) regular past tense requiring increased phonologic complexity (e.g., from *look* to *looked*), (b) plurals, (c) possessives, (d) pronouns. Talkative and expressive when with family, friends, and familiar adults.
4. *Academic achievement:* Grade level or above performance in all areas.

C. Psychosocial data

1. *Age:* 6 years, 4 months.
2. *Gender:* Male.
3. *Family dynamics:* Parents have expressed worry and anxiety about their son's speech. Discipline, as judged by the clinician, is sometimes inflexible.
4. *Individual behavioral characteristics:* Sam is discouraged and thinks he cannot make sounds. He is starting to become frustrated when asked to repeat words by older children or adults. Although he is not negative, hostile, or manipulative, in reaction to increased teasing he is beginning to withdraw in social situations.

III. Data assessments

A. Intelligibility assessment

1. *Quantitative:* No quantitative measure obtained.
2. *Qualitative:* Intelligibility moderately reduced for specific words and phrases, but overall can be mostly understood with careful listening. Distinctive and noticeable difference in speech.
3. *Related causal correlates factors:* According to parent report, it can be surmised that the child experienced some unintelligibility problems in his preschool years.

B. Dynamic assessment

1. Capability

   a. *Error stimulability:* Can easily produce /t/ and /d/ sounds in imitated citation forms (level IIA–syllables and words). Can easily produce /sp/, /sm/, and /sn/ sounds in imitated citation forms and about 50% of requested spontaneous production (level IIA–syllables and words). Can produce /st/ and /sk/ with salient auditory and graphic visual demonstration (level IIB–syllables). Cannot produce /l/, /r/, or the rhotic vowels and rhotic diphthongs (level III).
   b. *Discrimination of erred sounds:* Specific confusions with w/r, which also show up in reading and writing.
2. Focus
   a. *Attention:* There is a lot of inattention and off-task behavior. Sometimes Sam does not seem to listen in a conversation.
   b. *Motivation and effort:* He is reluctant to try what he considers difficult.
   c. *Self-monitoring:* He seems highly aware of his errors, except for /r/ but does not make an attempt to correct them.

C. Severity assessment
   1. *Quantitative:* PCC 82%, indicating mild severity.
   2. *Qualitative:* The overall judgment is moderate severity given overall perception in the context of his communicative efforts.
   3. *Related causal correlates factors:* Age, frustration, and parental pressure are factors in increasing the perception of severity.

D. Clinical decisions
   1. *Diagnostic conclusions:* Sam has a moderate speech delay with a history of previous unintelligibility. Although he can now mostly be understood by a wide range of listeners, his misarticulations are prominent and noticeable and related to consistent fronting, cluster reduction, and liquid simplification. Specific language form errors are present in his speech; however, the vocabulary, length, complexity, and content of his communications do not suggest a general language problem. His frustration level is increasing, exacerbated by peers who are teasing him and contributing to increased social withdrawal.
   2. *Treatment implications:* Sam's clinical profile suggests initial work with "focus." He needs encouragement that he can learn "clear speech" and strategies to handle teasing from peers. Work with the parents can reassure them about the increased potential for a positive prognosis with understanding, support, and home activities oriented toward success. Since he is stimulable on /k/ and /g/ and specific *s-* clusters, a cognitive-linguistic approach would facilitate generalization to continuous speech activities. A parallel "production"-oriented focus is suggested initially for

errors involving liquid simplification, which should transition into a cognitive-linguistic focus after production of /l/ and /r/ are stabilized. After a contrasting program and use of /k, g, l, r/ and /s, r, l/ clusters in short-play scenarios requiring correct production to effect "meaning," verbal expression activities can facilitate generalization and maintenance of "intelligibility" to continuous speech activities and general conversation.

CONCLUSION

The concept of differential diagnosis has evolved from differentiation of major disorder categories (Darley 1964; Lynch 1978), to differentiation of subgroups (Shriberg and Kwiatkowski 1994), to differentiation of individual characteristics within a specific disorder classification. A differential diagnosis framework accommodates all three viewpoints and offers several clinical advantages over a more typical diagnostic task checklist. Specific advantages can be of service to clients, to clinicians, and to the advancement of our knowledge base. From a client's perspective, a comprehensive assessment framework increases the likelihood that accurate and specific diagnoses will be made and that treatment will be effective and efficient. From a clinician's perspective, the proposed framework can provide a means to align research with clinical practice—that is, as an individual clinician endeavors to apply new research findings and to expand practices based on continuing education experiences. A basic framework provides for principled integration of state-of-the-art clinical practices. From the perspective of professional knowledge, the integration between clinical practice and research contributes to an evolving tapestry that will form the basis of service delivery to children with developmental phonologic disorders in the next century.

Acknowledgments

Both chapter authors contributed equally and should be considered coauthors without any ranking. We wish to thank Dennis Ruscello for his exceptional editing and involvement above and beyond the call of duty.

REFERENCES

Arndt WB, Shelton RL, Johnson AF, Furr ML. (1977) Identification and description of homogeneous subgroups within a sample of misarticulating children. *Journal of Speech and Hearing Research* 20, 263–292.

Bain BA. (1994) A framework for dynamic assessment in phonology: stimulability revisited. *Clinics in Communication Disorders* 4, 12–22.

Bankson NW, Bernthal JE. (1990) *Bankson-Bernthal Test of Phonology (BBTOP)*. Chicago: Riverside.

Bernhardt B, Stoel-Gammon C. (1994) Nonlinear phonology: introduction and clinical application: tutorial. *Journal of Speech and Hearing Research* 37, 123–143.

Bernthal JE, Bankson NW. (1993) *Articulation and Phonological Disorders* (3rd ed). New Jersey: Prentice-Hall.

Bernthal JE, Bankson NW. (1994) *Child Phonology: Characteristics, Assessment, and Intervention with Special Populations*. New York: Thieme.

Bishop DVM, Adams C. (1990) A prospective study of the relationship between specific language impairment, phonological disorders and reading retardation. *Journal of Child Psychology and Psychiatry* 31, 1027–1050.

Bishop DVM, Edmundson A. (1987) Language-impaired 4-year-olds: distinguishing transient from persistent impairment. *Journal of Speech and Hearing Disorders* 52, 156–173.

Blache SE. (1982) Minimal Word Pairs and Distinctive Feature Training. In M Crary (ed), *Phonological Intervention: Concepts and Procedures*. San Diego: PRO-ED.

Blache SE. (1989) A Distinctive Feature Approach. In NA Creaghead, PW Newman, WA Secord (eds), *Articulation and Phonological Disorders* (2nd ed) (pp. 361–382). New York: Macmillan.

Carrow-Woolfolk E. (1985) *Test for Auditory Comprehension of Language-Revised*. Allen, TX: DLM Teaching Resources.

Carter ET, Buck M. (1958) Prognostic testing for functional articulation disorders among children in the first grade. *Journal of Speech and Hearing Disorders* 23, 124–133.

Costello J. (1975) Articulation instruction based on distinctive features theory. *Language, Speech, and Hearing Services in Schools* 6, 61–71.

Costello J, Onstine J. (1976) The modification of multiple articulation errors based on distinctive feature theory. *Journal of Speech and Hearing Disorders* 41, 199–215.

Crary MA. (1993) *Developmental Motor Speech Disorders*. San Diego: Singular.

Creaghead NA, Newman PW, Secord WA. (1989) *Articulation and Phonological Disorders* (2nd ed). New York: Macmillan.

Curtis JF. (1970) The acoustics of nasalized speech. *Cleft Palate Journal* 7, 380–396.

Darley FL. (1964) *Diagnosis and Appraisal of Communication Disorders*. Englewood Cliffs, NJ: Prentice-Hall.

Deputy PN. (1984) The need for description in the study of developmental verbal dyspraxia. *Australian Journal of Human Communication Disorders* 12, 3–13.

Deputy PN. (1992, November) Interactive Component Model of Remediation of Phonologic Disorders. Poster session presented at the meeting of the American Speech-Language-Hearing Association, San Antonio, TX.

Deputy PN, Shine RE. (1994, November) Integrating Treatment Approaches for Phonologic/Articulatory Problems and Disorders. Short course presented at the meeting of the American Speech-Language-Hearing Association, New Orleans.

Deputy PN, Nakasone H, Tosi O. (1982) Analysis of pauses occurring in the speech of children with consistent misarticulations. *Journal of Communication Disorders* 15, 43–54.

Deputy PN, Weston A, Ruscello DM. (1997, November) Using a Framework for Differential Diagnosis of Developmental Phonological Disorders. Short course presented at the meeting of the American Speech-Language-Hearing Association, Boston.

Diedrich WM. (1983) Stimulability and articulation disorders. *Seminars in Speech and Language* 4, 297–311.

Dinnsen DA, Elbert M. (1984) On the Relationship Between Phonology and Learning. In M Elbert, DA Dinnsen, G Weismer (eds), *Phonological Theory and the Misarticulating Child* (ASHA Monograph No. 22). Rockville, MD: American Speech-Language-Hearing Association.

Dodd B. (1995) *Differential Diagnosis and Treatment of Children with Speech Disorders.* San Diego: Singular.

DuBois E, Bernthal J. (1978) A comparison of three methods for obtaining articulatory responses. *Journal of Speech and Hearing Disorders* 43, 205–305.

Dunn LM, Dunn LM. (1981) *Peabody Picture Vocabulary Test-Revised.* Circle Pines, MI: American Guidance Service.

Dworkin JP, Culatta RA. (1980) *Dworkin-Culatta Oral Mechanism Examination.* Nicholasville, KY: Edgewood Press.

Elbert M, Gierut J. (1986) *Handbook of Clinical Phonology: Approaches to Assessment and Treatment.* Austin, TX: PRO-ED.

Felsenfeld S, McGue M, Broen PA. (1995) Familial aggregation of phonological disorders: results from a 28-year follow-up. *Journal of Speech and Hearing Research* 38, 1091–1107.

Ferguson C, Macken M. (1983) The Role of Play in Phonological Development. In K Nelson (ed), *Child Language IV* (pp. 256–282). Hillsdale, NJ: Lawrence Erlbaum.

Fey ME, Cleave PL, Ravida AI, et al. (1994) Effects of grammar facilitation on the phonological performance of children with speech and language impairments. *Journal of Speech and Hearing Research* 37, 594–607.

Gordon-Brannan M. (1994) Assessing intelligibility: children's expressive phonologies. *Topics in Language Disorders* 14, 17–25.

Guyette T, Dietrick W. (1981) A Critical Review of Developmental Apraxia of Speech. In N Lass (ed), *Speech and Language: Advances in Basic Research and Practice* (Vol. 5, pp. 1–49). New York: Academic Press.

Hall PK. (1994) The Oral Mechanism. In JB Tomblin, HL Morris, DC Spriestersbach (eds), *Diagnosis in Speech-Language Pathology* (pp. 67–98). San Diego: Singular.

Hall PK, Jordan LS, Robin DA. (1993) *Developmental Apraxia of Speech: Theory and Clinical Practice.* Austin, TX: PRO-ED.

Hargrove PM, McGarr NS. (1994) *Prosody Management of Communication Disorders.* San Diego: Singular.

Hayden DA. (1994) Differential diagnosis of motor speech dysfunction in children. *Clinics in Communication Disorders* 4, 119–141.

Hodge M. (1996, February) Speech Intelligibility Measures of Young Children with Dysarthria. Paper presented at the Eighth Biennial Conference on Motor Speech, Amelia Island, FL.

Hodge M, Hancock H. (1994) Assessment of developmental apraxia of speech: a procedure. *Clinics in Communication Disorders* 4, 102–108.

Hodson BW. (1986) *The Assessment of Phonological Processes–Revised.* Austin, TX: PRO-ED.

Hodson BW, Paden EP. (1981) Phonological processes which characterize unintelligible and intelligible speech in early childhood. *Journal of Speech and Hearing Disorders* 46, 369–373.

Hodson BW, Paden EP. (1991) *Targeting Intelligible Speech* (2nd ed). Austin, TX: PRO-ED.

Hoffman PR, Norris JA, Monjure J. (1990) Comparison of process targeting and whole language treatments for phonologically delayed preschool children. *Language, Speech, and Hearing Services in Schools* 21, 102–109.

Howell J, Dean E. (1995) *Treating Phonological Disorders in Children: Metaphon-Theory to Practice* (2nd ed). London: Whurr Publishers.

Ingram D. (1981) *Procedures for the Phonological Analysis of Children's Language.* Austin, TX: PRO-ED.

Ingram D. (1989) *Phonological Disability in Children.* Jersey City: Whurr Publishers.

Ingram D. (1997) The Categorization of Phonological Impairment. In BW Hodson, ML Edwards (eds), *Perspectives in Applied Phonology* (pp. 19–41). Gaithersburg, MD: Aspen.

Johnson JP, Winney BL, Pederson OT. (1980) Single word versus connected speech articulation testing. *Language, Speech, and Hearing Services in Schools* 11, 175–179.

Kaufman AS, Kaufman NL. (1990) *Kaufman Brief Intelligence Test.* Circle Pines, MI: American Guidance Service.

Kelso JAS, Munhal KG. (1988) *R.H. Stetson's Motor Phonetics: A Retrospective Edition.* Boston: Little, Brown.

Kent RD. (1992) Speech Intelligibility and Communicative Competence in Children. In AP Kaiser, DB Gray (eds), *Enhancing Children's Communication: Research Foundations for Intervention* (Vol. 2, pp. 223–239). Baltimore: Brookes Publishing Co.

Kent RD, Miolo G, Bloedel S. (1994) The intelligibility of children's speech: a review of evaluation procedures. *American Journal of Speech-Language Pathology* 3, 81–93.

Kwiatkowski J, Shriberg LD. (1993) Speech normalization in developmental phonological disorders: a retrospective study of capability-focus theory. *Language, Speech, and Hearing Services in Schools* 24, 10–18.

Locke JL. (1980a) The inference of speech perception in the phonologically disordered child. Part I: a rationale, some criteria, the conventional tests. *Journal of Speech and Hearing Disorders* 45, 431–444.

Locke JL. (1980b) The inference of speech perception in the phonologically disordered child. Part II: some clinically novel procedures, their use, some findings. *Journal of Speech and Hearing Disorders* 45, 445–468.

Lowe RJ. (1994) *Phonology: Assessment and Intervention Applications in Speech Pathology.* Baltimore: Williams & Wilkins.

Lynch J. (1978) Evaluation of Linguistic Disorders in Children. In S Sing, J Lynch (eds), *Diagnostic Procedures in Hearing, Speech, and Language* (pp. 327–378). Baltimore: University Park Press.

Madison CL. (1979) Articulatory stimulability reviewed. *Language, Speech, and Hearing Services in the Schools* 10, 185–190.

Masterson J, Pagan F. (1993) *Interactive System for Phonological Analysis.* San Antonio: Psychological Corporation.

McDonald E. (1964) *Articulation Testing and Treatment: A Sensory Motor Approach.* Pittsburgh: Stanwix House.

McNutt JC, Hamayan E. (1984) Subgroups of Older Children with Articulation Disorders. In RG Daniloff (ed), *Articulation Assessment & Treatment Issues* (pp. 51–70). San Diego: College-Hill Press.

McReynolds LV, Engmann DL. (1975) *Distinctive Feature Analysis of Misarticulations*. Baltimore: University Park Press.

Meitus IJ, Weinberg B. (1983) *Diagnosis in Speech-Language Pathology*. Baltimore: University Park Press.

Milisen R. (1954) A rationale for articulation disorders. *Journal of Speech and Hearing Disorders Monograph Supplement 4*.

Minick N. (1987) Implications of Vygotsky's Theories for Dynamic Assessment. In C Lidz (ed), *Dynamic Assessment: An Interactional Approach to Evaluating Learning Potential* (pp. 116–140). New York: Guilford Press.

Monsen RB, Moog JB, Geers AE. (1988) *CID Picture SPINE*. St. Louis: Central Institute for the Deaf.

Morris SR, Wilcox KA, Schooling TL. (1995) The Preschool Speech Intelligibility Measure. *American Journal of Speech-Language Pathology* 4, 22–28.

Morrison JA, Shriberg LD. (1992) Articulation testing versus conversational speech sampling. *Journal of Speech and Hearing Research* 35, 259–273.

Nation JE, Aram DM. (1984) *Diagnosis of Speech and Language Disorders* (2nd ed). San Diego: College-Hill Press.

Parsons CL, Crary MA. (1984) Developmental verbal dyspraxia [special issue]. *Australian Journal of Human Communication Disorders* 12.

Paul R, Shriberg LD. (1982) Associations between phonology and syntax in speech-delayed children. *Journal of Speech and Hearing Research* 25, 536–546.

Pendergast K, Dickey ST, Selmar J, Soder A. (1984) *Photo Articulation Test*. Austin, TX: PRO-ED.

Pollock KE. (1991) The identification of vowel errors using traditional articulation or phonological process test stimuli. *Language, Speech, and Hearing Services in Schools* 22, 39–50.

Powell TW, Elbert N, Dinnsen DA. (1991) Stimulability as a factor in the phonological generalization of a factor in the phonological generalization of misarticulating preschool children. *Journal of Speech and Hearing Research* 34, 1318–1328.

Richardson S. (1983) Differential diagnosis in phonological disorders. *Folia Phoniatrica* 35, 66–80.

Riley G, Riley J. (1985) *Oral Motor Assessment and Treatment: Improving Syllable Production*. Austin, TX: PRO-ED.

Robbins J, Klee T. (1987) Clinical assessment of oropharyngeal motor development in young children. *Journal of Speech and Hearing Disorders* 52, 271–277.

Roberts JE, Clark-Klein S. (1994) Otitis Media. In JE Bernthal, NW Bankson (eds), *Child Phonology: Characteristics, Assessment, and Intervention with Special Populations* (pp. 182–198). New York: Thieme.

Schmitt LS, Howard BH, Schmitt JF. (1983) Conversational speech sampling in the assessment of articulatory proficiency. *Language, Speech, and Hearing Services in Schools* 14, 210–214.

Shine RE. (1989) Articulatory Production Training: A Sensory-Motor Approach. In NA Creaghead, PW Newman, WA Secord (eds), *Articulation and Phonological Disorders* (2nd ed) (pp. 335–358). New York: Macmillan.

Shriberg LD. (1986) *Programs to Examine Phonetic and Phonologic Evaluation Records (PEPPER)*. Hillsdale, NJ: Lawrence Erlbaum.

Shriberg LD. (1994) Five subtypes of developmental phonological disorders. *Clinics in Communication Disorders* 4, 38–53.

Shriberg LD. (1997) Developmental Phonological Disorders: One or Many? In BW Hodson, ML Edwards (eds), *Perspectives in Applied Phonology* (pp. 105–131). Gaithersburg, MD: Aspen.

Shriberg LD, Kent RD. (1995) *Clinical Phonetics* (2nd ed). Boston: Allyn & Bacon.

Shriberg LD, Kwiatkowski J. (1980) *Natural Process Analysis*. New York: Wiley.

Shriberg LD, Kwiatkowski J. (1982a) Phonological disorders I: a diagnostic classification system. *Journal of Speech and Hearing Disorders* 47, 226–241.

Shriberg LD, Kwiatkowski J. (1982b) Phonological disorders III: a procedure for assessing severity of involvement. *Journal of Speech and Hearing Disorders* 47, 256–270.

Shriberg LD, Kwiatkowski J. (1988) A follow-up study of children with phonologic disorders of unknown origin. *Journal of Speech and Hearing Disorders* 53, 144–155.

Shriberg LD, Kwiatkowski J. (1994) Developmental phonological disorders I: a clinical profile. *Journal of Speech and Hearing Research* 37, 1100–1126.

Shriberg LD, Aram DM, Kwiatkowski J. (1997b) Developmental apraxia of speech: II. Toward a diagnostic marker. *Journal of Speech, Language, and Hearing Research* 40, 286–312.

Shriberg LD, Austin D, Lewis BA, et al. (1997a) The Percentage of Consonants Correct (PCC) metric: extensions and reliability data. *Journal of Speech, Language, and Hearing Research* 40, 708–722.

Shriberg LD, Gruber FA, Kwiatkowski J. (1994b) Developmental phonological disorders III: long-term speech-sound normalization. *Journal of Speech and Hearing Research* 37, 1151–1177.

Shriberg LD, Kwiatkowski J, Gruber FA. (1994a) Developmental phonological disorders II: short-term speech-sound normalization. *Journal of Speech and Hearing Research* 37, 1127–1150.

Shriberg LD, Kwiatkowski J, Rasmussen C. (1990) *The Prosody-Voice Screening Profile*. Tucson, AZ: Communication Skill Builders.

Shriberg LD, Kwiatkowski J, Rasmussen C, et al. (1992) *The Prosody-Voice Screening Profile (PVSP): Psychometric Data and Reference Information for Children* (Tech. Rep. No. 1). Tucson, AZ: Communication Skill Builders.

Shriberg LD, Smith AJ. (1983) Phonological correlates of middle-ear involvement in speech-delayed children: a methodological note. *Journal of Speech and Hearing Research* 26, 283–296.

Singh S, Polen S. (1972) The use of a distinctive feature model in speech pathology. *Acta Symbolica* 3, 17–25.

Smit AB. (1994) Speech Sound Disorders. In JB Tomblin, HL Morris, DC Spriestersbach (eds), *Diagnosis in Speech-Language Pathology* (pp. 179–199). San Diego: Singular.

Smit AB, Hand L, Freilinger JJ, et al. (1990) The Iowa articulation norms project and its Nebraska replication. *Journal of Speech and Hearing Disorders* 55, 779–798.

St. Louis KO, Ruscello DM. (1987) *Oral Speech Mechanism Screening Examination, Revised*. Austin, TX: PRO-ED.

Stampe D. (1969) The acquisition of phonetic representation. Papers from the Fifth Regional meeting of the Chicago Linguistic Society 433–444.

Stampe D. (1973) A dissertation on natural phonology. Ph.D. diss., University of Chicago.

Stoel-Gammon C, Dunn C. (1985) *Normal and Disordered Phonology in Children*. Austin, TX: PRO-ED.

Stoel-Gammon C, Stone JR. (1991) Assessing phonology in young children. *Clinics in Communication Disorders* 1, 25–39.

Trost-Cardamone JD, Bernthal JE. (1993) Articulation Assessment Procedures and Treatment Decisions. In KT Moller, CD Starr (eds), *Cleft Palate: Interdisciplinary Issues and Treatment* (pp. 307–336). Austin, TX: PRO-ED.

Tyler AA, Sandoval KT. (1994) Preschoolers with phonological and language disorders: treating different linguistic domains. *Language, Speech, and Hearing Services in Schools* 25, 215–234.

Tyler AA, Watterson KH. (1991) Effects of phonological versus language intervention in preschoolers with both phonological and language impairment. *Child Language Teaching and Therapy* 7, 141–160.

Velleman SL, Strand K. (1994) Developmental Verbal Apraxia. In JE Bernthal, NW Bankson (eds), *Child Phonology: Characteristics, Assessment, and Intervention with Special Populations* (pp. 110–139). New York: Thieme.

Wechsler D. (1991) *Wechsler Intelligence Scale for Children* (3rd ed). San Antonio, TX: The Psychological Corp.

Weiss AL. (1995) Conversational demands and their effects on fluency and stuttering. *Topics in Language Disorders* 15, 18–31.

Weston AD, Shriberg LD. (1992) Contextual and linguistic correlates of intelligibility in children with developmental phonological disorders. *Journal of Speech and Hearing Research* 35, 1136–1332.

Weston AD, Shriberg LD, Miller JF. (1989) Analysis of language-speech samples with SALT and PEPPER. *Journal of Speech and Hearing Research* 32, 755–766.

Whitehurst GJ, Fischel JE. (1994) Practitioner review: early developmental language delay: what, if anything, should the clinician do about it? *Journal of Child Psychology and Psychiatry* 35, 613–648.

Yorkston KM, Strand EA, Kennedy MRT. (1996) Comprehensibility of dysarthric speech: implications for assessment and treatment planning. *American Journal of Speech-Language Pathology* 5, 55–66.

Zimmerman IL, Steiner VG, Pond RE. (1992) *Preschool Language Scale-3*. San Antonio, TX: The Psychological Corp.

6

Differential Diagnosis for Fluency Disorders

Gordon W. Blood

This chapter is concerned with disturbances in fluency. For most individuals, disruptions in speech and the accompanying temporary loss of control are an infrequent nuisance or temporary source of embarrassment. For other individuals who live with chronic fluency disturbances, the disturbance can pervade every aspect of their lives and become a disabling handicap. Fluency disorders are disturbances of both perception and production. They occur in children, adolescents, and adults and can be developmental or acquired. Fluency disorders can lead to changes in overt speech behaviors, attitudes, and feelings about general communication, and expectations about self. Fluency disorders affect the quality of an individual's life. Often they are related to the listener's perceptions, self-perceptions, expectations, and judgments of "loss of control." Individuals with fluency disorders show great variability. Some persons manifest severe disfluencies characterized by complete blockages of the airstream and respiratory distress. Other individuals with fluency disorders manifest few overt speech changes while living a life of constant guilt, fear, and vigilance in anticipation of a fluency breakdown or failure.

Fluency is not a binary entity. A critical concept in the assessment of fluency disorders is the notion of a "fluency continuum." This idea stresses the blending of fluent and disfluent speech. On one end of the continuum is very fluent speech, characterized by no breaks or disintegration in the forward movement of speech. The other endpoint of the fluency continuum is very disfluent speech, marked by the presence of multiple breaks and severe disintegration in the forward movement of speech. For most of the population, their place on the fluency continuum remains relatively stable over the life span. Changes on the continuum can accompany high emotional occurrences, neurologic disease and disorders, psychological disturbances, the use of medications, or transitional periods in development. Borden (1990) explained a subtyping system for adults who stutter using a two-tiered continuum system. She suggested that the first tier contained the "core behaviors," or the neurophysiologic events associated with stuttering. The second tier included the "reactive components" of the disorder. The core behavior was associated with the events necessary for stuttering to occur. She asserted that as researchers and practitioners peel away more and more of the "reactive" and learned behaviors, they will probably move higher up in the nervous system to interactions among the neurophysiologic components of phonation. Her subtyping is based on a continuum system and is important for the diagnosis of stuttering. Subtyping or subgrouping provides information about the coping strategies that people use to deal with fluency disorders.

Differential diagnosis in the area of fluency disorders rests on definitions of stuttering and cluttering and the classification (subtyping) of individuals with fluency disorders. Distinguishing subtypes of individuals with fluency disorders is a complex task. The literature supports the overt and covert features of the disorder, clonic and tonic subgroups, and interiorized and exteriorized individuals who stutter (Bloodstein 1995; Douglas and Quarrington 1952; Van Riper 1982). St. Onge (1963) described organic, psychogenic, and speech phobic subgroups in persons who stutter, while Preus (1981) reported on the heterogeneity and subgroups of individuals with different types of stuttering. Kidd and colleagues (1978) proposed that subgroups of individuals who stutter could be formed on the basis of genetic factors. Other authors have suggested that certain anatomic sites (e.g., laryngeal area, supplementary motor area) be used to classify individuals who stutter or manifest fluency disorders (Caruso et al. 1987; Conture et al. 1977; Starkweather 1987). Blood (1988) suggested subtypes of individuals who stutter based on the results of cerebral dominance testing, while Watson and Alfonso (1987) encouraged the use of severity of stuttering for subtyping. Yairi (1990) indicated that groups could be established based on a network of factors, including gender, age at onset, and dominant overt symptom. Suspected etiology of fluency disorders has also been used to subtype individuals displaying disfluencies. Three classifications include idiopathic, neurogenic, and psychogenic.

Approximately 3 million Americans, or about 1% of the population, are described as individuals who stutter (Starkweather and Givens-Ackerman 1997). Their position on the fluency continuum tends to be marked by variable cycles of disfluent periods. Stuttering includes (1) the motor behaviors associated with fluent and disfluent speech, (2) the antecedents and consequences of the disfluent speech, (3) any accompanying emotional responses to the disorder, and (4) belief systems developed as a result of the disorder. Therefore, the evaluation of stuttering and other fluency disorders should include four components: (1) the speech behavior, (2) the emotional disturbance observed in physiologic responses, (3) negative or ambivalent beliefs about stuttering, and (4) perceived loss of control (Blood 1993a, 1995a; Perkins et al. 1991; Van Riper and Emerick 1984). The protocol described in this chapter is appropriate for adolescents and adults and is designed to provide a comprehensive assessment for individuals with fluency disorders.

It should be noted that a number of excellent summaries and tutorials have been published about differential diagnosis in children who stutter. A great deal of the research in stuttering and fluency disorders is devoted to prevention and treatment of stuttering in children. Numerous books have identified protocols for distinguishing children who stutter from children who do not stutter (Conture 1990; Ham 1986, 1990; Starkweather et al. 1990; Wall and Myers 1995). In addition, numerous articles and programs have been published for differentiating incipient stuttering behaviors from normal nonfluencies. The literature also includes summaries of case strategy selections for children with fluency disorders based on differential diagnosis and developmental differences between children who stutter and children who do not stutter (Adams 1977, 1980; Blood 1988; Bloodstein 1960; Cooper 1982; Cooper and Cooper 1985; Curlee 1980; Gregory and Hill 1984; Pindzola and White 1987; Riley 1980; Van Riper 1982; Yairi and Ambrose 1992a, b). Six commonly used protocols for differentiating normal disfluencies from stuttering disfluencies have been compared and contrasted (Gordon and Luper 1992a, b). A detailed discussion of the general format, criteria, clinical data-collection procedures, documentation, and use of quantification was provided. Researchers and practitioners are referred to these reviews, as well as the excellent sources previously mentioned, to supplement differential diagnosis of fluency disorders in preschool and school-age children.

NEED FOR DIFFERENTIAL ASSESSMENT OF FLUENCY DISORDERS IN ADOLESCENTS AND ADULTS

Stuttering is an interesting disorder in terms of assessment. Some aspects of the disorder, such as identification of noticeable disfluent behaviors, dramatic stuttering moments, or obvious physical characteristics timed with the moment of stuttering, are relatively straightforward in terms of analysis. Other features of the diagnosis, however, are much more complex. For example, some disfluencies are associated with certain neurologic disorders and progressive diseases (Brown and Cullinan 1981; Duffy 1995). At other times, disfluencies can occur as the result of stage fright, severe communication phobias, or after serious emotional trauma (Deal 1982). Fluency disorders can be associated with certain developmental stages and the demands on individuals in relationship to their present physical, emotional, cognitive, and linguistic capacities (Culatta and Leeper 1988). Stuttering can sometimes be confused with cluttering.

Cluttering has been defined as a "speech disorder characterized by the individual's unawareness of their disorder, short attention span, disturbances in perception, articulation, and formulation of speech accompanied by an excessive speed of delivery ... a verbal manifestation of Central Language Imbalance" (Weiss 1964, p. 1). Daly (1981) reported that less than 5% of subjects examined were individuals with the clinical disorder of pure cluttering, while 55% were diagnosed as individuals with pure stuttering, and more than 40% were diagnosed as having cluttering-stuttering symptoms. Cluttering can sometimes be mistaken for stuttering, or, if differential diagnosis of fluency disorders is not completed, cluttering can masquerade as part of a central auditory or language-processing disorder.

The assessment of fluency disorders, specifically stuttering, becomes more challenging because of the episodic and cyclical nature of the problem. Although there are numerous theories posited about the etiology and maintenance of the disorder, no single theory provides a full explanation for stuttering. Consequently, assessment must include an examination of the potential influences of a number of factors.

This chapter presents guidelines for the differential diagnosis of fluency disorders. The goals of the assessment are (1) to identify the fluency disorder and (2) to determine the relative influence of behavioral, physiological, social, attitudinal, and emotional factors in the development, acquisition, and maintenance of the disorder.

POTENTIAL DIAGNOSES

To make a differential diagnosis in fluency disorders, the clinician must examine several factors. This factorial model for differential diagnosis is presented in Table 6.1. This model assumes that cluttering and stuttering frequently overlap and often can be observed in the same person. It also assumes that just because a rare psychogenic fluency disturbance is identified, neurogenic components cannot be eliminated

Table 6.1
Multifactorial model for differential diagnoses of fluency disorders

Factors	*Stuttering*	*Cluttering*	*Neurologic or Cortical*	*Psychological Disorder or Trauma*
Etiology	Idiopathic	Frequently associated with inherited conditions Organic	Bilateral, diffuse, or multifocal lesion sites (e.g., left hemisphere, basal ganglia)	Emotional or personality problems; may show an attitude of incongruous lack of concern, in contrast with the severity of the impairment
Factor 1: History				
1. Onset	Gradual; 24–48 mos	No specific onset, usually in childhood or adulthood	Sudden (stroke) Gradual (extrapyramidal disease) Usually adults	Sudden, severe symptoms in adolescents or adults
2. Family history	Significant subgroup	Significant subgroup	No	No
3. Childhood history	Yes	Yes, depending on age at onset	No	No
4. Duration of the disorder	Persistent after 12 yrs of age	Persistent	Persistent or transient (few days)	Persistent or transient
5. Medical history of psychogenic episodes, depression, etc.	No	No	Possible, not common	Yes
6. Medication usage (theophylline, antidepressant, antiseizure)	No	No	Yes	Yes

Table 6.1
Continued

Factors	*Stuttering*	*Cluttering*	*Neurologic or Cortical*	*Psychological Disorder or Trauma*
Factor 2: Stuttering and nonstuttering behaviors				
1. Rate of speech	Reduced because of disfluencies or rapid rate part-word repetitions	Tachylalia (rapid rate of delivery)	Palilalia (rapid repetition of whole words)	Slow rate
2. Concomitant accessory behaviors	Yes	No	Depending on duration	Usually none
3. Locus of disfluencies	Initial phonemes	Initial phonemes	Initial and medial phonemes	Initial phonemes or stressed syllable, often severe
4. Adaptation effect	Yes	No; may observe increase in disfluencies	No (stroke) Yes (extrapyramidal)	Sometimes
5. Disfluencies	Part-word repetitions Tense pauses Dysrhythmic phonations	Part-word, word, and phrase repetitions Interjections Revisions	Word repetitions Interjections Revisions	Part-word repetitions of the initial, stressed syllable Unvoiced prolongations Tense pauses
6. Difficulty initiating speech	Yes	Random Difficulty throughout utterances	Yes, may have difficulty throughout utterances	Yes, even automatic speech is stuttered

Factor 3: Client's level of awareness				
1. Awareness of disfluencies	Yes	No	Yes, but without significant anxiety	Yes
2. Avoidance behaviors	Yes	No	Yes	No avoidance No attempt to inhibit stuttering
3. Speaking under communicative stress	Worsens speech	Improves speech	Worsens speech	Patterns of speech not affected by different speaking situations
Factor 4: Concomitant problems				
1. Speech, language, writing, and reading	Sometimes	Distortions in articulation Linguistic problems Attention-span disorders	Sequelae to insult, language,writing, apraxia, dysarthrias, aphasia, etc.	Possible, not common
2. Academic difficulties	No	Yes, language-dependent skills	No	Possible, not common
3. Reduced general motor coordination	No	Yes	Associated with lesions, aphasia, seizure disorders	No
Factor 5: Previous facilitating techniques and treatments				
1. Treatments	Fluency enhancement techniques Delayed auditory feedback Conventional speech therapy	Client awareness Motor speech analysis Delayed auditory feedback worsens speech Auditory processing skills (Daly 1993;	Pacing boards Self-monitoring Delayed auditory feedback Biofeedback and relaxation Pharmacological treatment (Brady 1991; Helm 1979;	Psychotherapy Conventional speech therapy (i.e., modifying stuttering block by means of easy onset of voice)

Table 6.1
Continued

Factors	*Stuttering*	*Cluttering*	*Neurologic or Cortical*	*Psychological Disorder or Trauma*
	(i.e., modifying stuttering block by means of easy on-set of voice, light contacts, etc.) Counseling techniques Desensitization techniques Cognitive-behavioral techniques Pharmacological techniques (Bloodstein 1995; Brady 1991; Ham 1986; Ingham 1984; Van Riper 1982)	Myers and St. Louis 1992; St. Louis et al. 1985)	Helm-Estabrooks 1986; Rosenbeck et al 1978; Whitney and Goldstein 1989)	Spontaneous recovery Delayed auditory feedback, singing, and choral reading worsens speech (Mahr and Leith 1992; Roth et al. 1989)

as a part of the problem. Finally, the model has assumed an idiopathic etiology for a "typical stuttering disorder." Experienced clinicians are aware that certain histories, onsets, behaviors, disfluencies (e.g., part-word repetitions, dysrhythmic phonations and tense pauses, and prolongations), attitudes, and treatment responses can help to differentiate among a large group of people who have fluency disorders. No two people who stutter are exactly alike. Skilled clinicians use the data collected during the diagnostic to direct their questions to develop a complete picture of the individual with a fluency disorder.

Identifying the Overt Speech Problem

The first step in the diagnostic process is to identify the overt speech problem augmented with a detailed description of behaviors. This is followed by a broad set of scales measuring attitudes and cognitions held by the client with a fluency disorder. Much of this information can be acquired (1) during a precise diagnostic interview, (2) from detailed observations, (3) in responses to self-report measures, and (4) as information from other professionals working with the client.

The first factor that can be examined in the model requires information about history. This includes information about the onset of stuttering; duration of the disorder; and family, childhood, and medical history. At the next level, the stuttering and nonstuttering behaviors must be evaluated. These behaviors include rate of speech, locus of disfluencies, adaptation effect, types of disfluencies, concomitant accessory behaviors, and difficulties initiating speech. The third level deals with the client's level of awareness of the disorder, which is composed of awareness of disfluencies, avoidance behaviors, and the effects of speaking under communicative stress. The fourth factor is associated with concomitant problems in speech, language, reading, central processing, and academics and reduced general motor coordination. A final factor examines the effects of previous and current treatment options. Information about these five factors significantly impacts diagnosis and treatment. Examination of Table 6.1 shows the difficulty of differential diagnosis in the area of fluency disorders. It is common for clients to display a variety of responses that cut across a number of diagnostic categories. Sometimes this makes assignment to a distinct category (i.e., stuttering, cluttering, neurologic or cortical disorder, psychological disorder, or trauma) difficult. It is also possible to display a stuttering disorder of idiopathic origin and still have other psychological problems. The stuttering may not be part of the depressive condition but may contribute to the client's overall negative state of well-being. All of these factors and topics should be addressed during the assessment of individuals who present fluency disorders. The clinician should have enough information from this type of assessment to determine the severity of the fluency problem; the presence of a significant distortion in attitudes or beliefs about fluency disorders; the effects of communicative stress on the problem; the relationship of family histories to the fluency disorders; and directions about idiopathic, psychogenic or neurologic etiologies.

Diagnostic Interview

The purpose of diagnosis is to identify the presence of the problem and then discover what variables contribute to the maintenance or exacerbation of symptoms. The interview is part of the diagnostic process in which an individual is assigned to a classification on the fluency continuum. The interview should provide data for the initial determination of the problem. The questions asked by the clinician should continue to specify different target behaviors, a group of symptoms, and situations associated with the fluency disorder. This process leads to testing a number of hypotheses on which treatment decisions will be based.

Procedures for Gathering Information

After demographic data are obtained, a structured interview using direct questions should be employed. Initially, the interview will help to identify symptoms. A number of useful protocols have been developed (Conture 1990; Cooper and Cooper 1985; Ryan 1974). If time permits, a semi-structured interview can also be incorporated using open-ended questions. This allows greater flexibility, and experienced clinicians can follow the client's clues. The experienced clinician seeks to determine which symptoms or problems covary with the fluency disorder. A series of direct follow-up questions then helps to test the clinician's hypothesis. This format results in identifying social, psychological, and environmental variables associated with the disfluencies. The structured interview has a number of appealing features. These include efficiency, covering a list of specific content areas, and developing a framework for treatment.

Obtaining the Diagnostic Information: A Diagnostic Interview Ladder

Differential diagnosis requires the clinician to compare the results of his or her assessment to the symptoms of the client to make an appropriate diagnosis. Although there are numerous protocols and hundreds of questions that could be asked to discover relevant information about the fluency disorder, the diagnostic interview ladder is composed of eight rungs that assess general topic areas. These areas are intentionally broad to give the clinician flexibility for further investigation based on a client's individual needs and time constraints. Initially, the clinician allows the client time to describe the problem in his or her own words. The clinician then needs to direct a series of questions to the client in eight areas: reason for referral; definition and presenting complaint; client's perception of the problem; onset, development, and progression of the disorder; medical history; interpersonal and social history; educational and vocational history; and concomitant speech and other problems (Figure 6.1).

The first rung on the diagnostic interview ladder is to determine the referral source. This information can provide directions for other questions during the interview. The information provided by a neurologist, other speech-language pathologist, parent, teacher, psychologist, or client can have implications for the diagnosis. For example, the adult who was referred by a neurologist and has a history of sudden onset of disfluency following a cerebral vascular accident (Brookshire 1989) would be evaluated differently from an adolescent who has a history of a gradual onset and concomitant phonologic disorder and is showing signs of tension and prolongations.

The second step deals with the nature of the presenting complaint by the client. To rule out other problems and correctly identify the fluency disorder and the influencing factors, it is important that the clinician thoroughly understand what the client is saying. Issues surrounding the present symptoms, severity, types of disfluencies, and rate of speech are addressed. The clinician needs to allow the client to explain the disorder in his or her words. It is important at this time to clarify any diagnostic labels or words that the client uses. It is also important that the clinician use this part of the interview to establish a baseline of the client's knowledge about fluency disturbances and the symptoms. It is usually beneficial to explain the model for assessment to the client. Clients should be aware that fluency disturbances are multidimensional problems that require the conduction of at least a four-stage assessment of speech behavior, attitudes and beliefs about stuttering, emotional responses and feelings about stuttering, and perceived loss of control.

The third rung deals with self-identification and self-perceptions about fluency and fluency disruptions. Awareness is a critical diagnostic feature for classifying persons who stutter from persons who clutter. When evaluating adults who stutter, self-perception needs to be

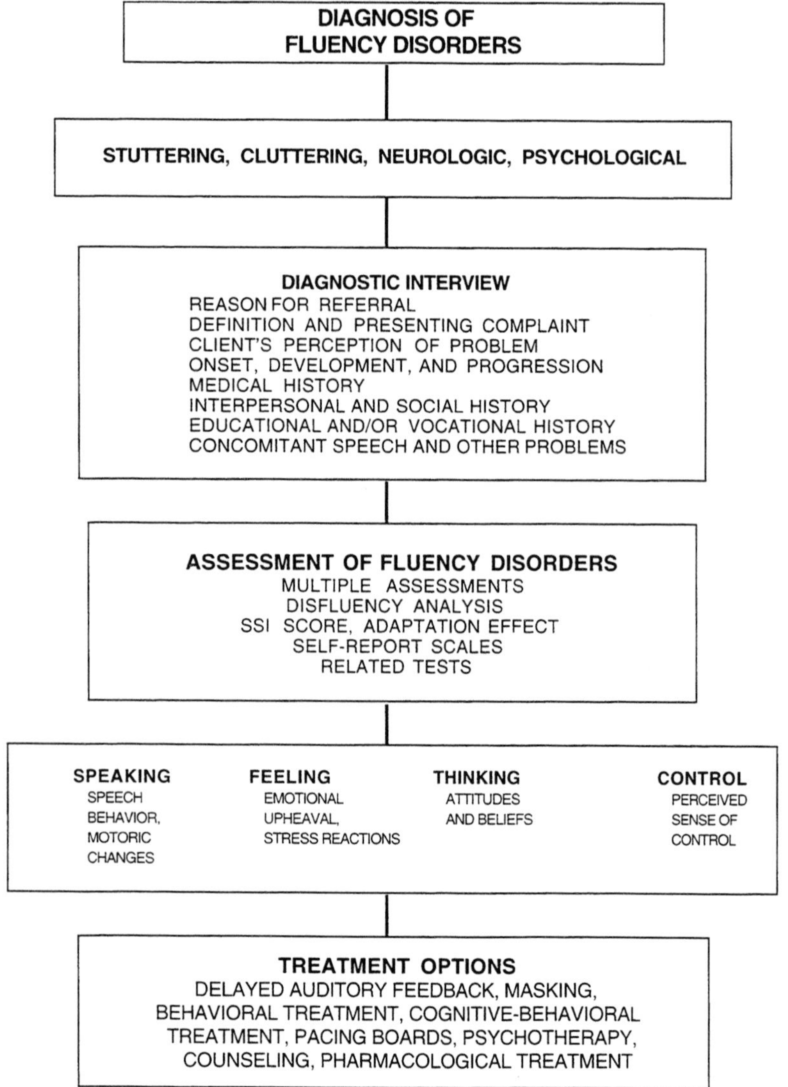

Figure 6.1 An overview of a protocol for interview questions and assessment techniques for fluency disorders. (SSI = Stuttering Severity Instrument.)

compared with clinicians' perceptions of the disorder. Perception of the disorder in terms of chronicity, attribution, etiology, and usefulness of treatment should be explored. Clients' perceptions about the degree of secondary struggle and avoidance also need to be assessed.

The next step is to assess the development and progression of the disorder. Inquiries should be made about the onset of the disorder, past severity of the disorder, detailed progression of the disorder, relapses and remissions, and present status.

The fifth rung on the diagnostic ladder refers to medical history. Information about the general health of the client is essential in differential diagnosis. Identification of rapid onset of disfluent speech following illnesses, history of neurologic disease (Andy and Bhatnagar 1991; Helm-Estabrooks 1986), or recent psychosomatic episodes is essential for differential diagnosis (Deal 1982; Duffy 1989; Mahr and Leith 1992; Roth et al. 1989). Similarly, the use of medications or recreational drugs and hospitalizations for physical or psychological problems provide vital information.

The sixth step on the diagnostic interview ladder is social history. When evaluating adolescents with fluency disorders, this stage of the interview becomes an excellent avenue for questioning about peer relationships, self-esteem, and parental and teacher relations. For adults, it is important to determine the impact of the disorder on the perceptions of the client's peer relationships, social activities, and family interactions. The influence of the disorder on marital status, children, other people living in the home, frequency of participation in social activities, or hobbies should also be ascertained. It is unusual that the quality of the client's life is not influenced by a fluency disorder.

The seventh rung on this ladder refers to educational and vocational history. These questions help to determine if the problem is situation dependent. Does the adolescent stutter more at school or home? Does he or she stutter less in the classroom, during after-school activities, or at sports camp? Is his or her stuttering less with a specific teacher or coworker? How does he or she stutter when asked to perform verbally? Questions for the adolescent with a disorder would focus on issues relating to peer pressures, parental demands, academic pressures, social activities, first-time employment ventures, and popularity. The adult interview should contain questions about occupational choices, success, and satisfaction. The relationship of the disorder to career goals and the impact of stuttering on promotions and retention of employment could also be addressed.

The eighth rung focuses on concomitant problems. Blood and Seider (1981) suggested that concomitant problems in children could not only complicate assessment but confound effective treatment. If the adolescent has a learning disability, reduced intelligence, voice or other speech disorders, or neurologic disturbance, identification of stuttering or cluttering may be obscured and compromised. This may also suggest that treatment needs would have to be prioritized for maximum communication gains. The identification of concomitant problems in adults highlights the importance of the fluency problem and its urgency in individuals' lives. If clients are dealing with the effects of physical illnesses (e.g., metastatic brain tumors, supranuclear palsy, Parkinson's disease, dialysis, dementia [Helm-Estabrooks 1986]), psychological disorders, anxiety or depression states, marital issues, or other serious problems, then stuttering behavior may be a lower priority for treatment. This piece of diagnostic information is invaluable in determining the time and type of treatment. Figure 6.2 provides a number of possible questions that could be used for each rung of the diagnostic ladder.

The results of the questions to the interview, coupled with the behavioral and attitudinal assessment, help to determine the best treatment for clients with fluency disorders. The diagnostic interview provides information about factors 1, 3, 4, and 5 from the model in Table 6.1.

ASSUMPTIONS AND OBJECTIVES OF THE BEHAVIORAL ASSESSMENT

The diagnostic session(s) should produce reliable, valid, and practical data. The assessment should provide data about what the person does in particular situations. Assessment of stuttering and nonstuttering behaviors is determined by a number of assumptions about human behavior. The first assumption is that symptoms should be defined in observable and measurable terms. The rate of speech used by clients who stutter, the language of responsibility adults employ to characterize a moment of stuttering, and the reports recounted by adolescents about their fluency problems should all be observable and measurable. The second assumption indicates that assessments should be duplicated over time. Most researchers and practitioners agree that disfluencies are not a stable behavior, rather they are situation and context dependent. That means that multiple and repeated assessment in a number of different situations is necessary for acquiring reliable data. A number of authors have suggested that repeated assessments or ongoing assessments provide more complete pictures of the clients' disorders (Blood 1988, 1995a, b; Costello 1983; Hillis 1992; Ingham 1984). A third assumption is that the specific stuttering behaviors and nonstuttering behaviors can interact with the environmental conditions. Speech-language therapists should accurately assess the impact of the physical and social stimuli in affecting the speech behavior. The interactions between behavioral, attitudinal, and environmental components become critical. The sampling of multiple environments and factors is crucial for a valid diagnosis of the fluency disturbance. A fourth assumption is that a relationship exists between the assessment and the treatment. The

Reason for referral

Who referred you to the clinic?
Why do you think Dr., Ms., Mr. ____________ made the referral?
Why did you come to the clinic today? (For a self-referral)

Definition and presenting complaint

Can you describe in your own words what you think the problem is?
How do you define or describe a fluency disorder? Stuttering? Cluttering?
Can you describe what happens when you stutter? Clutter?
Does this problem affect only your speech or does it also involve feelings? Attitudes? Sense of control?

Client's perception of the problem

Do you have any theories about what caused your stuttering?
What is your understanding or knowledge about your speech problem, its causes, gender ratios, number of people with the problem, etc.? How much information do you have about stuttering? Cluttering?
How and where did you learn that information?
How do you feel about your speech problem? Are there any related attitudes or emotions?
On a scale of 1 (no problem) to 10 (one of your biggest problems), how would you rate your speech?
How do you think other people perceive your speech (e.g., coworkers, employer, supervisor, friends, family members)?
Have you been enrolled in previous treatments? For how long?
What were the most beneficial techniques or strategies you learned in these treatments?
What were the least beneficial techniques or strategies?
What techniques or strategies are you currently using?
Why are you seeking treatment at this time?

Onset, development, and progression

When did this fluency problem begin?
Does any member of your family have a fluency problem?
Is your speech getting better, worse, or staying about the same?
Are there places or situations in which the problem is better? Worse?
Are there times when the problem is better? Worse?
Do you have periods of relapses and remissions in your stuttering?
Can you describe what happens when you are in remission? When you have relapsed?

Figure 6.2 Diagnostic ladder questions. Some practical questions for interviewing adolescents and adults who stutter.

results of the assessment should naturally lead to plans for managing the disorder. The selection of target behaviors and the evaluation of the outcome of treatment are directly linked to the results of the appraisal (Ingham and Costello 1985).

Medical history

How is your general health?
Have you ever been diagnosed or hospitalized for any medical, physical, or psychological conditions?
Do you have any chronic health problems?
Is your current problem related to a medical condition (e.g., stroke, degenerative disease, medications, seizures)?
Are you presently taking any prescribed medications?

Social history

Does your speech affect your social relationships with others (e.g., spouse, family members, peers, strangers)? In what ways?
How does your fluency problem affect your participation in social activities?
How does this problem affect the frequency of social activities?
Do you avoid certain people or situations because of your speech?
Could you provide an example of this behavior (e.g., avoiding talking on the telephone)?

Educational and vocational history

Does this problem occur more or less at school? At work?
Does your speech affect your popularity at school or work? Is this important?
Are there certain people (e.g., teachers, employees, supervisors, classmates) with whom the fluency problem occurs more often?
Are there certain people (e.g., teachers, employees, supervisors, classmates) with whom the problem occurs less often?
Does the problem worsen with time pressures in school or work?
Does the speech problem worsen in some situations (e.g., oral presentations, peer pressures during conversations, asking for days off at work)?
How has your speech influenced your career choices?
How does this speech problem influence your satisfaction on the job?

Concomitant problems

Do you have any additional speech, language, or hearing problems?
Have you ever been told you had learning disabilities, reading problems, or educational problems?
Do you have any other problems that may affect treatment for your fluency problem (e.g., loss of loved ones; problems with spouse, children, or siblings; medical problems; anxiety; depression)?

Figure 6.2 *Continued.*

OBTAINING THE SPEECH SAMPLES

To identify the individual's place on the fluency continuum and determine the perceptual severity of the disorder, speech samples must be obtained. Costello and Ingham (1984) suggested that multiple samples are the best way to obtain a representative picture of the client's stuttering. Multiple samples taken over a number of sessions (at least two baseline data collections) provide a more realistic picture of the individual's problem. It has been my experience that individuals seek assessment and treatment during times of crisis, when their stuttering is at its worst. Adolescents who stutter are not brought to the clinic during their periods of relative fluent speech but during times when parental concern is heightened by the presence of severe stuttering behaviors. Clients also tend to associate the evaluation of their speech with high stress and increased emotional arousal. This can result in a more severe placement on the fluency continuum and confound the results of treatment. In light of these observations, assessment requires evaluation of the client's speech at different times and in different environments.

Typically, a number of speech samples are obtained from the client with the clinician. Ryan (1974) recommended that a clinician tape record 5-minute samples of speech in (1) oral reading, (2) conversation with the clinician, and (3) talking on a topic (monologue). Two additional 5-minute speech samples should also be recorded for adolescents and adults: one while making a telephone call and the other while the client talks with the clinician outside the speech clinic environment. For each of these five samples, at least 200 words should by recorded. However, as observed by Conture (1990), time constraints for people with severe stuttering may warrant less than 100-word samples. A 100-word sample can provide sufficient information for analysis of disfluencies. Samples should be obtained early in the week and the diagnostic should be completed later in the week, at which time a second set of samples are obtained. The appendix at the end of this chapter provides an explanation of the disfluency categories and one method for recording disfluencies.

Larger samples of 200 words are recommended because it is then possible to discard the first and the last 50 words in each sample to improve the representation of the client's speech. One set of the five samples should be obtained early in the week in which the evaluation is being conducted, and a second set obtained later in that week. Figure 6.3 provides a summary of the Assessment of Fluency Disorders (Blood 1993b). Each of the speech samples are analyzed on a number of factors, including the number and percentage of stuttering moments, the frequency of stuttering and nonstuttering disfluencies, the duration of the longest stuttering moments, overall speaking rate, naturalness ratings, and obvious concomitant behaviors.

The Speaking Rate is calculated by determining the total number of words spoken in 1 minute using a stopwatch. The total number of stuttering and nonstuttering disfluencies are counted after a transcript of the audiotaped or videotaped speech sample has been made. It is important to note that using this system, clients can have more than one disfluency on a word. For instance, they may say "buh-buh-buh-

Client____________________ Clinician____________________ Date________

Multiple assessments: Circle one ---------- Assessment time 1 2 3

Analysis	Task 1 Monologue	Task 2 Reading	Task 3 Conversation in Clinic	Task 4 Conversation Out of Clinic	Task 5 Telephone
1. Total number Of words spoken					
2. Speaking rate: total number of words per minute					
3. Total number of stuttering disfluencies (A + B + C)					
4. Total number of nonstuttering disfluencies (D + E + F + G + H)					
5. Total number of stuttering (3) and nonstuttering (4) disfluencies					
6. Percentage of stuttered words (total number of stutterings divided by total number of words spoken)					
7. Mean duration of the three longest blocks					
8. Naturalness rating scale (1 = natural to 10 = unnatural)					
9. Obvious concomitant behaviors (e.g., facial grimaces, arm swinging, eye blinks, lip smacking, jaw movements)					
10. Fluency condition (e.g., delayed auditory feedback, masking, shadowing)					

Disfluency type	**Frequency**	**Disfluency type**	**Frequency**
A. Part-word repetitions	______	E. Phrase repetitions	______
B. Dysrhythmic phonations	______	F. Revisions	______
C. Tense pauses	______	G. Interjections	______
D. Word repetitions	______	H. Recoils	______

Total disfluencies ______

Stuttering Severity Instrument **Severity rating:** Very mild, Mild, Moderate, Severe, Very severe
Frequency score _____; Duration score _____; Physical concomitants score _____; Rating score _____

Adaptation effect (number of words stuttered)
Percentage _____ Time 1 _____ Time 2 _____ Time 3 _____ Time 4 _____ Time 5 _____

Figure 6.3 Assessment of Fluency Disorders. (Adapted from GW Blood. [1993b] Assessment of fluency disorders: a protocol for diagnosing stuttering in adolescents and adults. Unpublished manuscript. The Pennsylvania State University.)

baseball" with tension. This would be evaluated as a part-word repetition and a tense pause. The coding procedure consists of underlining the word(s) where the disfluency occurred and then placing the letters from the disfluency categories above the word. In this example the letters *a* and *c* would be placed above the word *baseball* in the transcription. This means that two types of disfluencies (i.e., part-word repetitions and tension or tense pauses) occurred on that one word. This system has been described in detail by numerous authors for assessment of fluency in adults and school-age children (Thompson 1983). Figure 6.4 provides examples of transcription coding and analyses for a number of different disfluencies.

The calculation of rate and identification of disfluency types can help in differentiating stuttering from cluttering. According to Dalton and Hardcastle (1989), the differential diagnosis between stuttering and cluttering is at a phonetic feature level. They suggested that transition smoothness, pausing, rhythmic patterning, and regulation of tempo are central to the evaluation. Data from this part of the assessment could show that persons who stutter demonstrate a reduced rate due to a large number of disfluencies, part-word or syllabic repetitions involving struggle, dysrhythmic phonations, and tension behaviors. In contrast, persons who clutter would be more apt to show excessively rapid speech rate, syllable repetitions often lacking in variation, and little or no tension and struggle.

The next calculation is the percentage of disfluent words. The total number of stuttering and nonstuttering disfluencies is used for the numerator and the total number of words spoken is used for the denominator. This number is multiplied by 100%. On the Assessment of Fluency Disorders (Blood 1993b) (see Figure 6.3), this is represented by item 5/item 1 × 100%. Some clinicians prefer to use only the total number of stuttering disfluencies for the numerator, or item 3/item 1 × 100%. The mean duration of the three longest stuttering behaviors is computed by adding the three longest stuttering disfluencies and dividing by 3. Self-rating by individuals who stutter on the dimension of speech naturalness has been reported as an important component of a fluency analysis (Ingham et al. 1989). Therefore, a subjective naturalness rating is also made by the clinician on a scale of 1 (natural-sounding speech) to 10 (unnatural-sounding speech). The clinician also identifies, either during direct observation or from a videotape, the obvious concomitant or associated behaviors. These usually include such apparent acts as head jerks, lip smacking, leg and arm movements, hair pulling, eye blinking, tongue protrusion, and so on. These actions must be associated with the moments of stuttering to be included. Finally, some fluency-facilitating conditions should be evaluated. Authors have recommended the use of

1. Part-word repetition in a sentence (one disfluency)
   A
   She saw the school and wa-wa-wanted to go home.

2. Part-word repetition and tense pause on two different words in a sentence (two disfluencies on two different words)
   C A
   She saw the school and wa-wa-wanted to go home.

3. Part-word repetition and tense pause on the same word in a sentence (two disfluencies on the same word)
   A+C
   She saw the school and wa-wa-wanted to go home.

4. Word repetition in a sentence (one disfluency)
   D
   She saw saw the school and wanted to go home.

5. Phrase repetition and tense pauses on two different words in a sentence (two disfluencies on two different words)
   E C
   She saw the, she saw the school and wanted to go home.

6. Interjection and part-word repetition on two different words in a sentence (two disfluencies on two different words)
   G A
   She um, um, er saw the school and wa-wa-wanted to go home.

7. Part-word repetition, dysrhythmic phonation, and tense pause on the same word in a sentence (three disfluencies on the same word)
   A+B+C
   She saw the sch-sch-school and wanted to go home.

8. Part-word repetition, dysrhythmic phonation, and tense pause on the same word in a sentence with an interjection and word repetition on other words in the sentence (five disfluencies)
   A+B+C D G
   Sh-sh-sh-e saw the school and wanted to to go um well, er um home.

Figure 6.4 Examples for transcribing and coding using disfluency categories. Each disfluency is identified, the place of the disfluency is identified by the underlining of the word or words, and the category is identified by the letter placed above the underlined word(s). (A = part-word repetition; B = tense pauses; C = interjections; D = word repetitions; E = phrase repetitions; F = hesitations; G = dysrhythmic phonation.)

a single subject ABAB paradigm during the diagnostic protocol (Blood 1988; Costello and Ingham 1984). This paradigm consists of A (1 minute of baseline), B (1 minute of trial treatment), A (1 minute of baseline), and B (1 minute of trial treatment) to determine the effects of a number of fluency-enhancing conditions. The clinician may try the ABAB paradigm with the delayed auditory feedback, masking noise, slowed rate, gentle onset, or other fluency-enhancing techniques. The purpose of this part of the assessment is to determine which strategies enhance fluency and which strategies are best suited for the client.

In addition to these analyses, the Stuttering Severity Instrument (SSI) (Riley 1980) and a measure of adaptation to stuttering are obtained. The SSI is used to evaluate the severity of the client's stuttering. The SSI evaluates stuttering frequency, duration, and physical concomitants. Total scores, percentiles, ranks, and severity ratings of very mild to very severe can be determined. The Adaptation Task (Johnson and Knott 1937; Van Riper and Hull 1955) is determined by having the client read the same paragraph five times. Ham (1986) found that frequency levels observed during the adaptation task can provide information about individuals' responses and flexibility to possible stress situations. He also suggested that the adaptation task provided a good opportunity to observe patterns and changes in clients' disfluencies, severities, and personal reactions during reading. This part of the assessment provides information about factor 2 (stuttering and nonstuttering behaviors) from the model in Table 6.1.

OBJECTIVES OF THE ATTITUDINAL AND BELIEF ASSESSMENT

A comprehensive assessment of fluency disorders includes the assessment of the client's attitudes, perceptions, and beliefs about the disorder. A series of standardized tests can be administered to the client. These tests provide information about the locus of control, assertiveness, communication apprehension, communication attitudes, expectations and perceptions about struggle, and avoidance and expectancy behaviors.

The Locus of Control of Behavior (Craig et al. 1984) is a 17-item Likert-type scale used to measure an individual's locus of control of behavior. The client is asked to score each statement on a six-point scale, ranging from 0 (strongly disagree) to 5 (strongly agree). Scores higher than 29.8 indicate externality or an external locus of control. Clients with a high score may be more likely to relapse after treatment for stuttering terminates, because they think that they are not in control of their new speech patterns. This information can also provide insight into disorders of a psychogenic etiology.

The Personal Report of Communication Apprehension (McCroskey 1978) is a standardized, self-administered rating scale of communication apprehension. The client is asked to score each of 25 statements regarding communication with others on a five-point scale, ranging from 1 (strongly agree) to 5 (strongly disagree). Individuals scoring above 88 are high in communication apprehension. Individuals scoring below 58 are low in communication apprehension. This test helps to provide additional information about the client's awareness of the disorder and his or her response to communicative stress. Persons who clutter may have little or no awareness and very little communicative apprehension, while individuals suffering disfluencies resulting from a stroke may be acutely aware of the communication problem and fearful to speak in conversations or public. This test provides objective data for differentiating stuttering from cluttering.

The Assertiveness Scale (Rathus 1973) is a 30-item self-report scale that presents a valid and reliable assessment of assertiveness or social boldness. Subjects endorse scores from +3 ("very descriptive of me") to –3 ("extremely nondescriptive of me"). During reliability checks, scores ranged from +60 to –70. The higher the score (i.e., closer to +90), the more assertively the client behaves. The lower the score (i.e., closer to –90), the more nonassertively the client behaves. This particular scale does not measure aggressiveness. This scale addresses the issues of awareness of the disorder and coping strategies (e.g., approach and avoidance). Sometimes, persons with long-term fluency problems have confronted so much embarrassment, harassment, and humiliation that they choose to avoid speech and nonspeech situations. Their lack of social boldness can be a result of their negative interactions during communication. Treatment protocols should include counseling and experiences that could change these feelings and attitudes created by the chronic fluency disturbance.

The Stutterer's Self-Rating of Reactions to Speech Situations (SRS)–Avoidance Scale (Darley and Spriestersbach 1978) is a 40-item self-report scale that provides a means to evaluate the client's avoidance behavior using a five-point scale. Scores are averages for all items and range from 1 (no avoidance) to 5 (great avoidance). This provides good information about awareness and long-term coping strategies. The results help the clinician determine the extent of the attitudinal problem. It may be that a person who is disfluent as the result of head trauma suffers no negative attitudes or beliefs and has learned to "cope" with the disfluencies as a concomitant to the neurologic disorder. Sometimes, the sudden onset of disfluent speech is so traumatic and disturbing that clients disclose extremely negative evaluations about themselves and their speech. This information needs to be included in the decisions for treatment.

The Self-Efficacy Scale for Adult Stutterers (Ornstein and Manning 1985) is based on the work of Bandura (1977) and was developed to estimate a client's confidence for entering and maintaining fluency in a variety of situations. Subjects are asked to complete 40 items dealing with their confidence in (1) approaching a situation and (2) maintaining a self-defined level of fluency in a situation. Subjects rate their approach and performance expectations on a 10 (quite certain) to 100 (very certain) decile scale. An overall average score can be obtained. The higher the number (percentage), the more confident the client is, or the more likely it is that he or she will approach a particular situation. This scale is particularly helpful for determining the client's beliefs and expectations about the fluency disorder. This becomes critical for successful treatment. It may be that clients with neurologic degenerative diseases who have great expectations and confidence for acquiring fluent speech need to be guided to more realistic expectations and counseling. The scale also provides information about individuals with chronic stuttering problems and their need for desensitization, problem-solving techniques, counseling, or relaxation regimens.

The Speech Locus of Control (McDonough and Quesal 1988) is an eight-item scale designed to determine an individual's speech locus of control (i.e., internal versus external). The individual is asked to answer each of the items as either true or false. A higher score indicates a greater external speech locus of control. Adult norms are 5.4 (standard deviation = 1.3) for persons who stutter and 3.0 (standard deviation = 1.9) for persons who do not stutter. As a group, individuals who stutter show a more external locus of control. This can provide information about treatment outcome. It can also be used during treatment to see if clients are assuming responsibility for their disorder.

The Modified Erickson Scale of Communication Attitudes (Andrews and Cutler 1974; Erickson 1969) is a 24-item scale designed to assess an individual's attitude toward interpersonal communication. Items are answered as either true or false. The higher the score, the poorer the communication attitude. People who stutter generally score between 9 and 24 (mean = 19.22). Scores for people who do not stutter range between 1 and 21 (mean = 9.14). People who clutter tend to have a carefree attitude toward their disfluency. This scale can help to differentiate people who stutter from people who clutter.

The Perceptions of Stuttering Inventory (Woolf 1967) was designed to assess an individual's perceptions of struggle, avoidance, and expectancy. The 60-item scale with 20 items in each category (i.e., struggle, avoidance, and expectancy) is completed by the individual with a fluency disorder by marking items "characteristic" of their problem at the present time. Total scores for the three categories are obtained by summing the endorsed items. Scale scores can be used to evaluate and determine progress toward treatment goals dealing with struggle, avoidance, and expectancy in stuttering.

OBJECTIVES OF THE ASSOCIATED PROBLEMS ASSESSMENT

In the final section of the diagnostic evaluation, the relationship between the fluency disorder and other concomitant problems is assessed. A typical evaluation should include a screening for hearing, voice, articulation, phonology, oral peripheral exam, central processing abilities, and receptive and expressive language. This is an important part of the differential diagnosis. For example, the literature in cluttering suggests that people who clutter may have associated weaknesses in linguistic encoding of one's thoughts, as well as language and learning disabilities (Myers and St. Louis 1992). In persons with neurologic disorders, the need for consultation with other health-care professionals is often warranted. Concomitant problems can reveal early signs of general degenerative disorders or highlight the use of medicines that might be contributing to the disorder.

PRACTICAL PROBLEMS

This chapter provides a method for the systematic assessment of fluency disorders for adolescents or adults. It reviews the importance of the diagnostic interview, as well as the accumulation of objective and subjective data. One practical problem that needs to be addressed is concerns about interview data. The clinician assumes that the client is providing accurate and actual data. Distorted perceptions and misunderstood questions can make it difficult to differentially diagnose a fluency disorder. A second practical problem that should be mentioned is that the behavior observed during the assessment may not be representative of the client's "typical" behavior. This is why multiple assessments are critical. Adolescents may not want to show any awareness or reveal anything about their feelings at the initial session. Clients with other neurologic disorders may not be able to deal with another problem at the time of the assessment and refuse to recognize the fluency disturbance or acknowledge the need for treatment. A third pragmatic issue is confidentiality during the diagnostic. Some clients may not want to discuss personal issues that impact the fluency disorder in the first session. Whether it includes teasing by classmates, rejection for a job promotion, or inability to confront their disorder, revelations about a fluency disorder can be difficult to share with a "clinical stranger." This can be especially true of adolescents who are reluctant and fearful about sharing personal information. The clinician should establish ground rules for confidentiality and privacy at the beginning of the diagnostic.

CONCLUSION

In summary, fluency disorders are a fascinating area to assess and treat in adolescents and adults. Inexperience, lack of education, and inadequate performance by the clinician during the assessment can have a significant impact on the information obtained and consequently the description of the client with a fluency disorder. Continuing education and specialization in fluency disorders by clinicians increase the likelihood of reliable diagnosis. When a clinician establishes a good working relationship and a professional environment anchored in realistic changes during the diagnostic, the stage is set for successful treatment.

REFERENCES

Adams MR. (1977) A clinical strategy for differentiating the normally nonfluent child and the incipient stutterer. *Journal of Fluency Disorders* 2, 141–148.

Adams MR. (1980) The Young Stutterer: Diagnosis, Treatment, and Assessment of Progress. In WH Perkins (ed), *Strategies in Stuttering Therapy. Seminars in Speech, Language, and Hearing* (pp. 289–299). New York: Thieme-Stratton.

Andrews G, Cutler J. (1974) Stuttering therapy: the relation between changes in symptom levels and attitudes. *Journal of Speech and Hearing Disorders* 39, 309–311.

Andy O, Bhatnagar S. (1991) Thalamic-induced stuttering (surgical observations). *Journal of Speech and Hearing Research* 34, 796–800.

Bandura A. (1977) Self-efficacy: toward a unifying theory of behavioral change. *Psychological Review* 84, 191–215.

Blood GW. (1988) Stuttering. In M Hersen, C Last (eds), *Child Behavior Therapy Casebook* (pp. 165–177). New York: Plenum Press.

Blood GW. (1993a) Treatment efficacy in adults who stutter: review and recommendations. *Journal of Fluency Disorders* 18, 303–318.

Blood GW. (1993b) Assessment of fluency disorders: a protocol for diagnosing stuttering in adolescents and adults. Unpublished manuscript. The Pennsylvania State University.

Blood GW. (1995a) POWER^2: relapse management with adolescents who stutter. *Language, Speech, and Hearing Services in Schools* 26, 169–179.

Blood GW. (1995b) A behavioral-cognitive therapy program for adults who stutter: computers and counseling. *Journal of Communication Disorders* 28, 165–180.

Blood GW, Seider R. (1981) The concomitant problems of young stutterers. *Journal of Speech and Hearing Disorders* 46, 31–33.

Bloodstein O. (1960) The development of stuttering: I. Changes in nine basic features. *Journal of Speech and Hearing Disorders* 25, 219–237.

Bloodstein O. (1995) *A Handbook on Stuttering* (5th ed). San Diego: Singular Publishing Group.

Borden GJ. (1990) Subtyping Adult Stutterers for Research Purposes. In J Cooper (ed), *Research Needs in Stuttering: Roadblocks and Future Directions* (pp. 58–62). ASHA Reports. Rockville, MD: American Speech-Language-Hearing Association.

Brady JP. (1991) The pharmacology of stuttering: a critical review. *American Journal of Psychiatry* 148, 1309–1316.

Brookshire RH. (1989) A Dramatic Response to Behavior Modification by a Patient with Rapid Onset of Dysfluent Speech. In N Helm-Estabrooks, JL Aten (eds), *Difficult Diagnoses in Adult Communication Disorders* (pp. 3–12). Boston: Little, Brown.

Brown G, Cullinan WL. (1981) Word-retrieval difficulty and disfluent speech in adult anomic speakers. *Journal of Speech and Hearing Research* 24, 358–365.

Caruso AJ, Gracco VL, Abbs JH. (1987) A Speech Motor Control Perspective on Stuttering: Preliminary Observations. In HFM Peters, W Hulstijn (eds), *Speech Motor Dynamics in Stuttering* (pp. 245–255). New York: Springer-Verlag.

Conture EG. (1990) *Stuttering* (2nd ed). Englewood Cliffs, NJ: Prentice-Hall.

Conture EG, McCall GN, Brewer DW. (1977) Laryngeal behavior during stuttering. *Journal of Speech Hearing Research* 20, 661–668.

Cooper EB. (1982) A disfluency descriptor digest for clinical use. *Journal of Fluency Disorders* 2, 355–358.

Cooper EB, Cooper CS. (1985) *Personalized Fluency Control Therapy Kit*. Hingham, MA: Teaching Resources.

Costello JM. (1983) Current Behavior Treatments for Children. In D Prins, RJ Ingham (eds), *Treatment of Stuttering in Early Childhood: Methods and Issues* (pp. 69–112). San Diego: College-Hill Press.

Costello JM, Ingham RJ. (1984) Assessment Strategies for Stuttering. In R Curlee, WH Perkins (eds), *Nature and Treatment of Stuttering: New Directions* (pp. 303–334). San Diego: College-Hill Press.

Craig A, Franklin J, Andrews G. (1984) A scale to measure the locus of control of behavior. *British Journal of Medical Psychology* 57, 173–180.

Culatta R, Leeper L. (1988) Dysfluency isn't always stuttering. *Journal of Speech and Hearing Disorders* 53, 486–487.

Curlee RF. (1980) A Case Selection Strategy for Young Disfluent Children. In WH Perkins (ed), *Strategies in Stuttering Therapy. Seminars in Speech, Language, and Hearing* (pp. 3–19). New York: Thieme-Stratton.

Dalton P, Hardcastle WJ. (1989) *Disorders of Fluency and Their Effects on Communication*. London: Edward Arnold.

Daly DA. (1981) Differentiation of stuttering subgroups with Van Riper's developmental tracks: a preliminary study. *Journal of the National Student Speech-Language Hearing Association* 9, 89–101.

Daly DA. (1993) Cluttering: Another Fluency Syndrome. In RF Curlee (ed), *Stuttering and Related Disorders of Fluency*. New York: Thieme.

Darley FL, Spriestersbach DC. (1978) *Diagnostic Methods in Speech Pathology* (2nd ed.). New York: Harper & Row.

Deal JL. (1982) Sudden onset of stuttering: a case report. *Journal of Speech and Hearing Disorders* 47, 301–304.

Douglas E, Quarrington B. (1952) The differentiation of interiorized and exteriorized secondary stuttering. *Journal of Speech and Hearing Disorders* 17, 377–385.

Duffy JR. (1989) A Puzzling Case of Adult Onset Stuttering. In N Helms-Estabrooks, JL Aten (eds), *Difficult Diagnoses in Adult Communication Disorders* (pp. 13–21). Boston: Little, Brown.

Duffy JR. (1995) *Motor Speech Disorders: Substrates, Differential Diagnosis, and Management*. St. Louis: Mosby–Year Book.

Erickson RL. (1969) Assessing communicative attitudes among stutterers. *Journal of Speech and Hearing Research* 12, 711–724.

Gordon PA, Luper HL. (1992a) The early identification of beginning stuttering I: protocols. *American Journal of Speech-Language Pathology* 1, 45–53.

Gordon PA, Luper HL. (1992b) The early identification of beginning stuttering II: problems. *American Journal of Speech-Language Pathology* 2, 24–37.

Gregory HH, Hill D. (1984) Stuttering Therapy for Children. In WH Perkins (ed), *Stuttering Disorders* (pp. 77–94). New York: Thieme-Stratton.

Ham R. (1986) *Techniques for Stuttering Therapy.* Englewood Cliffs, NJ: Prentice-Hall.

Ham R. (1990) *Therapy for Stuttering: Preschool Through Adolescence.* Englewood Cliffs, NJ: Prentice-Hall.

Helm NA. (1979) Management of palilalia with a pacing board. *Journal of Speech and Hearing Disorders* 44, 350–353.

Helm-Estabrooks N. (1986) Diagnosis and Management of Neurogenic Stuttering in Adults. In KO St. Louis (ed), *The Atypical Stutterer* (pp. 193–217). Orlando, FL: Academic.

Hillis JW. (1992) Ongoing assessment in the management of stuttering: a clinical perspective. *American Journal of Speech-Language Pathology* 2, 24–37.

Ingham RJ. (1984) *Stuttering and Behavior Therapy: Current Status and Experimental Foundations.* San Diego: College-Hill Press.

Ingham RJ, Costello JM. (1985) Stuttering Treatment and Outcome Evaluation. In JM Costello (ed), *Speech Disorders in Adults* (pp. 189–223). San Diego: College-Hill Press.

Ingham RJ, Ingham JC, Onslow M, Finn P. (1989) Stutterers' self-ratings of speech naturalness: assessing effects and reliability. *Journal of Speech Hearing Research* 32, 419–431.

Johnson W, Knott JR. (1937) Studies in the psychology of stuttering: I. The distribution of moments of stuttering in successive readings of the same materials. *Journal of Speech Disorders* 2, 17–19.

Kidd K, Kidd J, Records M. (1978) The possible cause of the sex ratio in stuttering and its implications. *Journal of Fluency Disorders* 3, 13–23.

Mahr G, Leith W. (1992) Psychogenic stuttering of adult onset. *Journal of Speech and Hearing Research* 35, 283–286.

McCroskey JC. (1978) Validity of the PRCA as an index of oral communication apprehension. *Communication Monographs* 45, 192–203.

McDonough A, Quesal R. (1988). Locus of control orientation of stutterers and nonstutterers. *Journal of Fluency Disorders* 13, 97–106.

Myers FL, St. Louis KO. (1992) *Cluttering: A Clinical Perspective.* Kibworth, Great Britain: Far Communications, Inc.

Ornstein A, Manning W. (1985) Self-efficacy scaling by adult stutterers. *Journal of Communication Disorders* 18, 313–320.

Perkins WH, Kent RD, Curlee RF. (1991) A theory of neuropsycholingustic function in stuttering. *Journal of Speech and Hearing Research* 34, 734–752.

Pindzola R, White D. (1987) A protocol for differentiating the incipient stutterer. *Language, Speech, and Hearing Services in Schools* 17, 2–15.

Preus A. (1981) *Identifying Subgroups of Stutterers.* Oslo, Norway: Universitetsforlaget.

Rathus SP. (1973) A 30-item scale for assessing assertive behavior. *Behavior Therapy* 4, 398–406.

Riley GD. (1980) *Stuttering Severity Instrument for Children and Adults.* Tigard, OR: C.C. Publications.

Rosenbek J, Messert B, Collins M, Wertz R. (1978) Stuttering following brain damage. *Brain and Language* 6, 82–86.

Roth C, Aronson A, Davis L Jr. (1989) Clinical studies in psychogenic stuttering of adult onset. *Journal of Speech and Hearing Disorders* 54, 634–646.

Ryan BP. (1974) *Programmed Therapy for Stuttering in Children and Adults*. Springfield, IL: Thomas.

Schwartz HD, Conture EG. (1988) Subgrouping young stutterers: preliminary behavioral observations. *Journal of Speech Hearing Disorders* 31, 62–71.

Starkweather CW. (1987) *Fluency and Stuttering*. Englewood Cliffs, NJ: Prentice-Hall.

Starkweather CW, Givens-Ackerman J. (1997) *Stuttering*. Austin, TX: PRO-ED.

Starkweather CW, Gottwald SR, Halfond MM. (1990) *Stuttering Prevention: A Clinical Method*. Englewood Cliffs, NJ: Prentice Hall.

St. Louis KO, Hinzman AR, Hull FM. (1985) Studies of cluttering: disfluency and language measures in young possible clutterers and stutterers. *Journal of Fluency Disorders* 10, 151–172.

St. Onge K. (1963) The stuttering syndrome. *Journal of Speech and Hearing Research* 6, 279–289.

Thompson J. (1983) *Assessment of Fluency in School-Age Children: Resource Guide*. Danville, IL: The Interstate Printers & Publishers, Inc.

Van Riper C. (1973) *The Treatment of Stuttering*. Englewood Cliffs, NJ: Prentice-Hall.

Van Riper C. (1982) *The Nature of Stuttering* (2nd ed). Englewood Cliffs, NJ: Prentice-Hall.

Van Riper C, Emerick L. (1984) *Speech Correction Principles and Methods*. Englewood Cliffs, NJ: Prentice-Hall.

Van Riper C, Hull CJ. (1955) The Quantitative Measurement of the Effect of Certain Situations on Stuttering. In W Johnson, RR Leutenegger (eds), *Stuttering in Children and Adults*. Minneapolis: University of Minnesota Press.

Wall M, Myers F. (1995) *Clinical Management of Childhood Stuttering* (2nd ed). Austin, TX: PRO-ED.

Watson B, Alfonso PJ. (1987) Physiological bases of acoustic LRT in nonstutterers, mild stutterers, and severe stutterers. *Journal of Speech and Hearing Research* 30, 434–447.

Weiss DA. (1964) *Cluttering*. Englewood Cliffs, NJ: Prentice-Hall.

Whitney J, Goldstein H. (1989) Using self-monitoring to reduce disfluencies in speakers with mild aphasia. *Journal of Speech and Hearing Disorders* 54, 576–586.

Williams DE, Silverman FH, Kools J. (1968) Disfluency behaviors of elementary school stutterers and nonstutterers: the adaptation effect. *Journal of Speech and Hearing Research* 11, 622–630.

Woolf G. (1967) The assessment of stuttering as struggle, avoidance and expectancy. *British Journal of Communication Disorders* 2, 158–171.

Yairi E. (1990) Subtyping Child Stutterers for Research Purposes. In J Cooper (ed), *Research Needs in Stuttering: Roadblocks and Future Directions* (pp. 50–57). ASHA Reports. Rockville, MD: American Speech-Language-Hearing Association.

Yairi E, Ambrose N. (1992a) A longitudinal study of stuttering in children: a preliminary report. *Journal of Speech Hearing Research* 35, 755–760.

Yairi E, Ambrose N. (1992b) Onset of stuttering in preschool children: selected factors. *Journal of Speech and Hearing Research* 35, 782–788.

Appendix

DISFLUENCY CATEGORIES

Disfluency categories (types) A–G were taken from Williams et al. (1968), and include a modified version of a form-type analysis developed by Johnson (1961). Category H, a frequently occurring disfluent behavior, was described by Van Riper (1971).

A. Part-word repetitions: Repetitions of parts of words, syllables, and sounds. No distinction is made between sound and syllable repetitions (Johnson 1961) (e.g., ruh—ruh—run, ba—ba—baby).

B. Dysrhythmic phonations: The kind of phonation that disturbs or distorts the normal rhythm or flow of speech. The disturbance may or may not involve tension; may be a prolonged sound, accent, or timing that is noticeably unusual; improper stress, break, or another speaking behavior not compatible with fluent speech (Williams et al. 1968) (e.g., fffffffish, befffffore).

C. Tension and tense pauses: Disfluency judged to exist between words, part-words, and non-words when at the point in question there are barely audible manifestations of heavy breathing or muscular tightening. "The same phenomena within a word ... would place the word in the category of dysrhythmic phonation" (Williams et al. 1968, p. 624) (e.g., He c—ame home from—school).

D. Word repetitions: Repetitions of whole words, including words of one syllable. A part-word repetition, or an interjection, does not nullify a word repetition (Johnson 1961) (e.g., I—I was going—uh—going [a word repetition + an interjection]).

E. Phrase repetitions: Repetitions of two or more words (Johnson 1961) (e.g., I was—I was going).

F. Revisions: Instances in which the content of a phrase is modified, or in which there is grammatical modification. Also, change in pronunciation of a word (Johnson 1961) (e.g., I went—I was going, the later—latter).

G. Interjections of sounds, syllables, words, or phrases: Extraneous sounds, such as uh, er, hmmm, and extraneous words, such as well, which are distinct from sounds and words associated with the fluent text (Johnson 1961) (e.g., She went—uh—to school).

H. Recoil: This includes a broken word followed by repetition or revision of the preceding word or phrase, and completion of the original broken word (Van Riper 1991) (e.g., He put the stri—he put the string, This bi—this big).

7

Differential Diagnosis of Voice Pathology

Joseph C. Stemple

The management of voice disorders follows one of several paths depending on the results of the diagnostic voice evaluation. These paths include medical, surgical, behavioral, psychological, or any treatment combination thereof. To choose the right path, differential diagnosis involving many different professionals may be required. The diagnostic process related to voice disorders is similar to assembling the parts of a complicated jigsaw puzzle. From patient to patient, many parts are similar, but when one inappropriate part is forced into place, the entire puzzle is violated, leading to an incorrect diagnosis and possibly ineffective treatment. Using the vast knowledge of others with different areas of expertise expands one's ability to view the entire puzzle and to make the pieces fit smoothly into place. This is the essence of differential diagnosis.

CASE 7.1

A 46-year-old father of two teenage sons was referred for a voice evaluation due to chronic hoarseness of 3 months duration. As a sales representative for a major plastics corporation, the hoarseness was not only an inconvenience but also a threat to his livelihood. The onset of the hoarseness was sudden. The patient had undergone triple bypass surgery and was required to be on a ventilator for 9 hours after surgery. In addition, the patient had been placed on a diuretic and another blood pressure medication 2 weeks after the surgery. When the ventilator tube was removed, his voice was severely dysphonic but improved to near normal within hours and remained normal for about 2 weeks. Feeling the pressure to return to work, the patient began making telephone sales calls from home and within a day began experiencing a greater level of hoarseness. In fact, within another week he developed a severe breathy dysphonia that then persisted.

Results of the laryngologic evaluation revealed a suspected paresis of the left true vocal fold. The stroboscopic evaluation, however, demonstrated normal abduction and adduction for respiration but an unusual closure pattern during phonation, as the arytenoid cartilage movement was asymmetric. This result was inconsistent with the diagnosis of paresis. Direct light observation of the larynx using a rigid endoscope revealed significant posterior larynx tissue change suggesting the possibility of gastroesophageal reflux burn.

While taking the patient's history, it became evident that other factors might have been contributing to his hoarseness. Apparently, the surgery could not have come at a more inopportune time. He was paid on commission and was under extreme financial pressure, as the date for payment of his eldest son's college tuition was fast approaching. In addition, his 14-year-old son was not handling his father's illness well. Having lost his mother to uterine cancer 7 years before, he was acting out and had begun to perform poorly in school.

This patient had been a robust, energetic, hard-driving individual. By all accounts, he was a good father who provided well—physically and emotionally—for his sons. However, the person who came for the voice evaluation appeared to be fatigued and depressed—a beaten man. What is your diagnosis?

Diagnosis

Case 7.1 clearly describes just how complex the diagnostic process can become. Does the patient have a voice problem associated with a neurologic deficit of the left vocal fold caused by the surgery or the ventilation tube? Is the problem one of voice overuse in his weakened physical condition, or does he have symptoms caused by reflux? Are the new blood pressure medications contributing to his hoarseness, or is he simply stressed and depressed as a result of his financial and current family situation? The key to understanding this case is in understanding all of the potential etiologic factors. Indeed, a differential diagnosis involving the speech-language pathologist, otolaryngologist, neurologist, gastroenterologist, internist, psychologist, and psychiatrist may be necessary to successfully evaluate and treat this hoarseness.

Finally, and not unusually, the vocal difficulties experienced by the patient in Case 7.1 were determined to be the result of a combination of problems, including the negative effects of reflux, dehydrating medications, and depression. The patient's voice problem was successfully rehabilitated.

Voice problems arise under many conditions, and, as a result, numerous etiologic factors can play a role in their development. The traditional definition explains that a voice disorder exists when a person's quality, pitch, and loudness differ from people of similar age, gender, cultural background, and geographic locations (Aronson 1980; Boone 1977; Greene 1972; Moore 1971). In other words, when the acoustic and aerodynamic properties of voice are so deviant that they draw attention to the speaker, a voice disorder may be present. A voice disorder may also be present when the structure, function, or both of the laryngeal mechanism no longer meets the voicing requirements established for the mechanism by the speaker. These demands include vocal difficulties that are not readily recognized by others (e.g., the negative effects of vocal fatigue) but are reported to be present by the owner of the voice. Successful management of a voice disorder is dependent on the individual's recognition of the problem and acceptance of the need for improvement (Stemple et al. 1995).

Successful management of a voice disorder is also dependent on a clear understanding by the speech-language pathologist of the myriad of etiologic possibilities that lead to the development of the disorder. Sometimes the causes are easily identified (e.g., vocal nodules are present in the shouting child). At other times, finding the contributing causes of the disorder requires the skill of an experienced diagnostician and the diagnostic contributions of other professionals. To enhance the successful outcome of the search, it is advantageous for those seeking the answers to be familiar with as many etiologic factors as possible as well as the roles of other medical professionals who can aid in the diagnostic process. In this chapter, etiologic factors associated with the development of voice disorders are described, as is the differential diagnostic process by which these factors can be discovered.

CAUSES OF VOICE DISORDERS

As described by Stemple and colleagues (1995), the causes of voice disorders fall into four major categories: (1) vocal misuse, (2) medically related etiologies, (3) primary disorder etiologies, and (4) personality related etiologies. The task of the speech-language pathologist is to use a systematic diagnostic process to ferret out the most likely contributing factors associated with the development of the voice disorder. Indeed, the voice qualities of many voice disorders from many causes can have the same perceptual, acoustic, and aerodynamic properties. While much can be gleaned with the trained clinical ear, the type of voice pathology cannot be diagnosed by perceptual means alone.

Treatment approaches and strategies for improvement vary considerably depending on the cause or causes of the deviant voice production. For example, the voice quality of an adult female with vocal nodules may have similar perceptual qualities to a female suffering with gastroesophageal reflux disease and subsequent acid burn of the posterior larynx. The treatment strategies, however, would be totally different. The following sections examine the various etiologic categories and discuss the causative factors as related to the advantages of differential diagnosis.

Vocal Misuse

Vocal misuse refers to functional voicing behaviors that contribute to the development of laryngeal pathologies. These include behaviors of vocal abuse and the use of inappropriate vocal components.

Traditionally, speech-language pathologists have concentrated most of their voice diagnostic efforts in the evaluation of vocal misuse. This is the etiologic category most associated with behavioral issues for which the profession is well prepared to treat. However, when the view of the problem stops at the behavioral level, much diagnostic information is lost. This may explain why some in speech-language pathology profess displeasure in the outcomes of voice therapy. Table 7.1 lists the more common forms of voice abuse and the inappropriate use of the components that make up voice production. Even with these well-known etiologic factors, the diagnostic process can be aided by others outside of the profession of speech-language pathology.

Discovering the frequency and severity of abusive vocal behaviors can often be aided by family, friends, teachers, coworkers, and others close to the patient. Voice pathologists are wise to use whatever resources possible to gain a broader awareness of the patient's vocal behaviors. The patient often has a much different view of these behaviors than do others. The expertise of singing instructors and vocal coaches can be helpful in the evaluation of the use of vocal components. Singers and actors often use their professional voices differently than their everyday speaking voices. Evaluation of the professional voice can be aided by these voice professionals. Speech-language pathologists should not hesitate to use their expertise.

Medically Related Etiologies

Medically related etiologies refer to medical or surgical interventions that directly cause voice disorders and medical or health conditions and treatments that indirectly contribute to the development of voice disorders (Table 7.2). Focal and regional influences of the head, neck, upper back, and throat can influence laryngeal status. In addition, whole-body or systemic influences can also affect the larynx and voice production. These influences can stem from endocrine, immunologic,

Table 7.1
Etiologies of vocal misuse

Vocally abusive behaviors
Shouting
Loud talking
Screaming
Vocal noises
Coughing
Throat clearing
Inappropriate vocal components
Respiration: shallow, nonsupportive, breathy, residual air
Phonation: hard glottal attacks, glottal fry, diplophonia
Resonation: hypernasal, hyponasal, assimilative nasality, cul-de-sac nasality
Pitch: too high, too low, monotone
Loudness: too loud, too soft, lacks inflection
Rate: too fast, too slow, monotonous

and cardiac disorders, as well as respiratory and gastrointestinal diseases and disorders. Each of these disorders can also have associated pharmacologic agents that alter voice production. Differential diagnosis is essential when dealing with the causes associated with other medical problems. Etiologic factors and the roles played by other professionals in differential diagnosis of voice problems associated with medically related etiologies are examined in the following sections.

Focal and Regional Influences

The diagnostic process associated with direct laryngeal and oral surgeries is fairly self-explanatory. Careful study of the surgeon's operative report can clue the therapist in to the management procedures that are required. Since these surgeries are often ablative and disfiguring, other professionals may also be involved in evaluation of the whole individual, not just voice rehabilitation. These professionals can include a maxillofacial prosthodontist, oral or plastic surgeon, social service worker, psychiatrist, physical therapist, employment councilor, and psychologist. Speech-language pathologists must remember to treat the whole person and not just the communication problem. Improving the lot of the whole patient will most likely improve the voice disorder as well.

Indirect surgeries can also cause voice disorders. Thyroid, heart, carotid, and lung surgeries can all involve trauma to the vagus, superior

Table 7.2
Medically related etiologies

- Focal and regional influences
  - Direct surgery
    - Laryngectomy (total, hemi-, supraglottic)
    - Glossectomy
    - Mandible surgery
    - Palatal surgery
    - Other head and neck surgery
  - Indirect surgery
    - Thyroid surgery
    - Heart surgery
    - Carotid surgery
    - Lung surgery
    - Hysterectomy
  - Intubation
  - Mechanical trauma
  - Burns
- Systemic influences
  - Endocrine disorders
    - Virilization
    - Hyperthyroidism
    - Hypothyroidism
  - Immunologic disorders
    - Allergy
    - Arthritis
    - Infectious disease
    - Sjögren's syndrome
    - Lupus
  - Cardiac disease
  - Respiratory diseases
    - Asthma
    - Chronic obstructive pulmonary disease
    - Croup
  - Gastrointestinal disorders
    - Gastroesophageal reflux disease
    - Hiatal hernia
  - Pharmaceutical effects
  - Alcohol and drug abuse
  - Smoking

laryngeal, or recurrent laryngeal nerves. Diagnosis of a voice disorder can require the cooperation of any one of the surgical specialists associated with the surgeries, as well as an otolaryngologist. Even with this cooperation, the cases can be confusing and require in-depth evaluation.

CASE 7.2

A professional singer developed a mass involving the right lobe of her thyroid gland. After unsuccessful attempts to resolve the mass with medical treatment, the endocrinologist decided that surgery was necessary to cure the disease process. The surgeon gave the patient all of the typical warnings and possible outcomes of surgery, including the possibility of a right vocal-fold paralysis.

Surgery was routine and without suspected complications. When the patient awoke from the anesthesia, however, she was unable to produce voice above a whisper. Both the patient and the surgeon were alarmed. A laryngologic consult was ordered, and the results demonstrated decreased adduction of the left vocal fold. The diagnosis was left true vocal-fold paresis.

The surgeon and otolaryngologist could not explain how surgery involving the right lobe of the thyroid could possibly cause damage to the left recurrent laryngeal nerve. The patient was subsequently referred for a voice evaluation, including a laryngeal videostroboscopic examination of vocal fold function. The patient entered the evaluation somewhat distraught and gave her history in a whispered voice. It was noted during the interview that she spontaneously cleared her throat with strong phonation.

When viewed via videolaryngoscopy, the left fold tilted strangely in an abducted position as the patient attempted to produce voice in the strong whisper. She was told that the folds actually looked pretty good and that some movement could be seen. She was instructed to view the monitor as the folds were examined and try to bring the folds into a closer approximation. Within a few minutes, this was accomplished, and the patient was producing near normal voice.

Diagnosis

Case 7.2 represents a situation in which a successful differential diagnosis was dependent on the knowledge of the speech-language pathologist. The symptom did not fit the history, and the nonspeech voicing behavior (throat clearing) did not fit the symptom (aphonia). This patient had permitted her worst fears to come true due to the anxiety she felt about losing her voice. Follow-up psychological counseling was not necessary in this case. The consequences of misdiagnosing a vocal fold paralysis may have led to further surgical intervention, which of course would have had even more negative consequences.

A hysterectomy, especially if it involves both ovaries, can contribute to voice change due to hormonal changes. Many patients are not good historians and do not have a clear understanding of the possible results of their surgeries. Consultation with the patient's gynecologist or information from the patient's medical record may be necessary when determining the diagnosis of voice problems associated with this surgery, which can also potentially lead to emotional disturbances.

Direct traumas from intubation injuries, mechanical trauma, and inhalation irritations and burns can also contribute to voice disorders. Differential diagnosis of these injuries can be assisted by information obtained from anesthesiologists, emergency room physicians, and otolaryngologists.

Systemic Influences

Treatment of systemic disorders is the domain of the medical physician who diagnosed the disease or disorder. In fact, improvement of the voice component of the disorder is directly influenced by the success of the medical treatment. The speech-language pathologist often assumes the responsibility for diagnosing the voice components affected by the systemic disorder and planning the appropriate direct voice management to complement the medical treatment.

Endocrine Disorders

CASE 7.3

A 38-year-old elementary school teacher who had been teaching for 15 years was referred for evaluation and treatment due to chronic hoarseness and voice fatigue of 4 months duration. She indicated that she had never experienced vocal difficulties until this year, when during the summer she noticed a dry hoarseness associated with a cough. Her internist treated her with two courses of antibiotics that did not resolve the symptoms. Allergy testing provided negative results for both airborne and food allergies. She was placed on an antibiotic and given an inhaler, but neither seemed to relieve her symptoms.

After school started, the severity of her hoarseness increased, and her voice began to fatigue toward the end of the day. In fact, she reported that she was feeling very tired and losing weight, even though she was always hungry and ate an excessive amount of food. Results of the laryngeal examination revealed a mild bilateral vocal-fold edema and erythema. Otherwise, no mass lesions, paresis, or paralysis were noted.

Diagnosis

The patient was single and lived a quiet life. She was noted to be soft spoken and denied any forms of voice abuse except for the persistent, dry cough. In short, this voice disturbance did not fit the pattern of a behavioral voice disorder. The speech-language pathologist described the vocal symptoms to be a mild-to-moderate dysphonia characterized by a low pitch and a dry, breathy hoarseness. The patient's whole-body symptoms, including the cough, physical fatigue, and weight loss, were thought to be more important and were shared with the referring otolaryngologist. A subsequent referral was made to an endocrinologist, whose testing revealed the presence of hyperthyroidism. Once treated for this primary systemic disorder, the voice disorder also resolved.

Endocrine disorders, such as the hyperthyroidism in Case 7.3, can alter or limit voice quality and production. Endocrine glands secrete hormones that are responsible for body growth, sexual maturation and function, and chemical and emotional balance. As a general rule, hormonal imbalances produce the greatest effect on vocal pitch. Virilization is the abnormal secretion of androgenic hormones, resulting in male sexual characteristics in females. The vocal effects are low pitch, hoarseness, and occasional voice breaks (Aronson 1985; Colton and Casper 1990; Jafek and Esses 1986). Treatment with estrogen or other hormonal therapy can improve voice quality, but the pitch change is normally permanent.

Thyroid disorders affect many bodily functions, intellectual acuity, and emotional balance. Hyperthyroidism results from excessive secretions of the thyroid gland. Treatment requires either surgical excision or radioactive iodine treatment to slow the production of the thyroid gland. Hypothyroidism, or reduced thyroxin production, is often treated medically with thyroid replacement medications. Endocrinologists are the physicians with an expertise in endocrine disorders. As in Case 7.3, differential diagnosis was essential in resolving this voice disorder. Behavioral therapy would have eventually frustrated both the patient and the therapist.

Immunologic Disorders

Immunologic disorders that can create or exacerbate dysphonia include allergies, rheumatoid arthritis, infectious diseases, and other autoimmune disorders such as lupus and Sjögren's syndrome (Pennover and Shefer 1988).

Allergies

Allergies, which are commonly diagnosed and treated by allergists, can affect voice production due to associated inflammation and irritation of the pharynx, larynx, and nasal mucosa. Increased mucous production, nasal drainage, and congestion of the respiratory mucosa can alter vocal function. Vocal symptoms vary with the severity of the allergic response and can cycle with the seasons, pollen counts, and specific exposures (Stemple et al. 1995). In addition, medications used to treat the allergic symptoms can also negatively influence voice production through dehydration of the laryngeal mucosa.

CASE 7.4

A 32-year-old office clerk with known allergies had been experiencing a chronic hoarseness for more than 1 year. She was treating the allergy symptoms with an over-the-counter antihistamine. In addition to the dehydration caused by the medication, the patient also drank several cups of caffeinated coffee and several cans of caffeinated soda per day. Caffeine also has a dehydrating effect on the mucous membrane of the vocal folds. In consultation with her otolaryngologist, who was also a board-certified allergist, the patient was placed on a low-level prescription antihistamine. She was instructed to significantly decrease caffeine intake and was placed on a formal hydration program (64-oz water-based liquids per day). These procedures relieved the sensation of thick mucus experienced by the patient, which in turn decreased chronic, abusive throat clearing. These procedures improved her voice quality, with follow-up behavioral therapy conducted as a concurrent treatment.

Rheumatoid Arthritis

Rheumatoid arthritis is a chronic inflammatory disorder that disrupts the normal structure and function of synovial joints, including the cricoarytenoid and cricothyroid joints of the larynx. In my experience, the frequency of occurrence of laryngeal joint arthritis causing a voice disorder is limited. When affected, laryngeal function for both respiration and voice production can be compromised due to pain, swelling, and, in extreme cases, fixation of the joints (ankylosis) (Bienenstock et al. 1963).

Rheumatologists are specialists who treat arthritic conditions. Treatment usually involves use of medications such as anti-inflammatory and corticosteroid drugs. These drugs can have an additional adverse effect on the mucous membrane tissue lining of the vocal folds, as they tend to dehydrate respiratory tissues.

Infectious Diseases

Infectious diseases, whether viral or bacterial in origin, can also create or aggravate voice problems. Symptoms include chronic cough, irritation, edema, and eruptions of the mucous membranes of the pharynx and larynx, which can all contribute to the dysphonia. When the microorganism is treated with antibacterial medications prescribed by a physician, the associated dysphonia typically resolves (Shumrick and Shumrick 1988). Speech-language pathologists often see individuals in therapy who report the onset of dysphonia during an incident of upper respiratory infection. These are often individuals who have continued teaching, singing, selling, or lecturing during the acute phase of the disease, causing a strain to the laryngeal musculature or a more chronic laryngitis. When the acute infection is resolved, the voice remains dysphonic. The history of the onset explains the cause of the disorder, but the medical treatment does not, in this case, resolve the dysphonia. Voice therapy is necessary in these cases.

Candida is a yeast infection that can occur in the larynx, pharynx, and trachea. It is often troublesome to treat, especially if the patient is immunocompromised. Antifungal medications are the treatment of choice, with a prolonged course of many months often required for full therapeutic effect. *Candida* is also a common finding in patients with human immunodeficiency virus who exhibit symptoms of hoarseness, dry mouth, and mild chronic laryngitis due to a depressed immunologic system and repeated upper respiratory infections (Pennover and Shefer 1988).

CASE 7.5

A 45-year-old female professional singer was referred for evaluation and treatment with the diagnosis of chronic laryngitis. She reported experiencing the vocal symptoms of hoarseness, voice fatigue, loss of range, and lack of vocal power and flexibility for at least 6 months before being seen by the otolaryngologist 2 weeks before the voice evaluation. The laryngologic report described a moderate, bilateral vocal-fold edema and erythema. The folds appeared "vascular" with a slight thickening "in the typical nodular area."

The patient was a country-and-western singer who performed in the regional area 5 nights per week. Her schedule included late nights in noisy bars with the typical smoky environment. She was accompanied by a four-piece band, and she also played guitar. She was the featured entertainer in this group, which had gained in popularity during the past year.

The patient entered therapy with much anxiety. In addition to the vocal problems, she complained of oral and pharyngeal dryness and a constant feeling of "swollen glands." She had not been able to wear her contact lenses because her eyes were dry.

She was placed on a typical hydration program, instructed to use a vaporizer, and purchase a commercial steam inhaler. Traditional therapy measures, including vocal-hygiene counseling and environmental manipulation were provided. Direct voice therapy using vocal function exercises (Stemple 1993), were also provided. Though the patient was diligent in her cooperation and effort, therapy was not affecting a positive change.

Diagnosis

In spite of the hydration program, the patient continued to complain of oral-pharyngeal dryness and sensitivity of the submandibular glands. This led the speech-language pathologist to think that this was not the traditional voice misuse or abuse case. He discussed the case and all of the symptoms with the patient's otolaryngologist and internist. Blood-work studies were conducted, which led to identification of the primary etiology of the patient's voice disorder. Elevated B-cell activity and numerous autoimmune antibodies along with the patient's physical symptoms indicated that she had Sjögren's syndrome. Sjögren's syndrome is the second most common autoimmune disease after rheumatoid arthritis. It causes a decrease in the function of the exocrine glands, leading to dryness of the mucous membrane. Without this differential diagnosis and the appropriate medical treatment, voice therapy would not have been successful.

Cardiac Disease

Heart disease can also contribute to vocal difficulties due to the course of the left recurrent laryngeal nerve that loops around the aorta of the heart. In addition to the disease process, whole-body fatigue and respiratory compromise caused by the disease process can also contribute to voice change. Communication with the cardiologist for diagnosis of the condition and the planning of appropriate management may be necessary.

Respiratory Diseases

Respiratory diseases, as diagnosed by a pulmonologist, can contribute to voice disorders. The most common diseases include asthma, chronic obstructive pulmonary disease, and croup. Although voice quality is clearly a secondary concern relative to the ventilatory needs and airway preservation, any compromise of the respiratory power behind vocal-fold vibration has negative effects on phonation (Pillsbury and Postma 1986). Treatment for these disorders usually includes bronchodilators and inhaled steroids to suppress the symptoms of dyspnea and laryngeal edema, if present. As with other systemic diseases, improvement in voice production is generally commensurate with overall return of respiratory function.

Speech-language pathologists are frequently asked to participate in the differential diagnosis of vocal-fold dyskinesia. Vocal-fold dyskinesia occurs when patients adduct their folds during inspiration, causing shortness of breath, stridor, and occasional severe respiratory distress and loss of consciousness (Appelblatt and Baker 1981). These patients often have a previous diagnosis of asthma, are on many pulmonary medications, and have been hospitalized through emergency rooms multiple times for acute respiratory distress. Confounding factors to the diagnosis of respiratory distress include oxygen levels that approximate normal, even during the distress episodes, and pulmonary function tests that demonstrate results that are inconsistent with the acute distress symptoms. Differential diagnosis of this unusual functional disorder includes a complete pulmonary function work-up by the pulmonologist and observation of the activity of the vocal folds through videolaryngoscopy during quiet respiration, forced respiration, and after exercise. When inappropriate vocal-fold activity is identified, biofeedback training using the visual observation of the folds, as seen through videolaryngoscopy, is used to modify the behavior. Differential diagnosis is imperative for cases of vocal-fold dyskinesia.

Reflux Esophagitis

Numbers of patients are referred for voice evaluation, all of whom experience similar symptoms, including a thickness or lump feeling in the throat, chronic cough and throat clearing, occasional throat pain or burning, a bitter taste in the mouth, and a mild, dry hoarseness. Some patients report experiencing heartburn, but many do not. Often, when subjected to a differential diagnosis, these patients are found to suffer with gastroesophageal reflux disease (GERD) (Koufman et al. 1988). GERD can result in both dysphonia and throat pain. Irritation of the mucosa in the posterior larynx can be seen as erythema or hyperplasia of the interarytenoid rim of the glottis and of the vocal processes of the arytenoid cartilages. The acid reflux irritation can lead to the development of granuloma tissue or contact ulcers. Formal assessment of GERD is made by a gastroenterologist using a pH monitor over a 24-hour period. For this test, probes are placed in both the upper and lower esophagus to monitor acid levels at these sites. High levels can indicate reflux. Treatment for GERD involves changing dietary habits, losing weight, elimination of caffeine and alcohol, wearing loose clothing, elevating the head of the bed when sleeping, waiting to recline for 3–4 hours after eating, and the use of prescription or over-the-counter antacids. Again, without a proper diagnosis of GERD, the voice component of this disorder persists in spite of the best efforts of the speech pathologist and the patient.

PHARMACEUTICAL EFFECTS ON VOICE

Many of the systemic medical conditions are treated with drugs that can have an effect on voice production. It is important for the voice pathologist to be aware of these effects, as they can contribute to how the patient is treated in therapy. This important topic is too extensive to discuss in detail in this chapter but has been discussed thoroughly by Martin (1988), Sataloff (1995), and Benninger and colleagues (1993). In short, four drug actions that can affect voice production include influences on

1. *airflow*, including bronchodilators, which expand the diameter of bronchioles of the lungs to increase the oxygen and carbon dioxide exchange during respiration; (These medications are common for treatment of allergies, asthma, and other forms of upper-respiratory compromise.)
2. *fluid level in tissues*, especially diuretics, corticosteroids, and decongestants, which use chemical actions to reduce edema of tissues due to local inflammation;
3. *upper-respiratory secretions*, through the use of agents that reduce the secretions such as antihistamines, antitussives (for cough), and antireflux medications; and
4. *vocal-fold structure*, through long-term use of hormonal therapies, especially testosterone, which can result in permanent deepening of the pitch of the voice.

CASE 7.6

A 62-year-old automobile salesman had been experiencing a dry cough and mild hoarseness for a 2-month period. Given the profession, it was assumed that his mild vocal-fold edema and erythema were caused by voice misuse. In discussing this patient's history, however, it became evident that this was a lifelong salesperson who had never experienced vocal difficulties in the past. He was more concerned with the chronic cough and believed that the cough was causing the voice problem. He believed that if the cause for the cough could be identified, the hoarseness would likely resolve. He was correct.

Diagnosis

In taking the patient's medical history, the speech-language pathologist questioned him about his medications. The only medication taken daily was for high blood pressure. This was a medication he had taken for several years; however, during further discussion, it was reported that the medication dosage was increased at about the same time that his cough and hoarseness began. This was reported to the otolaryngologist, who in turn discussed this with the patient's internist. The result was that the medication was changed, the cough subsided, and the voice cleared within 1 week.

CASE 7.7

An opera major from the local conservatory sought an opinion related to mild hoarseness and a decrease in his upper range, which had begun only 2 weeks before the voice evaluation. This singer had never experienced vocal difficulties and was known as a fine talent. While taking the patient's history, it was discovered that this patient was an avid runner. He had strained a lower back muscle and had been given a muscle-relaxant by his family physician. The medication had a drying effect on the mucous membrane of the respiratory system. When the patient stopped taking the medication, his vocal symptoms resolved within 2 days.

CASE 7.8

A 46-year-old woman, a nonsmoker, presented with a chronic mild hoarseness of several months duration. By all accounts, this computer operator was not a voice abuser. She did admit to some stress in her home situation, for which she was receiving counseling. When no other etiologic factors could be identified, it was assumed that this patient's emotional status (i.e., stress) was a contributing factor; however, stress alone was not likely to have caused the edema and erythema that were observed in the vocal folds.

Diagnosis

With the patient's permission, her counselor, who turned out to be a psychiatrist, was consulted. This consultation revealed that the patient had neglected to provide some very important information, including the fact that she had been prescribed two different psychotropic drugs for depression. These drugs, which tend to cause mucosal dehydration, along with her emotional stress were the causes of this patient's vocal problems. Discovering these causes required the input of another professional.

Primary-Disorder Etiologies

Primary-disorder etiologies include embryologic, physiologic, neurologic, and anatomic disorders (Table 7.3), which have vocal changes as secondary symptoms of the primary disorder. Primary disorders require appropriate medical, surgical, educational, and rehabilitative interventions. The speech-language pathologist most often serves as a part of a diagnostic and treatment team attempting to aid in the diagnosis

Table 7.3
Primary-disorder etiologies

Cleft palate
Organic velopharyngeal insufficiency
Deafness
Cerebral palsy
Neurologic disorders
Trauma

and modification of the voice, swallowing, articulation, and language components of these various disorders.

Hypo- and Hypernasality

Occasionally, both speech-language pathologists and physicians confuse hyponasality (too little nasal resonance) with hypernasality (too much nasal resonance). The term *nasality* is meaningless unless defined in terms of amount and type of resonance. In speakers with hyponasality, the production of /m/ and /n/ sounds close to /b/ and /d/, respectively. The speaker sounds as if he or she has a cold or nasal congestion. Indeed, nasal congestion or other types of nasal obstruction (e.g., nasal polyps) may be identified by medical examination and x-ray. Treatment of hyponasality is provided by the physician.

The speaker with hypernasality is unable to attain velopharyngeal closure during speech, and /b/ and /d/ are likely to sound closer to /m/ and /n/, respectively. For the hypernasal speaker, both medical and speech-language management may be indicated. Diagnosis and treatment for most cases of hypernasality require a multidisciplinary team effort. Included in this category of hypernasality are cleft palate and organic velopharyngeal insufficiency, with their characteristic hypernasal vocal components. The diagnosis is assisted by videofluoroscopic studies, nasopharyngeal endoscopic studies, aerodynamic (pressure-flow) studies, or a combination of these, which help the speech-language pathologist assess the adequacy of velopharyngeal and pharyngeal function. See Chapter 8 for further discussion of velopharyngeal closure disorders.

Deafness

The vocal components of people who are deaf are frequently characterized by an inappropriate high pitch and a pharyngeal resonatory focus. People with severe hearing loss often present with a hypernasal resonance. In more subtle deficits, patients may talk either too loudly or softly depending on the type of hearing loss. The type and degree of hearing loss, of course, must be determined by an audiologist.

Cerebral Palsy

The voices of individuals with cerebral palsy vary widely because the neurologic damage is not related to one form of neurologic lesion (Greene and Mathieson 1989). Individuals presenting with cerebral palsy often speak with a labored, monotonous, and strained phonation with a limited frequency range. Control of intensity, due to positioning and respiratory support limitations, can also be problematic. Speech pathologists find it beneficial to work directly with the patient's physiatrist and physical therapist for seating, positioning, and posturing these patients in the most advantageous manner for voice support and production. Evaluation of these postural issues is essential in aiding the most effective voice production.

Neurologic Disorders

Many voice symptoms are present in a wide range of neurologic disorders. Neurologic disorders with associated voice symptom can be organized by lesion site as follows:

1. The upper motor neurons
2. The extrapyramidal system
3. The cerebellum
4. The lower motor neurons
5. The peripheral nervous system and myoneural junction

Differential diagnosis of the voice changes associated with these neurologic disorders often involves the cooperation of a neurologist, radiologist, otolaryngologist, and speech pathologist. The range and type of neurologic voice problems are as varied as the underlying dysarthrias that usually accompany the disorders. Characteristics of the changes in respiration, articulation, resonance, prosody, and voice have been described in detail by Aronson (1985), Sudarsky and colleagues (1988), Griffiths and Bough (1989), and Colton and Casper (1990). The classic audioperceptual attributes of voice production, for those who have neurologic disease, augmented with the neurologic and laryngologic examinations, as well as imaging and pressure-flow studies, determine the diagnosis.

Myasthenia gravis, for example, may initially present as an acquired hypernasal resonance deviation, decreased loudness, and, possibly, swallowing disorder. Initial identification of a possible neurologic problem is likely to be made by the speech-language pathologist.

The following case study discusses an example of the influence on speech and voice production and identification of another neurologic disorder.

CASE 7.9

An active 64-year-old homemaker and community volunteer was referred by an otolaryngologist with the complaint of "loss of power" in the voice. In fact, the chief complainer was not the patient, but rather her husband who said he was having progressive difficulty hearing and understanding his wife, especially with noisy backgrounds. His hearing might have been the problem, but his hearing and discrimination in noise proved to be excellent.

During the patient interview, she presented perceptually with a voice that was low in intensity and characterized by glottal fry phonation. She spoke rapidly but indicated that rapid speech had been a life-long habit. She did admit, however, that she occasionally noticed that her "tongue was getting tangled up." The patient indicated that she was very involved with her family, church, and community and that she was constantly talking in person, on the phone, during meetings, and in public. She used to sing in the church choir but had resigned from this, as she was losing the ability to control her singing voice. She attributed this to "old age." She admitted that, while her voice may be changing as she got older, she thought that the problem was a concern to only her husband. She agreed to come in for the evaluation to "get him off [her] back."

Indeed, results of the voice evaluation (including acoustic analysis, aerodynamic analysis, and videostroboscopy), along with the perceptual analysis, revealed that the patient was able to produce normal voice under the clinical conditions. It was noted, however, that connected speech, as opposed to the isolated vowels that were objectively tested, demonstrated bursts of short, rapid phrases with intensity decreasing at the end of the phrase as the breath stream was exhausted. In addition, mild dysarthria was noted, though it was difficult to tell whether this was caused by the rapid rate of speech. The patient appeared to be totally unaware of these speech characteristics.

In addition to the speech symptoms, three other observations were made during the voice evaluation. First, the clinician noticed that the patient's signature on the insurance form was written with an unsteady hand. Second, the patient appeared to have a rigidity in her facial features. At first it was thought that the patient's expression was somewhat dower because she really had no desire to take part in the evaluation. However, as she became more engaging during the course of the evaluation, her features remained somewhat expressionless. The third observation was noted as the patient moved around the various stations in the voice lab. Her balance was unsteady, and she constantly sought to steady herself by holding on to the table, the counter, or the back of a chair.

Diagnosis

The diagnostic signs that emerged from the evaluation were as follows:

1. Low intensity in conversation
2. Rapid rate of speech
3. Breathlessness at the end of a phrase
4. Mild dysarthria
5. Unsteady hand
6. Facial masking
7. Lack of balance
8. Inability to perceive these symptoms

It was the speech pathologist's impression that this patient demonstrated signs of neurologic involvement of an unknown etiology. Further medical evaluation was recommended. Although the patient was somewhat put off by the concerns, she agreed to discuss the matter further with her family physician.

A report regarding the findings was shared with the referring otolaryngologist, who in turn alerted her family physician to the concerns. A subsequent referral was made to a neurologist who ordered a magnetic resonance imaging (MRI) and conducted a complete neurologic evaluation. The radiologist reported that the results of the MRI were negative; however, the neurologic examination revealed mild hand tremor, bradykinesia (a slowness of movement in her arms and legs), and postural instability, along with the previously diagnosed speech symptoms. In short, this patient presented with the onset of Parkinson's disease, with the first symptom of consequence being the negative effect on speech and voice production. Differential diagnosis was necessary to identify and confirm the presence of this debilitating neurologic disease. The patient subsequently was treated medically and enrolled in the Lee Silverman Voice Therapy (LSVT) program (Ramig et al. 1995), which proved successful in improving her overall voice and speech production.

Peripheral Nerve Damage

Peripheral nerve damage to the vagus nerve or its branches and the recurrent and superior laryngeal nerves is fairly common during various head and neck surgeries (e.g., thyroidectomy, endarterectomy, spinal fusions) and some cardiac and lung surgeries. Approximately 30% of all vocal-fold paralyses are idiopathic. Diagnosis of a vocal-fold paralysis is made through routine visual examination by the otolaryngologist. Through indirect laryngoscopy, the otolaryngologist can see the movement or lack of movement of the fold. Stroboscopic observation during phonation of the folds enables the examiner to comment on the approximation of the folds and the stability of the vibratory pattern. In some cases, however, there may be question as to whether the vocal fold or folds are totally paralyzed or only partially paretic. In other cases, it may be unclear as to whether a paralysis exists or whether subluxation of the cricoarytenoid joint occurred due to trauma. In all cases of decreased vocal-fold abduction and adduction, it is important to understand that the only direct measure of nerve function is through the use of electromyography (EMG). EMG involves inserting an electrode directly into the muscles in question as a means of measuring the electrical activity of those muscles. This diagnostic procedure is normally performed by a neurologist or an otolaryngologist who is specially trained in EMG procedures.

Trauma

Trauma also is a cause of a voice disorder in the primary disorder category of etiologies. Blunt or penetrating injuries to the larynx often cause edema, fractured laryngeal cartilages, joint dislocations, and lacerations. These injuries can be caused by automobile accidents and sports-related injuries, stabbing and gunshot wounds, strangulation, or, on rare occasions, intubation injuries. Inhalation of flames, gases, and fumes and swallowing of caustic substances can also cause serious traumatic injury to the larynx. The primary concern related to severe trauma of the larynx is the establishment and maintenance of an adequate airway. Voice therapy follows recovery from the acute stage of the injury. In these cases, the speech-language pathologist must work closely with the otolaryngologist to obtain a complete description of the results of the injury. With this knowledge, reasonable goals and expectations for improvement can be established. Trauma cases often present with severe vocal consequences, and reasonable expectations for improvement must be established for both the patient and for the clinician. This can only be accomplished through direct cooperation with the otolaryngologist.

Personality-Related Disorders

The final etiologic category to be discussed as related to differential diagnosis of voice disorders is the category associated with personality issues, which include *environmental stress, conversion behaviors,* and *identity conflict.* Voice is a sensitive indicator of emotions, attitudes, and role assumptions (Morrison and Rammage 1994). Indeed, the way a person feels physically and emotionally is often directly reflected in the quality of voice. Resultant vocal symptoms may simply be the result of whole-body tension, which causes a more specific hypertonicity of the intrinsic and extrinsic laryngeal muscles, which in turn causes a tension dysphonia. On the other hand, the symptoms may be a sign of a much more serious underlying psychological disorientation. In either case, the tensions and stresses of everyday life can contribute directly to the abnormal functioning of the sensitive vocal instrument. The speech-language pathologist often plays the lead role in the differential diagnosis of these functional voicing disorders.

CASE 7.10

A 17-year-old high school student was referred by the otolaryngologist with the diagnosis of chronic hoarseness. An evaluation was the last of many attempts to determine the cause of this voice disorder. The young man first began experiencing hoarseness when he was 13 years old. His mother at first assumed that the hoarseness was related to his normal voice maturation but became concerned when the hoarseness persisted and worsened during the next year. She mentioned the hoarseness to her son's pediatrician when the son was 14 years old. Various medications, including antibiotics, nasal sprays, and antihistamines, were prescribed over the next year. The hoarseness persisted. At 15 years of age, allergy testing was conducted, which showed the patient to be sensitive to grass, dust, and molds. Allergy shots were begun and continued to the time of the voice evaluation. The hoarseness persisted. At 16 years of age, his mother sought the opinion of an otolaryngologist who identified sinusitis. A sinus irrigation was performed, and, when the patient remained dysphonic, a rhinoplasty to repair a deviated septum was performed. The young man remained dysphonic. In fact, his hoarseness over the years had caused him to become somewhat withdrawn. He was described as being very quiet in all situations, and he only spoke in school when he was forced to speak in a classroom situation.

At 17 years of age, his mother chose to try once more and sought the opinion of another otolaryngologist, who in turn referred him for a voice evaluation. The evaluation included the perceptual evaluation, acoustic and aerodynamic analysis of vocal function, and laryngeal videostroboscopy.

The patient presented with a moderate-to-severe dysphonia characterized by persistent glottal fry phonation, raspiness, and a cul-de-sac nasality. Acoustic analysis was significant only because the voice was so disturbed that reliable measures could not be taken. Aerodynamic analysis revealed normal airflow volumes, but airflow rates were very high. Stroboscopic observation of the vibration pattern of the vocal folds revealed an unusual parallel positioning of the folds, incomplete glottic closure, vibratory stiffness, and phase asymmetry.

Diagnosis

When these results were examined in total, it became evident that this young man presented with a functional falsetto. In his attempt to sound more normal, he attempted to lower the falsetto tone, which created the persistent raspiness that had for years been identified as hoarseness. During the evaluation session, laryngeal manipulation resulted in immediate modification of his voice. The patient quickly established normal voice production.

This was a case in which all of the appropriate diagnosticians were involved but not in a team orientation, which is important in differential diagnosis. It reminds one of the story of the elephant and the three blind men. Each had a completely different description of the elephant because each man was touching a different part of the elephant. The men did not bother to communicate with each other for a clearer understanding of the elephant's appearance. The pediatrician was treating symptoms with medication. The allergist was treating allergies. The otolaryngologist was treating sinus and nasal problems. All of these etiologies can be implicated in a voice disorder. However, because a differential diagnostic process was not conducted, this young man continued to experience vocal difficulties during the very important social development years. These difficulties ultimately influenced his personality.

Diagnosing personality-related voice problems is best accomplished in cooperation with an otolaryngologist. Most of the functional voice disorders present with symptoms that are out of proportion with the condition of the vocal mechanism. The otolaryngologist informs the speech-language pathologist of the appearance of the vocal folds. When the folds are essentially normal in the presence of aphonia or dysphonia, the disorder is most likely caused by a psychological disequilibrium. At times, the clinician may choose to seek the opinion of a psychiatrist, psychologist, or other mental health–care professional to confirm the suspected behavioral etiology. Neurologists may also be consulted during diagnosis of unusual dysphonias.

CASE 7.11

A young woman presented with symptoms similar to adductor spasmodic dysphonia and a physical complaint of leg weakness. Unlike cases of spasmodic dysphonia, however, her voice symptoms were intermittent. An EMG study conducted by a neurologist revealed normal leg muscle function. It was suspected that both her voice and leg symptoms were caused by psychogenic factors. Evaluation of her symptoms was being managed by her internist and referral was made to a psychologist for evaluation. At the same time, diagnostic voice therapy was conducted, which stabilized her voice production. Results of the psychological testing revealed a clinical depression and other psychosocial problems. This case again demonstrated the power and necessity of differential diagnosis.

CONCLUSION

Voice disorders present from a myriad of possible etiologic factors. Because of the complicated nature of voice evaluation, differential diagnosis is not only necessary but essential to the appropriate treatment planning for patients. Speech-language pathologists must be well versed in all of the etiologic factors that contribute to the development of voice disorders. Beyond this, the development of relationships with medical, mental health, educational, and other health care professionals is necessary for both the differential diagnosis and the management of the voice problem to be successful. The speech-language pathologist must develop the expertise necessary to become effective in interactions as a member of the diagnostic team.

REFERENCES

Appelblatt N, Baker S. (1981) Functional upper airway obstruction. *Archives of Otolaryngology* 107, 305–307.

Aronson A. (1980) *Clinical Voice Disorders: An Interdisciplinary Approach.* New York: BC Decker.

Aronson A. (1985) *Clinical Voice Disorders: An Interdisciplinary Approach* (2nd ed). New York: BC Decker.

Benninger M, Jacobson B, Johnson A. (1993) *Voice Arts Medicine: The Care and Prevention of Professional Voice Disorders.* New York: Thieme.

Bienenstock H, Ehrlich G, Freyberg R. (1963) Rheumatoid arthritis of the cricoarytenoid joint: a clinicopathologic study. *Arthritis and Rheumatism* 6, 48–63.

Boone D. (1977) *The Voice and Voice Therapy* (2nd ed). Englewood Cliffs, NJ: Prentice-Hall.

Colton R, Casper L. (1990) *Understanding Voice Problems: A Physiological Perspective for Diagnosis and Treatment.* Baltimore: Williams & Wilkins.

Greene M. (1972) *The Voice and Its Disorders* (3rd ed). Philadelphia: Lippincott.

Greene M, Mathieson L. (1989) *The Voice and Its Disorders* (5th ed). London: Whurr Publishers.

Griffiths C, Bough I Jr. (1989) Neurologic diseases and their effects on voice. *Journal of Voice* 3, 148–146.

Jafek B, Esses B. (1986) Manifestations of Systemic Disease. In C Cummings, J Fredrickson, L Harker, et al (eds), *Otolaryngology-Head and Neck Surgery* (pp. 1933–1941). St. Louis: Mosby.

Koufman J, Weiner G, Wu W, Castell D. (1988) Reflux laryngitis and its sequelae: the diagnostic role of ambulatory 24-hour pH monitoring. *Journal of Voice* 2, 78–89.

Martin F. (1988) Tutorial: drugs and vocal function. *Journal of Voice* 2, 338–344.

Moore P. (1971) *Organic Voice Disorders*. Englewood Cliffs, NJ: Prentice-Hall.

Morrison M, Rammage L. (1994) *The Management of Voice Disorders*. San Diego: Singular Publishing Group.

Pennover D, Shefer A. (1988) Immunologic Disorders of the Larynx. In M Fried (ed), *The Larynx: A Multidisciplinary Approach* (pp. 279–290). Boston: Little, Brown.

Pillsbury H, Postma D. (1986) Infections. In C Cummings, J Fredrickson, L Harker, et al. (eds), *Otolaryngology-Head and Neck Surgery* (pp. 1919–1931). St. Louis: Mosby.

Ramig L, Pawlas A, Countrymen S. (1995) *The Lee Silverman Voice Treatment (TLSVT): The Practical Guide to Treating the Voice and Speech Disorders in Parkinson's Disease.* Iowa City, IA: National Center for Voice and Speech.

Sataloff R. (1995) Medications and their effects on voice. *Journal of Singing* 52, 47–52.

Shumrick K, Shumrick D. (1988) Inflammatory Diseases of the Larynx. In M Fried (ed), *The Larynx: A Multidisciplinary Approach* (pp. 249–278). Boston: Little, Brown.

Stemple J. (1993) *Voice Therapy: Clinical Studies*. St. Louis: Mosby-Year Book.

Stemple J, Glaze L, Gerdeman B. (1995) *Clinical Voice Pathology: Theory and Management* (2nd ed). San Diego: Singular Publishing Group.

Sudarsky L, Feudo P, Zubick H. (1988) Vocal Aberrations in Dysarthria. In M Fried (ed), *The Larynx: A Multidisciplinary Approach* (pp. 179–190). Boston: Little, Brown.

8

Diagnosis of Velopharyngeal Disorders

Sally J. Peterson-Falzone

A speaker's velopharyngeal system comes into question (1) when something is heard in speech that may be indicative of a past or current problem in the function of the system or (2) when there is something in the speaker's medical history that may have interfered with velopharyngeal function. The "red flag" in the medical history can be either congenital or acquired and can be a physical inadequacy of tissue (e.g., cleft palate, congenitally short palate, traumatic loss of tissue in the palate or pharynx) or a deficiency in neuromotor control of the velopharyngeal mechanism.

When trying to diagnose a speaker who is referred with simply a "speech problem," the perceptual identification of inadequate function of the velopharyngeal system can be difficult. At the most basic level, the client may exhibit audible nasal air loss on the pressure consonants with consequent weakening of these phonemes, hypernasal resonance on vowels and vocalic segments, and possibly the use of "compensatory articulations" (e.g., glottal stops, pharyngeal fricatives, pharyngeal affricates) (Trost-Cardamone 1987). However, speakers may exhibit some of these patterns as a result of *previous* inadequacy of the velopharyngeal mechanism, making it difficult for the clinician to know if they are occurring as a result of current physical problems or as a residual of past problems.

The diagnostic process starts with the clinician's ear and proceeds to instrumentation-dependent studies as necessary or appropriate. Even when a client is referred because of a known physical difference (e.g., submucous cleft palate or repaired palatal cleft), the question is likely to be, "Is there a speech problem, and, if so, is it due to inadequate function of the velopharyngeal mechanism?" Some guidelines for making these judgments are provided in the section *Key Items in Making Perceptual Judgments*.

The availability of instrumentation for looking at the velopharyngeal system (e.g., x-rays) or for measuring the acoustic or aerodynamic consequences of velopharyngeal function depend on the professional setting and the availability of referral sources. Clinicians may be working in the public schools without immediate access to instrumentation; however, acoustic studies may be available at a nearby university, endoscopic examination may be available through a local otolaryngologist, radiographic studies may be available through a local orthodontist (for still cephalometric films), or a physician may arrange for videofluoroscopic studies. A word of caution: When the clinician refers a client for such studies, he or she should make every effort to accompany the client to the examination. The clinician should confer directly and on-site with the physician or other professional whose help is being sought. Otherwise, the clinician runs the risk of obtaining the wrong information.

Ideally, diagnosis and treatment planning for speakers with velopharyngeal inadequacy (VPI)* should always take place in an interdisciplinary setting where speech pathologists, otolaryngologists, dental specialists, and surgeons can examine the client together, and where any necessary studies can be obtained on-site. The American Cleft Palate–Craniofacial Association (1829 Franklin Street, Suite 1022, Chapel Hill, NC 27514. Telephone: 800-242-5338) maintains a directory of interdisciplinary cleft palate and craniofacial teams. Even if the nearest team is several hours' drive away, the assistance that can be received is worth the inconvenience.

AN OVERVIEW OF ETIOLOGIES OF VELOPHARYNGEAL DISORDERS

Structural

Cleft Palate

Clefts of the palate can occur with or without a cleft of the lip. The terminology used in differentiating types of clefts is based on the embry-

---

*Most of the literature uses the terms *velopharyngeal inadequacy, velopharyngeal incompetency,* and *velopharyngeal insufficiency* interchangeably. Trost (1981b) suggested using *incompetency* for deficiencies of movement, *insufficiency* for deficiencies of tissue, and *inadequacy* for cases of mixed or undiagnosed origin. Folkins (1988) pointed out that speech-language pathologists do not yet have the ability to always separate speakers on the basis of neuromuscular versus structural deficits. For purposes of simplicity, I am using *velopharyngeal inadequacy* as a generic or umbrella term and abbreviate it as *VPI* for ease in reading.

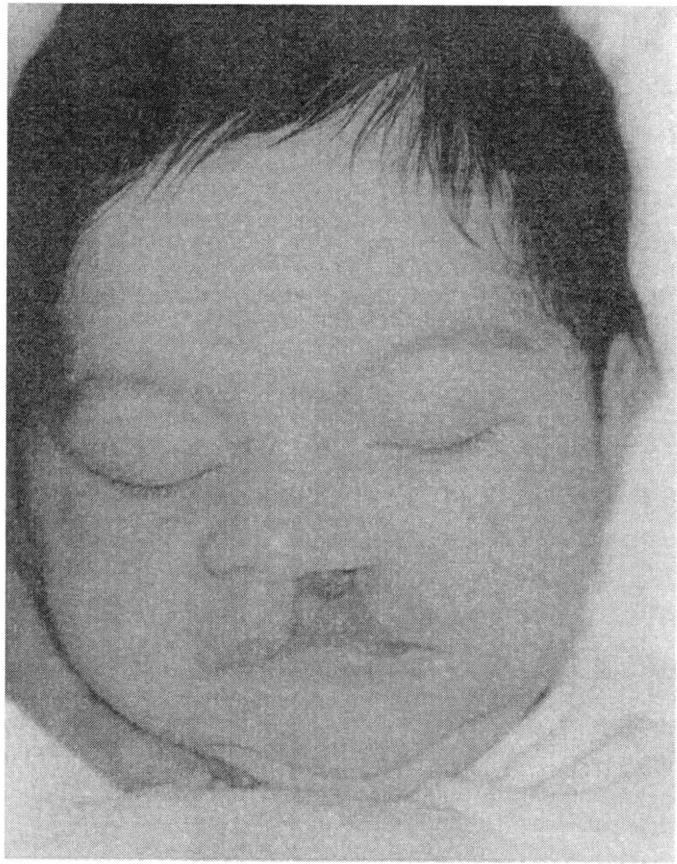

A

Figure 8.1 A. Frontal view of wide unilateral cleft with a Simonart's band in an 11-day-old infant.

ologic development of these structures and can be confusing. The embryonic structure called the *primary palate* becomes the *premaxilla,* a term that designates a wedge-shaped section in the anterior portion of the maxilla, with the posterior point of the wedge being the incisive foramen. The primary palate develops into the anterior portion of the hard palate, the portion of the alveolar ridge from which the four incisors erupt, and the medial portion of the upper lip. The remainder of the hard palate and all of the soft palate form from the embryonic secondary palate. Clefts of the lip and alveolus are often called *clefts of the primary palate* (Figure 8). Either unilateral or bilateral clefts of the primary palate can occur in isolation, with no involvement of the secondary palate, and have no bearing on the function of the velopha-

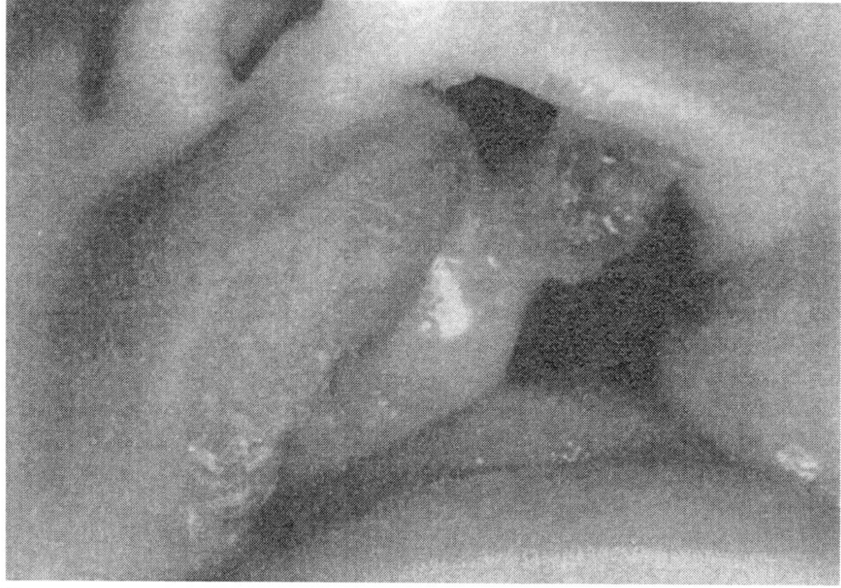

B

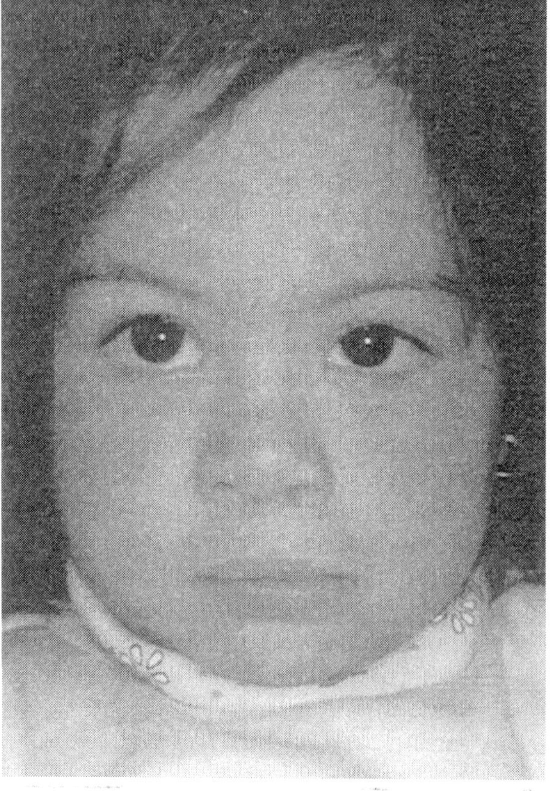

C

Figure 8.1 *Continued* B. Intraoral view of wide unilateral cleft with a Simonart's band in 11-day-old infant in Figure 8.1A. C. The same child at the age of 19 months.

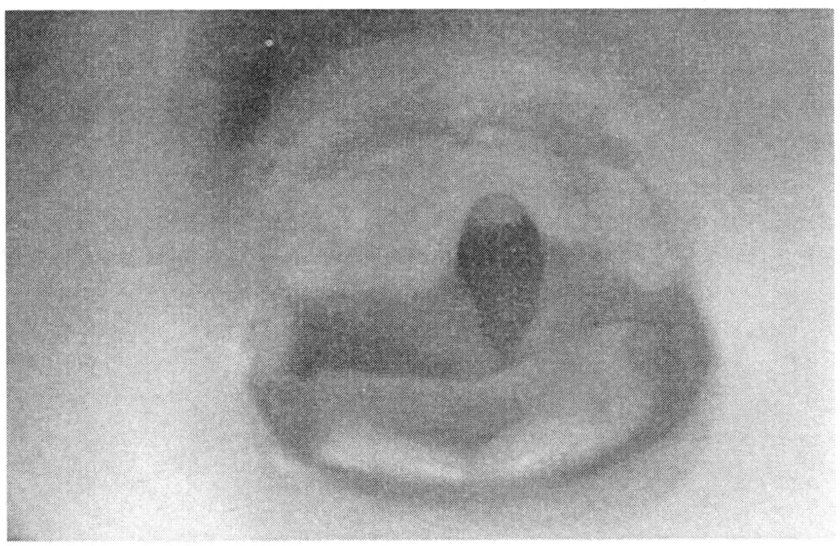

Figure 8.2 Complete cleft of the soft palate with extension into the hard palate in a 6-day-old infant.

ryngeal mechanism. A cleft of the secondary palate can be either an overt cleft or a submucous cleft. (There are also submucous defects of the lip and alveolus, but these do not affect speech and are in fact rarely reported, perhaps because they are rarely detected.) The extent of the defect can vary from a small defect in the uvula to a complete cleft extending all the way forward to the incisive foramen (Figure 8.2). If the cleft of the secondary palate is complete, it can be wide with a virtual horseshoe shape and little tissue mesial to the alveolar ridge.

An open cleft of the secondary palate is an obvious cause of inadequate velopharyngeal closure unless the defect is extremely small (i.e., not much more than a bifid uvula). After the cleft is surgically repaired, velopharyngeal function should be adequate for speech but in some cases is not. There are three ways in which surgical closure of the palate can fail:

1. Postoperative fistulae. The surgeon may fail to obtain complete closure of the tissues at the operating table,* or a fistula may open some time in the postoperative period (Figure 8.3). The effects of fistulae on speech vary with their size and position.

*In most cleft palate surgery done in the United States, the alveolar bony cleft is not closed surgically until midchildhood (i.e., 9 years of age or later). The defect is left open to allow for better growth of the anterior portion of the maxilla and so as not to interfere with orthodontic positioning of the maxillary segments. The intentional nonunion of the alveolar defect is technically a fistula but does not constitute a postoperative breakdown.

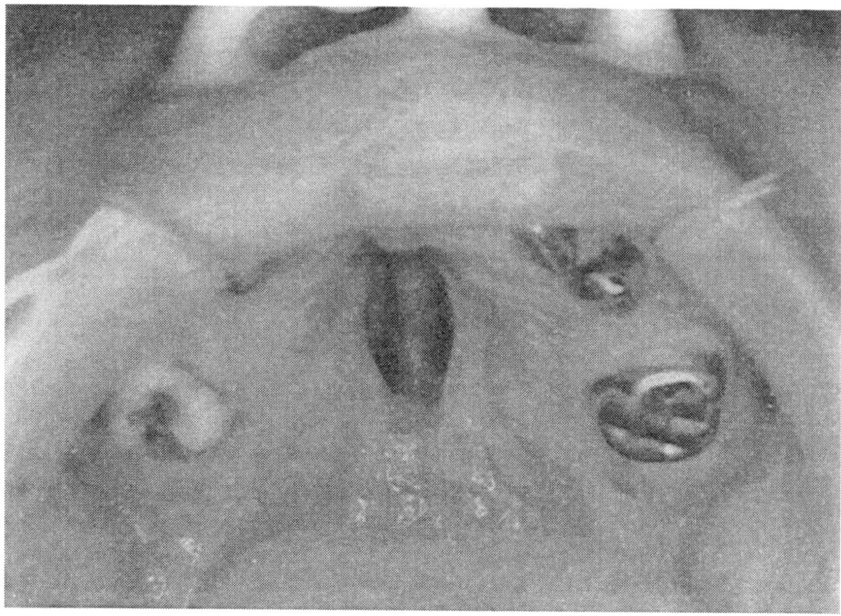

Figure 8.3 Large postoperative fistula in an adult. The structure seen in the midline of the fistula is the base of the vomer bone.

2. A repaired palate that is too short to reach the posterior pharyngeal wall.
3. A repaired palate that is inadequate in mobility.

Historically, about 66–75% of individuals with repaired clefts are reported to have adequate velopharyngeal function (Morris 1973). That number is climbing to the extent that success rates of the original palatal surgery are now often reported to be 80–90% or above (Peterson-Falzone 1993). Nevertheless, there is a percentage of patients for whom palate repair has not produced a fully adequate system and for whom the speech-language pathologist should address the various points presented in this chapter.

Submucous clefts are an enigma (Figure 8.4). The three intraorally visible signs of a submucous cleft are a bifid uvula, a dehiscence in the musculature of the soft palate, and a bony defect in the hard palate. These three do not always appear together: One can be present without the other two and two without the third. All three can be present, and velopharyngeal closure can still be adequate for speech. Furthermore, there can be a defect in the musculature on the nasal or upper surface of the velum that is not visible on the intraoral view but detectable via nasopharyngoscopy. This is sometimes

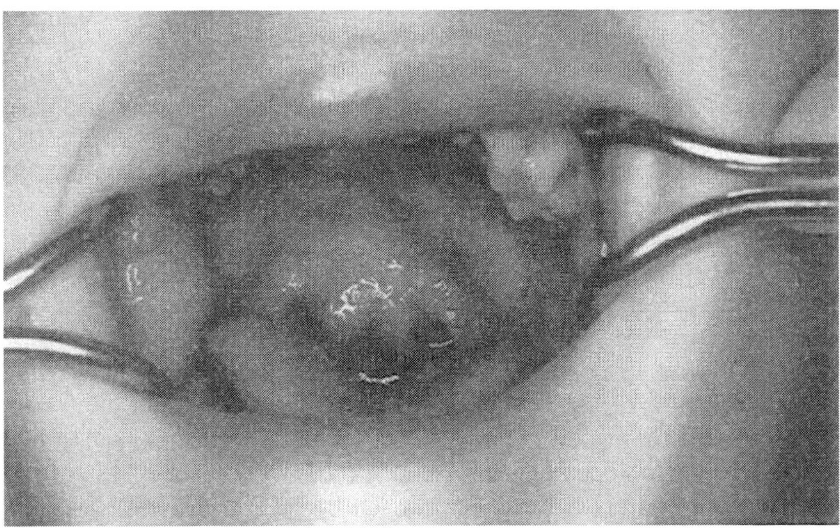

Figure 8.4 Submucous cleft of secondary palate, with bifid uvula and notch into the posterior border of the hard palate.

termed an *occult submucous cleft* and signifies an absence of normal muscular bulk on the upper surface (Croft et al. 1978). This is a situation in which the speech-language pathologist may be puzzled by obvious perceptual evidence of VPI in speech in the absence of an overt abnormality on the intraoral exam.

Noncleft Structural Abnormalities

Even without an overt or submucous cleft, speech can be hypernasal due to other structural problems of the velopharyngeal system. The palate may be congenitally short or the pharynx may be excessively deep. Either situation is essentially palatopharyngeal disproportion. In reviewing the literature on congenitally short palates, it is difficult to draw the line between those cases in which there is clear evidence of a submucous deformity and those in which there is not, primarily because, until the advent of nasopharyngoscopy, clinicians did not have a means of detecting more subtle submucous defects unless the patient was on the operating table. Sometimes the presence of a short palate is masked by a large adenoid pad or other architectural difference in the nasopharynx. An overly large adenoid pad may leave no nasopharyngeal airspace, causing *hyponasality*. Other causes for a lack of normal nasal resonance include various types of nasal obstruction and decreased nasopharyngeal depth. The latter occurs in syndromes in which there is a lack of normal forward growth of the midface. Speech becomes symptomatic for *hypernasality* when the adenoids are surgically removed or when they go through natural involution. (For a more thorough discussion of VPI in the absence of overt cleft palate, see Peterson-Falzone 1985.)

The tonsils can impede velopharyngeal closure if they are positioned between the velum and the posterior pharyngeal wall: Simple removal of the tonsils can cure the closure problem (MacKenzie-Stepner et al. 1987; Shprintzen et al. 1987). Certainly the possibility that enlarged tonsils can actually be impeding velopharyngeal closure indicates that a simultaneous tonsillectomy and secondary procedure on the palate, such as a pharyngeal flap, is an ill-considered approach to management (Argamaso et al. 1988).

Congenital abnormalities of the faucial pillars have been described in sporadic case reports since the late 1800s (see Peterson-Falzone 1985 for a list of references). Some of these reports described speech as being impaired but did not give details. Warren and colleagues (1978) described limitation of velar motion and hypernasal speech in three cases of posterior pillar webbing. However, on the intraoral view, the posterior pillars can appear to merge behind the uvula in individuals with normal speech (Peterson-Falzone 1985).

Insufficient velopharyngeal closure can be acquired as a result of surgical procedures such as removal of part or all of the maxilla or palate in the treatment of neoplastic disease and, occasionally, as a result of a poorly performed tonsillectomy or adenoidectomy. In addition, surgical advancement of the maxilla can lead to velopharyngeal inadequacy, a problem that has generally occurred more often in patients with repaired palatal clefts than in noncleft patients, although the overall reported incidence has been low, even in cases of substantial forward movement of the maxilla (Dalston and Vig 1984; Eskenazi and Schendel 1992; Kummer et al. 1989; Mason et al. 1980; Okazaki et al. 1993; Schwartz et al. 1979; Schwarz and Gruner 1976; Vallino 1990; Witzel and Munro 1977). Preoperative nasopharyngoscopic and videofluoroscopic studies of the velopharyngeal mechanism are now routinely used to help clinicians predict whether a particular patient is vulnerable to this problem.

Neurologic

Dysarthria

Either acquired or congenital neurologic disorders can cause problems in the neuromotor control of the velopharyngeal mechanism. The literature on velopharyngeal deficits attributable to neurologic etiologies is difficult to track because of the variety of forms in which the information is presented. Case descriptions in the medical literature often do not offer much detail on specific speech difficulties in individual patients. Articles on specific types of speech problems often include patients with different diseases, and, to make matters even more confusing, more than one name may be applied to a given disease or set of medical symptoms (e.g., Duffy [1995] listed six different names given to *orofacial dyskinesia*). In a table of neurologic disorders leading to various forms of dysarthria (i.e., flaccid, spastic, ataxic, hypokinetic, hyperkinetic, unilateral upper motor neuron), Duffy (1995) listed 23 degenerative diseases, four demyelinating diseases, three muscle diseases, and two neuromuscular junction diseases, as well as several dozen conditions classified as vascular, traumatic, neoplastic, toxic or metabolic, infectious, inflammatory, anatomic malformation, undetermined etiology, and "other." Duffy (1995) offered extensive detail on the speech symptomatology in each type of dysarthria, basing his information on the clusters of symptoms as originally conceptualized by Darley and colleagues (1969a, b, 1975) and their own clinical observations in several large series of patients at the Mayo Clinic. The following is a synopsis of Duffy's information specific to velopharyngeal function:

1. Flaccid dysarthria (velopharyngeal involvement dependent on site of damage in the final common pathway). Hypernasality, imprecise consonants, nasal emission, short phrases. In a unilateral involvement, the velum hangs lower on the side of the lesion and pulls toward the nonparalyzed side on phonation. The gag may be weak on the involved side.
2. Spastic dysarthria. Hypernasality, imprecise consonants (pressure consonants more severely impaired than in other types of dysarthria). The gag may be hyperactive, but the palate moves minimally or slowly on phonation.
3. Ataxic dysarthria. Abnormal resonance rare (predominantly an articulatory and prosodic disorder). Infrequent reports of hyponasality, presumably reflecting improper timing of velar and articulatory gestures. Oral exam often normal.
4. Hypokinetic dysarthria. Increased nasal airflow during non-nasal target productions. Reduced velocity and degree of velar movement during speech. Abnormal spread of nasalization across syllables.
5. Hyperkinetic dysarthria. May include palatopharyngeal myoclonus, which may have no detectable effect on speech. If apparent during connected speech, the listener may hear slow voice tremor and, less frequently, intermittent hypernasality.
6. Unilateral upper motor neuron dysarthria. Hypernasality heard in 11% of Mayo cases with this type of dysarthria (Duffy's own

observations). Duffy (1995) expressed surprise at this number because of the bilateral upper motor neuron supply to the tenth cranial nerve (CN X). As one possible explanation, he conjectured that the upper motor neuron supply to CN X may not always be completely bilateral in some individuals.*

Duffy (1995) stated that mixed dysarthrias account for more than 34% of all the dysarthric patients seen at the Mayo Clinic and that the most common mixture is flaccid plus spastic. In any patient with mixed dysarthria, the speech symptomatology, including problems in velopharyngeal function, would obviously depend on the particular types of dysarthria apparent in that patient.

Many clinicians have described patients with neuromuscular problems *apparently* affecting only the velopharyngeal system, with no observable problems in the rest of the motor-speech system (see Peterson-Falzone 1985 for a list of references). In 1956, Worster-Drought wrote, "[t]he most frequent example of congenital suprabulbar paresis† affecting a single peripheral organ, I believe to be that of paralysis or weakness of the soft palate; this may be accompanied by an increased jaw jerk‡ but by no other manifestation of the disorder. Paresis of the soft palate may also coexist with only a minor degree of weakness of the tongue or of the orbicularis oris ... I have come to regard an isolated congenital palsy of the soft palate as a manifestation of a mild form of congenital suprabulbar paresis."§ In addition, Johns (1985, p. 156) stated, "[i]n some cases, the palatal paresis or paralysis may be found in isolation; in others, with involvement of other muscle complexes of the oral-facial-pharyngeal-

---

*Duffy (1995) attributed motor innervation of the velum solely to the tenth (vagus) nerve. However, the majority of the motor innervation of the velar musculature comes from the pharyngeal plexus, which receives fibers from the ninth and tenth nerves. The cranial portion of CN XI also innervates the levator palatini and the musculus uvulae (Zemlin 1988). In addition, there is evidence that CN VII may be responsible for fine adjustments in velar position (Nishio et al. 1976a, b). The tensor palatini, which is generally considered not to play a key role in velopharyngeal closure, is innervated by the mandibular branch of CN V.

†The term *congenital suprabulbar paresis* was used as a synonym for cerebral palsy in some of the older literature.

‡A positive jaw jerk reflex is often present in spastic dysarthria (Duffy 1995); however, Duffy stated (p. 138) that spastic dysarthria" is generally not confined to a single component [of speech]."

§According to Duffy (1995), the only type of dysarthria that can result in abnormalities of movement at only one level of speech production is hyperkinetic dysarthria (an involuntary movement disorder), one clinical characteristic of which can be palatal myoclonus. He later stated that intermittent hypernasality can be heard infrequently in palatopharyngeal myoclonus.

laryngeal complex." For the practicing clinician, the possibility of an isolated neurogenic problem in the function of the velopharyngeal system is a dilemma, particularly since experts who specialize in motor disorders of speech have been unable to agree whether involvement of the velopharyngeal system in isolation is even neurologically possible. (Refer to Case 2 in the chapter appendix.)

Apraxia

There are few references to perceptual evidence of VPI in apraxia of speech, either as a result of acquired neurologic damage or in the controversial diagnosis of "developmental apraxia of speech" (Hall et al. 1993). In either case, if apraxia is conceptualized as a problem in the neuromotor programming of speech, it is conceivable that the programming for the nasal-nonnasal contrast could suffer, as well as the programming for other aspects of speech production. Inappropriate nasalization has been described in a few case studies of children with apraxia (Bowman et al. 1984; Dabul 1971; Hall et al. 1990; Weiss et al. 1987; Yoss and Darley 1974). In 1977, Itoh and colleagues described an adult apraxic patient who showed marked variation in velar movement and abnormal movement patterns, including inappropriate coordination of velar movements with the movements of other articulators; however, the report did not describe hypernasality or nasal emission in speech. Noll (1982) conjectured that the lack of mention of perceptual evidence of VPI in this speaker may have been due to the subtlety of the abnormalities of velar motion. However, neither Rosenbek (1985) nor Duffy (1995) mention problems in velopharyngeal control in their discussions of clinical findings in adult apraxia.

Mixed or Unknown Etiology

"Stress" Velopharyngeal Inadequacy

There have been several case reports of VPI in wind instrument players (Argamaso and Shprintzen 1983; Dibbell et al. 1979; Massengill and Quinn 1974; Peterson-Falzone 1985; Weber and Chase 1970), the inadequacy typically being manifest by onset of nasal air leakage after long hours of playing. Weber and Chase (1970) labeled this phenomenon *"stress velopharyngeal incompetence."* In most of the reported cases, speech is not affected. Some of these musicians had demonstrable structural defects, such as a submucous cleft or post-tonsillectomy scarring. Others may have had either a structural defect that was undetected or minor muscular weakness that became apparent only under sustained use of very high intraoral pressure. For this reason, speech-language pathologists cannot categorize this phenomenon as being either exclusively structural or neuromotor.

Phoneme-Specific Nasal Emission

Since the 1940s, there have been sporadic descriptions in the literature of speakers exhibiting nasal emission only on specific phonemes, with non-nasal production of the remainder of the pressure consonants (Beebe 1946; Berry and Eisenson 1942, 1956; Edwards and Shriberg 1983; Hall and Tomblin 1975; Lawson et al. 1972; Peterson 1975; Powers 1971; Van Dantzig 1940; Van Riper 1972; West and Ansberry 1968; West et al. 1937, 1947, 1957). Trost (1981a) coined the term *phoneme-specific velopharyngeal inadequacy,* and later modified the term to *phoneme-specific nasal emission,* using the latter term to encompass the perceptual impression of either nasal emission or posterior nasal frication. This is another velopharyngeal disorder of seemingly heterogeneous etiology because it can be heard in speakers (1) with previously treated clefts (and velopharyngeal systems that function well on everything except the identified phonemes) and (2) with no such clefts or other documented abnormalities of the velopharyngeal system (Peterson-Falzone and Graham 1990). In the former, it is not difficult to conceptualize this phenomenon as either (1) a residual behavior from earlier times when velopharyngeal closure for all pressure consonants was physically impossible or (2) the consequence of greater aerodynamic demands for stop plosives and fricatives, particularly the sibilants. In speakers for whom there is no history of previous anatomic problems, speech-language pathologists postulate a learned behavior of directing the airstream through the nose instead of through the mouth with no clear idea of why or how this happens. One possible contributing factor is early ear disease and hearing loss (Peterson-Falzone and Graham 1990), but this same speech behavior occurs in speakers for whom such a history cannot be documented. In any of these cases, the critical clinical information (and decision) is that traditional surgical or prosthetic treatment of the velopharyngeal system is unlikely to change the speech problem and that, in contrast to cases of true physical inadequacy of the velopharyngeal mechanism, speech therapy is not only likely to be beneficial but the only realistic approach to remediation. It is also important to note that speech therapy is also typically very effective, even in the first session. (Refer to Case 1 in the chapter appendix.)

GETTING STARTED IN THE DIAGNOSTIC PROCESS

Key Items in History Taking

In many nonmedical settings, speech-language pathologists are faced with the task of reconstructing medical histories for the client. What was the situation in infancy and early childhood, and what has transpired since that time? The client may have only a part of his or her medical history available. The extent to which the speech-language pathologist is able to find crucial information depends on what the parent of a child or what the adult patient is willing or able to share. The following is a list of points that can help in finding important information. These points are organized by the particular type of problem the patient presents, although many times that is not known before the history taking. Therefore, the speech-language pathologist may need to inquire about points in more than one "category" of patient.

I. In a patient with a known or suspected cleft:
  A. Family history of any type of cleft. Any individual with a cleft or other craniofacial defect should be examined by a geneticist or dysmorphologist (American Cleft Palate–Craniofacial Association 1993), who should also take a definitive genetic history and carry out any necessary testing. The speech-language pathologist may see the individual before this examination or consultation takes place.
  B. Neonatal problems in feeding, respiration, and weight gain. Be aware that, although clinicians always ask parents if there was a problem with nasopharyngeal regurgitation when their baby was feeding, a positive history for this behavior is not an automatic indication of a problem with the velopharyngeal system. Many noncleft babies exhibit nasal regurgitation, at least on a sporadic or temporary basis.
  C. Early history of ear infections or hearing loss. Certainly, a high number of noncleft babies exhibit ear disease, but children with both overt and submucous clefts of the secondary palate are known to have a higher vulnerability to ear disease than their noncleft peers.
  D. History of surgical interventions (e.g., palatal procedures, tonsillectomy, adenoidectomy). Try to obtain copies of operative reports to be certain of dates and procedures.
  E. Early history of speech and language development. Was speech late in developing? What did the parents hear from their child at 6, 12, and 18 months of age, and can they imitate what they were

hearing? If surgical procedures were done, was there a change in speech postoperatively?

II. In a patient with a known or suspected neuromotor disorder:*
   A. Prenatal and perinatal history. Any known maternal toxic conditions, physical traumas, or diseases; family history of neuromotor disorders; birth history and early development (e.g., Apgar scores, early hypo- or hypertonia); and early feeding and respiratory history.
   B. Childhood illnesses, particularly any that might have been associated with a high fever.
   C. Note any history of accidents or seizures.
   D. Early developmental history. Age at which the child turned over in the crib, sat assisted, sat unassisted, crawled, walked, and so on.
   E. Early history of speech and language development.
   F. Educational and therapy history. Placement in early intervention programs, including physical therapy, occupational therapy, and speech therapy, as well as school placement and achievement.
   G. Age of onset of speech problems and any nonspeech symptoms developing at the same time.
   H. Current medical status of the patient and ongoing treatments.

Key Items in Making Perceptual Judgments

There are four classic perceptual signs of inadequate function of the velopharyngeal mechanism that have been described in multiple references (McWilliams et al. 1990). What is difficult to understand is that virtually all of the perceptual stigmata of VPI can persist even after a speaker has been provided with a physically competent mechanism, most often the presumably compensatory articulations (Trost 1981a; Trost-Cardamone 1987; Trost-Cardamone and Bernthal 1993) that have a notorious reputation for destroying intelligibility. The following are classic perceptual signs of VPI:

1. Nasal emission on pressure consonants (in English, these are the stop plosives, fricatives, and affricates). Perceptually, the nasal air loss can be heard as either laminar airflow or nasal frication (turbulent airflow). The latter is more noisy to the listener and can have multiple sources. Nasal emission can be so mild that it is heard only intermittently or not at all, being detectable only with instrumentation such as pressure-flow devices. The clinician should note that nasal airflow that

*The reader is urged to consult current textbooks and references on neuromotor disorders of speech to learn important points of history-taking in dealing with these speakers.

is heard only inconsistently across all pressure consonants is not the same thing as a phoneme-specific nasal emission.

2. Weakening of the pressure consonants as a direct result of the nasal air loss. These consonants become more difficult for the listener to accurately identify simply because of the lack of normal oral air pressure and oral airflow.

3. Hypernasal resonance that can vary from mild to severe. Resonance deviations can be quite difficult for the beginning clinician to discriminate. Speakers with clefts often have structural deviations of the nose that lead to hyponasality. Other causes of hyponasality include an overly wide pharyngeal flap or an overly wide speech bulb. If a speaker has a pharyngeal flap (or a speech bulb) that is so wide that it does not allow adequate coupling of the oral and nasal cavities for normal nasal resonance but at the same time has inadequate movement of the pharyngeal musculature so that complete velopharyngeal closure is never achieved, the listener hears alternating hypo- and hypernasality. In a speaker who has an inadequately functioning velopharyngeal port but also some nasal obstruction, the perceptual impression may be one of "cul-de-sac" (literally, a blind-ended cavity) resonance.

4. Compensatory articulations (Trost 1981a; Trost-Cardamone 1987; Trost-Cardamone and Bernthal 1993), most often involving retrodisplacement of the place of articulation with manner of production being retained. Trost-Cardamone and Bernthal (1993) gave a thorough explanation of each of these articulations: glottal stops, pharyngeal stops, pharyngeal affricates, pharyngeal fricatives, velar fricatives, mid-dorsum palatal stops, and posterior nasal fricatives. Glottal stops, pharyngeal fricatives, and posterior nasal fricatives can occur both as replacements for normal oral pressure consonants and as coarticulations or simultaneous articulatory maneuvers (a fact that can be very confusing for the beginning clinician). For example, a speaker may simultaneously produce bilabial closure for intended /b/ but actually shut off the vocal airstream at the level of the glottis (glottal stop) instead of the labial valve. The result is that the listener sees a /b/ but hears a glottal stop. Trost-Cardamone's videotape (1987) is an excellent training program for learning to identify and discriminate all of these aberrant articulations.

It is worthwhile to point out that, to a certain extent, speech-language pathologists only presume that the maladaptive articulations just listed are compensatory. There is evidence that glottal placements occur more often in the prespeech vocalizations of babies and toddlers with clefts than in children without clefts (Chapman 1991; Chapman and Hardin 1992; O'Gara and Logemann 1988, 1990), but glottal stops do appear for a short period in the speech of normal babies in the second 6 months of life (Locke 1983; Stoel-Gammon 1988). Bzoch (1965) found no occurrence of glottal stops or pharyngeal fricatives in noncleft preschool children. However, there is no epidemiologic evidence regarding occurrence or lack of occurrence of the other compensatory articulations in noncleft speakers.*

Whether the underlying etiology of a velopharyngeal problem is structural or functional, there are some speakers for whom nasal air loss is inconsistent across all pressure consonants (i.e., not phoneme-specific). Morris (1972) suggested the acronym *SBNA* meaning "sometimes but not always" for the velopharyngeal closure in these speakers. Likewise, for the speaker who shows a consistent but small defect in velopharyngeal closure, Morris suggested the acronym *ABNQ*, meaning "almost but not quite." The function of the velopharyngeal mechanism can be marginal in the sense that closure is possible so long as the speaker is not fatigued; however, closure begins to break down as the speaker tires or as length or complexity of utterance increases. In neurologically involved speakers, any number of problems in neuromotor control can contribute to inconsistent closure.† In speakers with repaired clefts, one can envision a velum stretching to nearly its full length to reach the posterior pharyngeal wall and achieving this feat only inconsistently; there may also be a significant contribution of the pharyngeal walls (posterior, lateral, or both) to closure that begins to tire over time.

In addition to the classic perceptual stigmata associated with inadequate function of the velopharyngeal port, there is ample evidence that loss of a portion of the airstream through an incompetent port can lead to "overdrive" or hyperfunction of the laryngeal system, producing or contributing to the development of vocal nodules and abnormal laryngeal voice quality (McWilliams et al. 1990). This is not considered one of the classic signs of inadequate velopharyngeal closure because there are so many speakers without VPI who have laryngeal voice disorders; however, hoarseness, breathiness, or both is known to occur at a higher rate in speakers with VPI or a history of VPI than in other speakers

*Trost-Cardamone and Bernthal (1993) discussed several reports of the occurrence of nasal fricatives in the speech of noncleft individuals, in a pattern Trost (1981a) labeled phoneme-specific nasal emission. Since this phenomenon has been described in so many speakers with clefts or other anomalies of the velopharyngeal system, it is possible that nasal fricatives should not automatically be classified as compensatory articulations.

†Philips (personal communication, 1995) related an account of a 3-year-old child with a repaired cleft who exhibited inappropriate nasal airflow in speech, echolalia, disfluencies, difficulty in word retrieval, and slowed rate of speech. These behaviors occurred frequently but inconsistently. The neurologist to whom the speech pathologist had referred the child reported no abnormal findings but, at the special request of the speech pathologist, conducted an electroencephalogram that revealed seizure activity, although there were few other clinical signs. The speech problems disappeared when medication was introduced to control the seizures.

(McWilliams et al. 1990). Historically, hypernasality was often labeled a voice disorder, but this leads to confusion: Speakers with VPI can have true voice disorders (i.e., abnormal function of the laryngeal system) in addition to abnormal resonance.

Any of the perceptual signs of inadequate velopharyngeal function listed in this section can persist after a physically adequate velopharyngeal system has been restored through physical intervention. A young child who has had palatal repair past the optimum age in terms of acquisition of speech-production skills can persist in nasal direction of the airstream and in the use of compensatory articulations. For the clinician, the diagnostic decisions for a client at this young age depend on stimulability and the child's variability in productions in different stimulus situations (particularly if the child is so young that definitive imaging studies of the velopharyngeal system in speech are not possible). For older clients who have had velopharyngeal function physically restored long past childhood, all four of the classical stigmata of VPI can persist, in addition to abnormal laryngeal vocal quality. The diagnostic process in either of these situations becomes challenging, particularly because, if the wrong decision is made, the child or adult can be subjected to unnecessary secondary surgery.

The clinician is occasionally faced with the task of trying to decide if the nasal air loss heard in a particular speaker is due to inadequate velopharyngeal closure or an open oronasal fistula. If there is a fistula in the anterior portion of the hard palate, and the velopharyngeal mechanism is actually functioning well in speech, nasal air loss should be restricted to the anterior stops and fricatives. The velar stops should be free of such loss. Another way to discriminate the source of air loss is to temporarily occlude the fistula with a skin barrier material, such as that used to cover stomas, and carry out the perceptual assessment with the fistula both occluded and unoccluded (Reisberg et al. 1985).

VELOPHARYNGEAL MECHANISM ON THE ORAL EXAM

The visual examination of the oral cavity provides some usable information, but there are important limitations and precautions for the speech-language pathologist to keep in mind when conducting an oral exam. These include:

1. When beginning the oral examination, particularly with a young child, do not approach with a tongue depressor in full view as though it were a weapon, because a child (and many adults) might feel

a need to protect himself or herself, even when wanting to be cooperative. Begin by saying, "Put your teeth together—tight—don't let me in!" Use the tongue blade vertically to explore the buccal sulcus on each side. Look at the dentition and occlusion. Only after gaining the child's confidence, ask him or her to open "a little bit, not too much" and then gradually increase the access to the oral cavity with the child's cooperation.

2. Remember that under no circumstances is velopharyngeal closure observable on an oral examination. The closure takes place on the other (nonvisible) side of the velum not on the side that is seen in an oral exam. In addition, do not be fooled into thinking that an adequate assessment of the length of the velum in proportion to pharyngeal depth can be made on the direct intraoral view.

3. If a tongue blade is used to press down on the tongue while asking the client to say "ahh," the upward movement of the velum may be artificially inhibited because of the muscular link between the tongue and the velum (i.e., palatoglossus muscle).

4. Velopharyngeal movement as observed on gag is not a good indicator of movement during speech. Some speakers have a minimal gag response but very active velopharyngeal movement in speech. Others may have a gag that appears hyperactive but lack adequate or appropriate velopharyngeal movement in speech.

5. Observe the position and size of the tonsils. Remember that the upper poles of the tonsils may extend above your level of view, just as the lower poles will most likely be below your level of view. The adenoids are rarely seen on the direct intraoral view, because they are positioned behind the velum.

6. Some fistulae may be anterior in the mouth, and, in a small child, these may be hard to visually identify. Either place the child in a semi-supine position or contort your position if the child is upright. Ask the child or adult to "sniff hard" when looking for a fistula, because natural accumulations of mucous or food residue can easily obscure a patent opening.

7. No matter what the age or level of cooperation of the client, make observations of the oral cavity and the movement of the velum over a repetitive series of views. The behavior of even a normal velopharyngeal mechanism can appear quite different from one examination to another.

8. In observing the soft palate, look for symmetry and asymmetry both at rest and in function. If limited elevation of the velum is seen, is it possible that the upper poles of the tonsils are in the way? Is there an enlarged adenoid pad or other structural limitation in the space over which the velum would normally move in elevation? If so, it will not be seen on the oral examination because, like velopharyngeal closure itself,

the structural limitation will be behind the velum, out of view. Radiographic views will be needed to explore this possibility. Unilateral elevation of the velum may be seen in conditions involving abnormal development of one side of the face (e.g., hemifacial microsomia) or when there is a unilateral mechanical interference with movement, as in one enlarged tonsil.

9. Be on the alert for tremors, fasciculations (fast or slow), or signs of myoclonus in any observable part of the oral and pharyngeal musculature. These can be indicative of problems in neuromotor control.

As an adjunct to the oral exam, the speech-language pathologist may wish to try a few simple, noninvasive techniques for obtaining a gross index of velopharyngeal closure. A small mirror held beneath the nose during production of a sustained fricative or a short speech sample containing oral pressure consonants (not nasal consonants) fogs if nasal air is lost. It is wise to assess each side of the nose separately because of the prevalence of nasal obstruction in individuals with clefts. The See-Scape (The Speech Bin, Vero Beach, FL) is another means of detecting the presence or absence of nasal airflow. It consists of a nasal olive connected by flexible plastic tubing to a rigid tube containing a small piece of Styrofoam. If nasal airflow is present, the Styrofoam rises in the tube. Again, it is wise to assess both sides of the nose. It is also good to remember that small children may enjoy watching the Styrofoam rise in the tube and begin to purposefully direct the airstream through the nose after they see the result it produces. Some clinicians use flexible plastic tubing with a nasal olive simply to help them hear nasal air loss, placing the nasal olive at the end of the client's nose and the end of the tubing in the clinician's ear. The simple, nonelectronic earphones often used on airlines can be used in the same way. In using any of these crude approaches for detecting nasal air loss, the clinician must be careful that he or she is not actually detecting the normal airflow associated with nasal respiration or with production of nasal consonants. Finally, another gross index of velopharyngeal closure used by some clinicians is the "modified tongue-anchor" technique described by Fox and Johns (1970). Using a small piece of sterile gauze, the clinician gently holds the client's tongue tip outside the mouth and directs the client to close his or her lips around the tongue and inflate his or her cheeks. In theory, holding the tongue tip forward prevents the client from using the dorsum of the tongue to assist in velopharyngeal closure. If the client cannot inflate his or her cheeks, velopharyngeal function may be inadequate.

INSTRUMENT-DEPENDENT EVALUATION OF VELOPHARYNGEAL FUNCTION

Instrument-dependent evaluation of velopharyngeal function is generally designed either (1) to measure various consequences of the action of the system (e.g., nasal versus oral airflow, acoustic changes) or (2) to facilitate visualization of the system. In the first case, the "objective" measures serve to validate the clinician's perceptions and judgments. Although as Moll (1964) pointed out, all such objective measures are actually validated against listener judgments. In the second case, the clinician is seeking information that may be critical in making decisions about surgical or prosthetic management of the velopharyngeal system. A third category consists of indirect studies of movement of the system conducted for research purposes rather than for clinical diagnosis: electromyography, movement transduction, and photodetection. Photodetection is still being developed as a possible biofeedback approach and is discussed briefly in the section *Implications for Treatment* at the end of this chapter. For a thorough discussion of instrumental evaluation of velopharyngeal function, see Moon (1993).

MEASURING THE FUNCTION OF THE VELOPHARYNGEAL SYSTEM

Acoustic Instrumentation

Spectrography

Spectrography has been used since the 1940s to study the acoustic characteristics of hypernasality. (See McWilliams et al. 1990 for a detailed review of spectrographic studies.) The major characteristics of nasalization of vowels are (1) reduction in intensity of the first formant; (2) appearance of antiresonances (i.e., sharp drops in the intensity of a portion of the spectrum); (3) appearance of extra resonances, most notably between the first and second formants; and (4) a shift in the center frequencies of the vowel formants. Philips and Kent (1984) reported that spectrograms of nasalized vowels showed an extra "nasal formant" below the first formant, a weakening of intensity and a slight upward shift in frequency of the second formant, an overall reduction of energy, and an increase in formant band widths. Spectrographic equipment is generally found only in speech science or linguistic laboratories, as are the computer-assisted forms of spectrographic analysis. Clinical application is less popular today than it was decades ago, when there were fewer choices of methods for "objectifying" the clinician's perceptual judgments.

Nasometry

Historically, a number of approaches have been used to compare nasal sound pressure level to oral sound pressure. In the 1970s, the TONAR I and TONAR II (Fletcher 1970, 1972) came into clinical use. This was a noninvasive device that gave an index of "nasalance" of speech by measuring nasal sound pressure level and dividing that value by the overall sound pressure level of speech (oral plus nasal). With the increasing use of computer-assisted analyses of speech output, the early TONARs were replaced by the Nasometer (Kay Elemetrics, Pine Brook, NJ). This device consists of a nasal microphone and an oral microphone, which are separated by a horizontal shield. The output of the two microphones are fed into a computerized system that provides a readout of the "nasalance" ratio. The literature contains an increasing number of studies on the use of the Nasometer in clinical settings. In 1991, Dalston and colleagues compared measures of velopharyngeal function from the Nasometer, aerodynamic studies, and perceptual judgments and concluded that the Nasometer could be used "with considerable confidence in corroborating clinical impressions of hypernasality" (Dalston et al., p. 187). The Nasometer is appealing because of its noninvasive nature and because the computer readout is intriguing to children. Clinicians are currently investigating its potential use as a biofeedback device for improving velopharyngeal closure in cases of minimal or inconsistent VPI.

Accelerometry

An accelerometer is a vibration-sensitive device, essentially equivalent to a stethoscope. Moon (1993) pointed out that the use of vibration-sensitive devices on the nose as an approach to measuring velopharyngeal opening has been described since the 1940s. Horii (1980, 1983) described the use of two transducers, one on the nose and one over the thyroid lamina, to produce a ratio of nasal to laryngeal output. As Moon (1993) pointed out, small differences in placement of the transducer can significantly alter results, as can differences in the patency of the two sides of the nose (Moon 1990). To date, there have been only a few studies establishing correlations between accelerometric measurements and perceptual judgments of hypernasality, and some of these have used normal speakers simulating hypernasality rather than speakers with actual VPI. The reported correlations have been moderate to high (Horii 1980, 1983; Redenbaugh and Reich 1985). Like the Nasometer, accelerometry is appealing because of its noninvasiveness. However, the technical requirements are considerable, and the data yielded by the instrumentation are vulnerable to multiple sources of artifacts. Clinical application of the accelerometer has not reached the level of the Nasometer.

Aerodynamic Instrumentation

In 1964, Warren and Dubois developed a quantitative technique for measuring nasal air flow, nasal air pressure, and oral air pressure to calculate the cross-sectional area of the velopharyngeal port (Warren and Dubois 1964). This approach has been used in a lengthy series of studies on large numbers of speakers and has become the standard in aerodynamic investigation of velopharyngeal function. (For more complete references, see McWilliams et al. 1990; Moon 1993; Warren 1989.) Over the series of investigations carried out in Warren's laboratory, normal speakers did not demonstrate cross-sectional areas greater than 0.05 cm^2. Speakers with areas of 0.20 cm^2 or above could not create a pressure differential between the oral and nasal cavities (i.e., the coupling was so great that the two became essentially one cavity). In 1986, Warren suggested four categories of velopharyngeal function based on calculated cross-sectional areas of the port: (1) adequate velopharyngeal function (areas less than 0.05 cm^2), (2) adequate to borderline closure (0.05–0.09 cm^2), (3) borderline to inadequate closure (0.10–0.19 cm^2), and (4) inadequate closure (greater than 0.20 cm^2) (Warren 1986). It should be emphasized that these numbers are estimates of velopharyngeal port area size, not direct measurements. Correlations to other measures of velopharyngeal function have varied. Dalston and Warren (1986) reported their pressure-flow data to correlate at a level of $r = 0.80$ with listener judgments of nasality and $r = 0.74$ with nasalance scores from the TONAR II. However, McWilliams and colleagues (1981) reported an agreement rate of only 23% between categorization of VPI based on pressure-flow data and those derived from videofluoroscopic studies.

Warren (1979) developed a packaged version of his aerodynamic instrumentation that he named the *PERCI*, for "palatal efficiency rating computed instantaneously." PERCI was originally only a screening device that calculated the ratio between oral and nasal air pressures. This device was further developed into the PERCI-PC (Microtronics Corporation, Carrboro, NC), a hardware and software package with expanded capabilities: "This system is used to collect pressure-flow data and the software provides analysis modes for measuring the pressure, air flow, volume, sphincter area, resistance, conductance, and timing variables associated with palatal closure and breathing" (Warren 1989, p. 234). The PERCI-PC has become increasingly popular in clinical settings, despite the cost and the fact that training for the examiner is essential to correct use of the equipment.

It should be pointed out that, in addition to providing estimates of velopharyngeal port size, pressure-flow instrumentation has allowed clinicians and researchers to study other aspects of speech production (e.g., nasal resistance; respiratory volumes; oral port constriction; coordination of timing of activity of the respiratory, articulatory, and velopharyngeal systems), all of which can influence what the listener hears in speech.

IMAGING THE VELOPHARYNGEAL MECHANISM

Radiographic Approaches

Cephalometric Films

Cephalometric films are taken in nearly all orthodontists' offices in lateral, frontal (anterior-posterior [A-P]), and oblique views for purposes of studying the size and relationship of craniofacial structures. These still films are taken with the head in a fixed position and with a fixed x-ray tube-to-focal plane distance, so that the enlargement factor can be measured. Orthodontists use superimposed tracings from films taken on the same child over time to measure changes in size and position of structures resulting from growth and treatment (Figure 8.5). The lateral film is focused at the midsagittal plane and can be used to assess the size and relationship of velopharyngeal structures at rest and perhaps during production of a sustained vowel or fricative (although not during speech itself).

Beginning in the 1960s, reliance on still cephalometric films for images of the velopharyngeal system was gradually replaced first by lateral cinefluoroscopic studies, then by multiview cinefluoroscopy, and ultimately by multiview videofluoroscopy (see *Videofluoroscopy*). Clinically, cephalometric films are still used as a screening device in some settings. The advantages of these films are their relatively low cost, ease of accessibility, and the low radiation dosage of approximately 0.01 rads per film (Moon 1993). The disadvantages are that they cannot be used to study actual speech production, and they provide only a two-dimensional image of a multidimensional system.

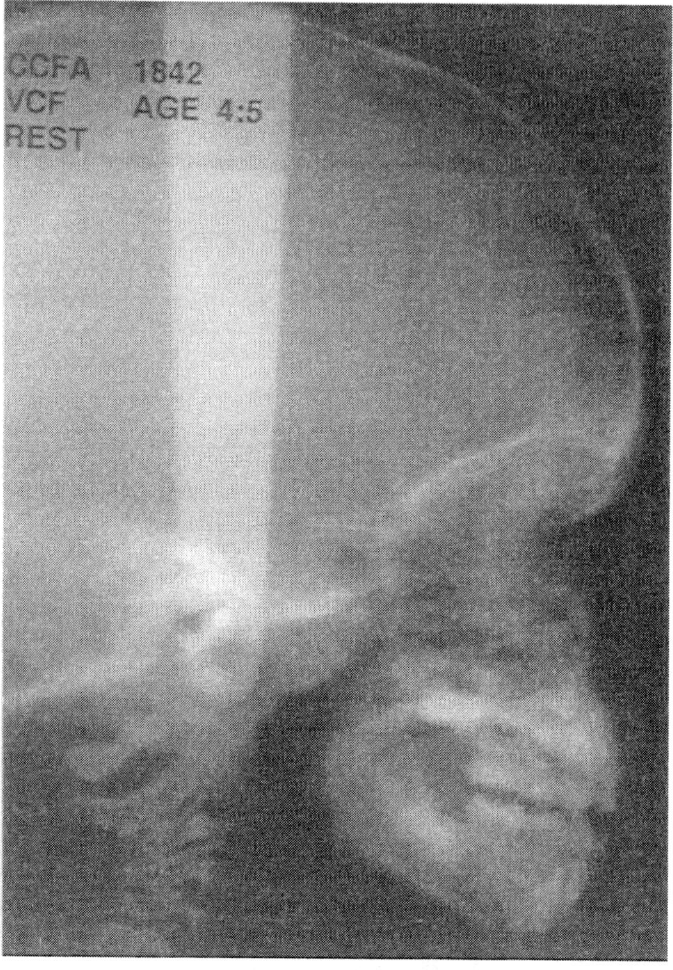

A

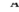

Figure 8.5 A. Lateral cephalometric films at rest in a child with velopharyngeal inadequacy secondary to abnormal pharyngeal depth. B. Lateral cephalometric films during sustained /s/ in the same child.

Videofluoroscopy

Currently, the most popular radiographic imaging technique for studying the velopharyngeal mechanism is multiview videofluoroscopy. The most commonly used views are the lateral, frontal, and base. The lateral view, like the lateral cephalometric film discussed in the previous section, is focused at the midsagittal plane. It allows the examiner to see movement of the velum and any anterior movement of the posterior pharyngeal wall, as well as movements of the tongue

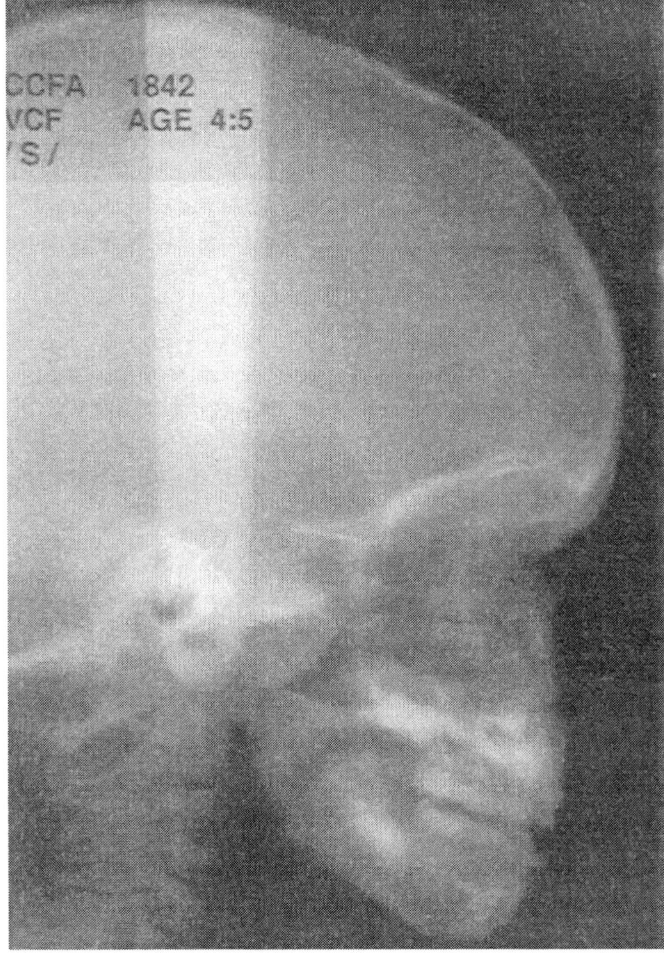

B

and mandible. In the frontal view, the examiner can see the amount and vertical level of inward movement of the lateral pharyngeal walls. The base view provides a horizontal or transverse picture of the system, showing the contribution of all of these structures (the velum, posterior pharyngeal wall, lateral pharyngeal walls) toward closure. It was this view that prompted Skolnick and colleagues (1973) to urge clinicians to "think sphincter" in conceptualizing velopharyngeal closure. Sometimes oblique views are used when asymmetric movement of the velum is suspected. Additional views include Towne's projection, which is an angled view from above that is used to more accurately image the velum approximating the adenoid pad, and Waters' projection, which is an angled view from below that is used for imaging lateral pharyngeal wall motion when bony structures interfere with seeing that motion in the straight-on frontal view (Witzel and Stringer 1990).

Multiview videofluoroscopy has provided a wealth of information about the function of the velopharyngeal system both in normal speakers and in speakers with various types of velopharyngeal problems. (For an extensive list of references, please see McWilliams et al. 1990; Peterson-Falzone 1988; Skolnick and Cohn 1989.) It was not until this imaging technique became easily accessible that it was learned, for example, that there are four basic patterns of velopharyngeal closure, categorized by the relative contribution of the velum and pharyngeal walls, in both noncleft and cleft palate speakers (Croft et al. 1981). The most common pattern of velopharyngeal closure in either normal or cleft speakers is coronal (i.e., the major or sole movement toward closure is in the velum itself). Additional patterns include sagittal (little contribution of the velum or posterior pharyngeal wall with closure accomplished by inward movement of the lateral pharyngeal walls), circular (approximately equal contribution from all components), and circular with Passavant's ridge. Small central deficits in closure had previously eluded standard lateral radiographic imaging and were not seen until the advent of the base or transverse view. Asynchronous movements of the components of the system could not be appreciated without multiple views nor could movements occurring at disparate vertical levels. In any of these three situations, speakers might previously have been labeled as exhibiting "functional" (physically inexplicable) VPI because prior imaging techniques could not detect the problem.

For obvious reasons, multiview videofluoroscopy has improved planning for physical intervention (surgical, prosthetic) and helped to identify speakers in whom very small or inconsistent deficits in closure may respond to behavioral therapy. The advantage of multiview videofluoroscopy is the amount of information that can be obtained on the individual patient. The disadvantage is the radiation dosage. Although the amount of radiation varies with the length of the study, the specific equipment, and the area exposed, the dosage estimates given by Skolnick and Cohn (1989) indicated that a multiview study could reach as much as 2.5 rads for a 3-minute study, which is more than 60% of the annual radiation limit for a small child.

Computed Tomography

Computed tomography (CT) imaging of the velopharyngeal system was first reported by Honjo and colleagues in 1984. The limitations at the time included the facts that (1) the images were restricted to viewing the system at rest or in prolongation of a phoneme (similar to the restrictions on still cephalometric films), (2) the level of velopharyngeal activity had to be predetermined to be certain that the obtained "slice" would capture the activity, (3) the activity had to be sustained for more than 3 seconds, (4) the speaker had to be in a supine position, and (5) the radiation dosage for a single slice varied from 0.5 to 3.0 rads. As the technology developed, motion picture, or cine CT, scans became available, reducing scan times and allowing for scanning of multiple slices simultaneously. As Moon (1993) described this technique, each scan represents a single frame in the cine CT, and the radiation dosage per scan is 0.1 rads (10 times that for a cephalometric film). Cine CT allows for visualization of all sides of the velopharyngeal system at different levels (Moon and Smith 1987) but is subject to problems in resolution due to the thickness of the imaging "slice" and other technical problems. As of this writing, there have been few reports on the use of cine CT in viewing the velopharyngeal system either in normal speakers or speakers with VPI. This is not surprising in view of the technologic constraints and the cost and relative inaccessibility of the equipment.

Nonradiographic Imaging of the Velopharyngeal System

Magnetic Resonance Imaging

Currently, the most exciting prospect in nonradiographic imaging of the velopharyngeal system is magnetic resonance imaging (MRI). MRI provides realistic soft-tissue images in a two-dimensional plane without the use of radiation. The first report of the use of MRI to study the speech mechanism appeared in 1987 (Baer et al. 1987), with subsequent reports in 1991 and 1992 (Baer et al. 1991; Moore 1992; Sulter et al. 1992). In 1993, Moon (p. 270) wrote, "[w]ith advances in technology, MRI will undoubtedly receive a great deal of attention as an alternative to radiographic imaging of the velopharyngeal mechanism." His words were prophetic: Since 1993, the technology has changed significantly to the extent that previous technical limitations (e.g., number of images per second, speaker position) are either no longer in effect or are destined for extinction. For example, previous technology had limited image acquisition to four images per second (which is far too slow to allow real-time imaging of speech), and studies could be obtained only with the subject in a supine position in an elongated tube. Image acquisition rates are now 40 per second in some laboratories. This far exceeds the number of images available in videofluoroscopy (Johns and Rohrich 1995). In addition, the technology allows the speaker to remain in an upright (seated) position with the head inside a relatively small "doughnut," instead of the entire body being encased in a tube. MRI allows clinicians to obtain multiple views of the velopharyngeal system in motion without radiation and without invasive endoscopes.

Endoscopy

Oral Endoscopy

In 1966, Taub described the use of a rigid endoscope with an angled viewing end for looking at velopharyngeal closure. The obvious limitations of the instrument were that speech samples were severely limited (typically to a sustained open vowel) with a rigid tube in the oral cavity, but the technique attracted interest because it did not involve radiation. A few studies of velopharyngeal function used this technique (Willis and Stutz 1972; Zwitman et al. 1974, 1976). Oral endoscopy was almost immediately supplanted by nasopharyngoscopy, but Karnell and Morris (1985) pointed out that some aspects of velopharyngeal function, particularly the contribution of anterior motion of the posterior pharyngeal wall, may be better appreciated on the oral as opposed to the nasal endoscopic view and advocated the use of both views in clinical practice.

Nasopharyngoscopy

In 1969, Pigott first reported on the use of a side-viewing rigid nasoendoscope to study velopharyngeal closure (Pigott 1969). This view from above the velopharyngeal port provided a transverse or horizontal image of the system without interfering with speech. Nasoendoscopy (or nasopharyngoscopy) soon became a major tool for evaluating the velopharyngeal system, with flexible fiberoptic endoscopes becoming more popular than rigid scopes because of patient comfort and compliance. There are now many different rigid and flexible scopes commercially available, each with different characteristics (e.g., diameter, angle of view, cone of acceptance, light-conducting capabilities). For complete discussions of types of equipment and for information on examination procedure, the reader is referred to Karnell (1994) and Shprintzen (1995a, b, 1997). (See Case 2 in the chapter appendix.)

Flexible fiberoptic nasopharyngoscopes have an adjustable tip, allowing the examiner to insert the scope into the nose and then angle the tip downward to obtain the transverse view of the velopharyngeal port. This is equivalent to the base view in videofluoroscopy. However, the tip can also be moved or rotated to different angles when the examiner wants to look at particular structures more closely; for example, to view each pharyngeal orifice of the eustachian tube or each lateral port on the side of a pharyngeal flap independently (Karnell 1994; Shprintzen 1995a, 1997). By extending the end of the scope down past the velum, the examiner can also examine the rest of the vocal tract, including the larynx (Karnell 1994; Witzel and Stringer 1990).

The image from either rigid or flexible endoscopy is typically recorded on videotape for purposes of record keeping, cross comparison among speakers, longitudinal comparisons in individual speakers, pre- and postmanagement comparisons, and so on. Because the procedure does not involve radiation, there is no "safety" limit to the length of examination or the number of times a given speaker can be examined. It can be used as a tool for biofeedback and has become a standard means of improving physical management (e.g., surgery, prosthetic treatment) of VPI (Shprintzen 1995b, 1997).

As with multiview videofluoroscopy, nasopharyngoscopy has taught clinicians much about the function of the velopharyngeal system both in normal speakers and in speakers with velopharyngeal problems. For extensive references that chronicle the contribution of this technology, see Karnell (1994) and Shprintzen (1995a, 1997).

Nasopharyngoscopy requires administration of a topical anesthetic and is an invasive procedure in the sense that it requires the insertion of a foreign body (the scope) into a body cavity (the nose). It should not be performed outside of a medical setting.

IMPLICATIONS FOR TREATMENT

The options for treating problems in velopharyngeal function should *not* be viewed as discrete, independent categories. They are often used in combination or sequentially, and the sequence varies with the particular problem(s) the speaker presents. That is why accurate diagnosis is so important.

Overall, the treatment options include

- Surgical management
  - Primary palatoplasty of clefts
  - A variety of surgical approaches to noncleft VPI
  - Secondary surgical procedures when the primary palatoplasty has not provided a functioning velopharyngeal mechanism (These procedures are essentially the same as those used in noncleft VPI.)
- Prosthetic management
  - Palatal plate with a pharyngeal bulb if an overt cleft is not to be closed surgically (Small palatal plates are also used to obturate palatal fistulae.)

    A pharyngeal bulb if the palate is short (e.g., repaired palate, submucous cleft palate that is short)
    A palatal lift if the palate is inadequate in mobility
  Behavioral management
    Approaches to changing muscle (i.e., mass, strength, endurance) (Starr 1993)
    Approaches to changing velopharyngeal muscle control (Starr 1993)
    Approaches to changing articulatory behaviors, which can have a secondary effect on behavior of the velopharyngeal system
    Approaches to changing respiratory or laryngeal behaviors to reduce the amount of hypernasality heard by the listener, although there is no direct effect on behavior of the velopharyngeal mechanism

Details on surgical and prosthetic management of velopharyngeal problems can be found in several comprehensive sources (Bardach and Morris 1990; McWilliams et al. 1990; Moller and Starr 1993; Shprintzen and Bardach 1995) and are not discussed here. Behavioral management of VPI is a broad and controversial topic that has intrigued clinicians for decades. Proponents of various approaches to achieving either increased strength or improved coordination (timing) of velopharyngeal closure were historically vague about their specific goal or why their approach might work. For comprehensive discussions of this topic, see Ruscello (1989), Starr (1993), and Tomes and colleagues (1997). This chapter includes only some approaches appearing (or still appearing) in current clinical reports.

Trost-Cardamone and Bernthal (1993) provided helpful guidelines for using the perceptual speech information to choose approaches to treatment. In condensed form, the following are those guidelines:

1. Compensatory articulations, no hypernasality, or nasal emission: articulation therapy to modify compensatory placements
2. Phoneme-specific nasal air emission: articulation therapy to eliminate pattern
3. Pervasive and moderate-to-severe hypernasality and nasal emission across phonetic contexts with no compensatory articulations: physical management (surgical or prosthetic), then postmanagement reassessment.
4. Compensatory articulations accompanied by nasal emission; marginal or adequate closure on orally articulated pressure consonants: four steps in treatment: (1) articulation therapy to modify compensatory placement, watching for changes in nasal emission as oral placements are established; (2) pre- and post-treatment

nasopharyngoscopy; (3) nasopharyngoscopy biofeedback to modify pharyngeal compensatory articulations, glottal compensatory articulations, or both; (4) speech-training appliance (e.g., speech bulb) to close velopharyngeal port and facilitate modification of compensatory articulations. (In this sequence, Trost-Cardamone and Bernthal [1993] appeared to suggest the third and fourth alternatives if therapy to modify compensatory placements *without* biofeedback or a speech bulb does not work.)

5. Mild nasal emission and hypernasality across phonetic contexts; no compensatory articulations: Nasopharyngoscopy biofeedback to modify velopharyngeal closure or combined nasopharyngoscopy and bulb reduction program to achieve velopharyngeal closure.

Trost-Cardamone and Bernthal (1993), along with many other clinicians writing about therapy for speakers with clefts, emphasized the importance of correcting compensatory articulations before making a decision that further physical management is necessary. In fact, McWilliams and colleagues wrote (1990, p. 378), "[c]ertainly it is the case that pharyngeal flap surgery, for example, should never be performed when the patient shows only glottal and pharyngeal speech articulation. . . Any such patient must have speech therapy first to teach appropriate placement for plosives and fricatives in order to assess adequacy of speech aerodynamics." This situation corresponds to the first item in the Trost-Cardamone and Bernthal guidelines. In the fourth item, Trost-Cardamone and Bernthal are stating that correcting compensatory articulations can actually eliminate nasal emission. From the work of Henningsson and Isberg (1986), it is known that the velopharyngeal mechanism behaves differently when speakers are using glottal articulations as opposed to oral articulations. In 1986, Hoch and colleagues advocated eliminating compensatory articulations before pharyngeal-flap or other physical management, even when nasal air loss was pervasive across all pressure consonants, including those produced without compensatory placements (Hoch et al. 1986). Note that this is quite different from the position taken by Trost-Cardamone and Bernthal (1993) or McWilliams and colleagues (1990). In fact, Trost-Cardamone and Bernthal did not directly address what the treatment decision should be or what the first step in treatment should be if the speaker is exhibiting both compensatory articulations and pervasive nasal emission.

As mentioned previously, nasopharyngoscopy has become a popular tool for biofeedback when a speaker is trying to learn to change the behavior of the velopharyngeal system, although application is limited to medical settings (Golding-Kushner 1995; Hoch et al. 1986; Witzel et al. 1989). Other forms of biofeedback in use or in development include the Nasometer, discussed in the section *Nasometry*, and the photodetector (Dalston 1982, 1989; Dalston and Keefe 1987). The photodetector consists of two small fiberoptic fibers inserted through the nasal cavity, one fiber acting as the light source and the other as the "detector" fiber. The ends are placed such that the light source fiber is below the velopharyngeal port and the detector fiber above the port. Movement toward velopharyngeal closure is "tracked" by the amount of light detected by the second fiber.* As of this writing, use of the photodetector as a feedback device is under study. With either the Nasometer or the photodetector, the feedback to the speaker is the analog signal or trace on an oscilloscope or computer screen, not an actual view of the velopharyngeal mechanism.

Use of any form of biofeedback about the behavior of the velopharyngeal mechanism should be limited to those cases in which there is an indication that the system is in fact capable of closure (i.e., the velum is long enough). However, even when there is *no* movement seen in the velopharyngeal system, biofeedback may be useful to see if movement (and perhaps velopharyngeal closure) is possible without surgery or a prosthesis.

One form of biofeedback that does not track the behavior of the velopharyngeal mechanism itself is palatography, which consists of a palatal plate embedded with electrodes that provide visual feedback of articulatory contacts. This technology has been used to modify articulatory contacts in cleft palate speakers (Michi et al. 1993). This device is commercially available as the Palatometer (Kay Elemetrics, Pine Brook, New Jersey).

The "bulb reduction" program mentioned by Trost-Cardamone and Bernthal (1993) is an approach to changing velopharyngeal behavior that has been described in the literature since the 1960s (Blakeley 1960, 1964, 1969; McGrath and Anderson 1990; Weiss 1971; Weiss and Louis 1972). The goal of the program is to stimulate increased motion of the pharyngeal walls; however, there are two different interpretations as to why increased movement is obtained. In the first interpretation, the presence of a large, obstructing bulb in the velopharynx completely eliminates any possibility of nasal emission. Although complete obstruction of the port does not in itself eliminate compensatory articulations, Trost-Cardamone and Bernthal (1933), like others before them, suggested the obstruction of the bulb may "facilitate" modification of those articulatory behaviors. If oral placements are learned and then maintained with a smaller bulb or no bulb at all, velopharyngeal

*A similar device called the velograph was described by Kunzel in 1982 and was also advocated as a means for patients to learn to control velopharyngeal muscle activity.

behavior has been successfully modified. The second interpretation focuses on the physical effect of a large bulb in the velopharynx "stimulating" the pharyngeal walls, producing motion where there was none or very little. Some clinicians view the bulb as providing resistance to mesial or anterior movement of the pharyngeal walls; others simply say the presence of the bulb against the pharyngeal walls stimulates movement without explaining why this occurs. Regardless of the proposed theoretical basis, or lack of a theoretical basis, clinicians have reported increased pharyngeal wall motion after placement of the bulb, further increments in motion as the bulb is reduced in size, and, in some cases, complete elimination of the bulb (Blakeley 1960, 1964, 1969; McGrath and Anderson 1990; Weiss 1971; Weiss and Louis 1972). Documentation of bulb-reduction programs and the results produced has been greatly improved through the use of endoscopy (Golding-Kushner et al. 1995).

In the realm of behavioral therapy for VPI, there were many older approaches for supposedly strengthening the musculature, including blowing, sucking, swallowing, and even electrical stimulation. There was little empirical evidence, however, that any of these were effective (Ruscello 1989; Starr 1993; Tomes et al. 1997). A more recent approach to strengthening velopharyngeal musculature, specifically the levator palatini, is Kuehn's (1991) resistance technique using continuous positive airway pressure (CPAP). In this approach, the resistance to upward movement of the velum is the heightened airway pressure delivered to the nasal cavities by the CPAP device. Kuehn (1991) set forth a detailed protocol for use over an 8-week period in a home-therapy program. The results varied in the first few patients subjected to the program, and an intercenter study is underway to determine the effectiveness of CPAP resistance therapy in speakers with various degrees of VPI.

As concluded by Tomes and colleagues (1997), the paucity of conclusive research regarding behavioral treatments of VPI could lead one to think that there is little hope of any of these procedures proving to be effective. However, as pointed out by those authors, there is a clinical need for noninvasive treatments, and the limited data that are in clinical reports suggest that certain speakers may have the potential for improving closure without surgery.

Finally, in the broad range of velopharyngeal problems covered in this chapter and in the current array of treatment approaches, it is tempting to think that, no matter what the specific nature of the velopharyngeal problem presented by the patient, there must be something that will cure the problem. That is not the case, particularly for a speaker who presents with neurologic problems. Both historically and currently, surgical approaches to "curing" VPI in neurogenically based disorders have been only partially satisfactory, a clinical finding that has led to a preference for prosthetic management with either a speech bulb or a palatal lift, depending on the velopharyngeal physiology in each patient (Johns 1985). Even in patients without known neurogenic disorders, lack of movement in the velopharyngeal system calls for caution in predicting the outcome of treatment. More recently, Witt and colleagues (1995) chronicled their experiences in trying to manage "black-hole" problems in velopharyngeal function, meaning velopharyngeal systems exhibiting little to no mobility in speech. Despite the prosthetic and surgical management options used with their 36 patients who had a "hypodynamic" velopharynx, the authors reported an overall success rate of 58.3% in primary treatment and 46.2% when secondary procedures were necessary. While the number of cases in this report was small, the frustration expressed by the authors (an interdisciplinary team using current diagnostic technology and a range of physical management approaches) was a reminder that fully functional velopharyngeal closure is not yet possible for every patient.

REFERENCES

American Cleft Palate–Craniofacial Association. (1993) Parameters for evaluation of cleft lip/palate or other craniofacial anomalies. *Cleft Palate–Craniofacial Journal* 30(Supplement 1), S1–S16.

Argamaso RV, Shprintzen RJ. (April 1983) Fanfare for a Pharyngeal Flap. Videotape presentation before the American Cleft Palate Association, Denver.

Argamaso RV, Bassila M, Bratcher GO, et al. (1988) Tonsillectomy and pharyngeal flap operation should not be performed simultaneously [letter to the editor]. *Cleft Palate Journal* 25, 176–177.

Baer T, Gore JC, Boyce S, Nye PW. (1987) Application of MRI to the analysis of speech production. *Magnetic Resonance Imaging* 5, 1–7.

Baer T, Gore JC, Gracco LC, Nye PW. (1991) Analysis of vocal tract shape and dimensions using magnetic resonance imaging: vowels. *Journal of the Acoustical Society of America* 90, 799–828.

Bardach J, Morris HL. (1990) *Multidisciplinary Management of Cleft Lip and Palate.* Philadelphia: Saunders.

Beebe HH. (1946) Sigmatismus nasalis. *Journal of Speech Disorders* 11, 35–37.

Berry MF, Eisenson J. (1942) *The Defective in Speech.* New York: Appleton-Century-Crofts.

Berry MF, Eisenson J. (1956) *Speech Disorders, Principles, and Practices of Therapy.* New York: Appleton-Century-Crofts.

Blakeley RW. (1960) Temporary speech prosthesis as an aid in speech training. *Cleft Palate Bulletin* 10, 63–65.

Blakeley RW. (1964) The complementary use of speech prostheses and pharyngeal flaps in palatal insufficiency. *Cleft Palate Journal* 1, 194–198.

Blakeley RW. (1969) The rationale for a temporary speech prosthesis in palatal insufficiency. *British Journal of Disorders of Communication* 4, 134–139.

Bowman SN, Parsons CL, Morris DA. (1984) Inconsistency of phonological errors in developmental verbal dyspraxic children as a factor of linguistic task and performance load. *Australian Journal of Human Communication Disorders* 12, 109–119.

Bzoch KR. (1965) Articulation proficiency and error patterns of preschool cleft palate and normal children. *Cleft Palate Journal* 2, 340–349.

Chapman KL. (1991) Vocalizations of toddlers with cleft lip and palate. *Cleft Palate–Craniofacial Journal* 28, 172–178.

Chapman KL, Hardin MA. (1992) Phonetic and phonologic skills of two-year-olds with cleft palate. *Cleft Palate–Craniofacial Journal* 29, 435–443.

Croft CB, Shprintzen RJ, Daniller A, Lewin ML. (1978) The occult submucous cleft palate and the musculus uvulae. *Cleft Palate Journal* 15, 150–154.

Croft CB, Shprintzen RJ, Rakoff SJ. (1981) Patterns of velopharyngeal valving in normal and cleft palate subjects: a multi-view videofluoroscopic and nasoendoscopic study. *Laryngoscope* 91, 265–271.

Dabul BL. (1971) Lingual incoordination-language delay. *California Journal of Communication Disorders* 2, 30–33.

Dalston RM. (1982) Photodetector assessment of velopharyngeal activity. *Cleft Palate Journal* 19, 1–8.

Dalston RM. (1989) Using simultaneous photodetection and nasometry to monitor velopharyngeal behavior during speech. *Journal of Speech and Hearing Research* 32, 195–202.

Dalston RM, Keefe MJ. (1987) The use of a microcomputer in monitoring and modifying velopharyngeal movements. *Journal of Computer Users in Speech and Hearing* 3, 159.

Dalston RM, Vig PS. (1984) Effects of orthognathic surgery on speech: a prospective study. *American Journal of Orthodontics* 86, 291–298.

Dalston RM, Warren DW. (1986) Comparison of TONAR II, pressure flow, and listener judgments of hypernasality in the assessment of velopharyngeal function. *Cleft Palate Journal* 23, 108–115.

Dalston RM, Warren DW, Dalston ET. (1991) Use of nasometry as a diagnostic tool for identifying patients with velopharyngeal impairment. *Cleft Palate–Craniofacial Journal* 28, 184–189.

Darley FL, Aronson AE, Brown J. (1969a) Clusters of deviant diagnostic patterns of dysarthria. *Journal of Speech and Hearing Research* 12, 462–496.

Darley FL, Aronson AE, Brown J. (1969b) Differential diagnostic patterns of dysarthria. *Journal of Speech and Hearing Research* 12, 246–269.

Darley FL, Aronson AE, Brown J. (1975) *Motor Speech Disorders*. Philadelphia: Saunders.

Dibbell DG, Ewanowski S, Carter WL. (1979) Successful correction of velopharyngeal stress incompetence in musicians playing wind instruments. *Plastic and Reconstructive Surgery* 64, 662–664.

Duffy JR. (1995) *Motor Speech Disorders: Substrates, Differential Diagnosis, and Management*. St. Louis: Mosby.

Edwards ML, Shriberg LD. (1983) *Phonology: Applications in Communicative Disorders*. San Diego, CA: College-Hill.

Eskenazi LB, Schendel SA. (1992) An analysis of Le Fort I maxillary advancement in cleft lip and palate patients. *Plastic and Reconstructive Surgery* 90, 779–786.

Fletcher SG. (1970) Theory and instrumentation for quantitative measurement of nasality. *Cleft Palate Journal* 7, 601–609.

Fletcher SG. (1972) Contingencies for bioelectric modification of nasality. *Journal of Speech and Hearing Disorders* 37, 329–346.

Folkins J. (1988) Velopharyngeal nomenclature: incompetence, inadequacy, insufficiency, and dysfunction. *Cleft Palate Journal* 25, 413–416.

Fox DR, Johns DF. (1970) Predicting velopharyngeal closure with a modified tongue-anchor technique. *Journal of Speech and Hearing Disorders* 35, 248–251.

Golding-Kushner KJ. (1995) Treatment of Articulation and Resonance Disorders Associated with Cleft Palate and VPI. In RJ Shprintzen, J Bardach (eds), *Management of Cleft Palate Speech* (pp. 327–351). St. Louis: Mosby.

Golding-Kushner KJ, Cisneros GJ, LeBlanc EM. (1995) Speech Bulbs. In RJ Shprintzen, J Bardach (eds), *Management of Cleft Palate Speech* (pp. 352–363). St. Louis: Mosby.

Hall PK, Tomblin JB. (1975) Case study: therapy procedures and remediation of a nasal lisp. *Language, Speech, and Hearing Services in Schools* 6, 29–32.

Hall PK, Hardy JC, LaVelle WE. (1990) A child with signs of developmental apraxia of speech with whom a palatal lift prosthesis was used to manage palatal dysfunction. *Journal of Speech and Hearing Disorders* 55, 454–460.

Hall PK, Jordan LS, Robin DA. (1993) *Developmental Apraxia of Speech: Theory and Clinical Practice*. Austin, TX: PRO-ED.

Henningsson GE, Isberg AM. (1986) Velopharyngeal movement patterns in patients alternating between oral and glottal articulation: a clinical and cineradiographical study. *Cleft Palate Journal* 23, 1–9.

Hoch L, Golding-Kushner KJ, Sadewitz V, Shprintzen RJ. (1986) Speech therapy. In BJ McWilliams (ed), *Seminars in Speech and Language: Current Methods of Assessing and Treating Children with Cleft Palates* 7, 313–325.

Honjo I, Mitoma T, Ushiro K, Kawano M. (1984) Evaluation of velopharyngeal closure by CT scan and endoscopy. *Plastic and Reconstructive Surgery* 74, 620–627.

Horii Y. (1980) An accelerometric approach to nasality measurement: a preliminary report. *Cleft Palate Journal* 17, 254–261.

Horii Y. (1983) An accelerometric measure as a physical correlate of perceived hypernasality in speech. *Journal of Speech and Hearing Research* 26, 476–480.

Itoh M, Sasanuma S, Ushijima T. (1977) Velar movements during speech in a patient with apraxia of speech. *Annual Bulletin of the Research Institute of Logopedics and Phoniatry, University of Tokyo* 11, 67–75.

Johns DF. (1985) Surgical and Prosthetic Management of Neurogenic Velopharyngeal Incompetency in Dysarthria. In DF Johns (ed), *Clinical Management of Neurogenic Communicative Disorders* (2nd ed) (pp. 153–177). Boston: Little, Brown.

Johns DF, Rohrich RJ. (April 1995) Functional Magnetic Resonance Imaging of the Velopharynx: Technique and Future Application. Presented before the American Cleft Palate-Craniofacial Association, Tampa.

Karnell MP. (1994) *Videoendoscopy: From Velopharynx to Larynx*. San Diego: Singular.

Karnell MP, Morris HL. (1985) Multiview endoscopic evaluations of velopharyngeal physiology in 15 normal speakers. *Annals of Otology, Rhinology and Laryngology* 94, 361–365.

Kuehn DP. (1991) New therapy for treating hypernasal speech using continuous positive airway pressure (CPAP). *Plastic and Reconstructive Surgery* 88, 959–966.

Kummer AW, Strife JL, Grau WH, et al. (1989) The effects of Le Fort I osteotomy with maxillary movement on articulation, resonance, and velopharyngeal function. *Cleft Palate Journal* 26, 193–199.

Kunzel H. (1982) First applications of a biofeedback device for the therapy of velopharyngeal incompetence. *Folia Phoniatrica* 34, 92–100.

Lawson LI, Chierici G, Castro A, et al. (1972) Effects of adenoidectomy on the speech of children with potential velopharyngeal dysfunction. *Journal of Speech and Hearing Disorders* 37, 390–402.

Locke JL. (1983) *Phonological Acquisition and Change*. New York: Academic Press.

MacKenzie-Stepner M, Witzel MA, Stringer DA, Laskin R. (1987) Velopharyngeal insufficiency due to hypertrophic tonsils: a report of two cases. *International Journal of Pediatric Otorhinolaryngology* 14, 57–63.

Mason RM, Turvey TA, Warren DW. (1980) Speech considerations with maxillary advancement procedures. *Journal of Oral Surgery* 38, 752–758.

Massengill R, Quinn G. (1974) Adenoidal atrophy, velopharyngeal incompetence and sucking exercises: a two-year follow-up case report. *Cleft Palate Journal* 11, 196–199.

McGrath CO, Anderson MW. (1990) Prosthetic Treatment of Velopharyngeal Incompetence. In J Bardach, HL Morris (eds), *Multidisciplinary Management of Cleft Lip and Palate* (pp. 809–815). Philadelphia: Saunders.

McWilliams BJ, Morris HL, Shelton RL. (1990) *Cleft Palate Speech* (2nd ed). Toronto: BC Decker.

McWilliams BJ, Glaser ER, Philips BJ, et al. (1981) A comparative study of four methods of evaluating velopharyngeal adequacy. *Plastic and Reconstructive Surgery* 68, 1–10.

Michi K, Yamashita Y, Imai S, et al. (1993) Role of visual feedback treatment for defective /s/ sounds in patients with cleft palate. *Journal of Speech and Hearing Research* 36, 277–285.

Moll KL. (1964) 'Objective' measures of nasality [letter to the editor]. *Cleft Palate Journal* 1, 371–374.

Moller KT, Starr CD. (1993) *Cleft Palate: Interdisciplinary Issues and Treatment*. Austin, TX: PRO-ED.

Moon JB. (1993) Evaluation of Velopharyngeal Function. In KT Moller, CD Starr (eds), *Cleft Palate: Interdisciplinary Issues and Treatment* (pp. 251–306). Austin, TX: PRO-ED.

Moon JB. (1990) The influence of nasal patency on accelerometric transduction of nasal bone vibration. *Cleft Palate Journal* 27, 266–270.

Moon JB, Smith WL. (1987) Application of cine CT technology to the assessment of velopharyngeal function. *Cleft Palate Journal* 24, 226–232.

Moore CA. (1992) The correspondence of vocal tract resonance with volumes obtained from magnetic resonance images. *Journal of Speech and Hearing Research* 35, 1009–1023.

Morris HL. (1972) Cleft Palate. In A Weston (ed), *Communicative Disorders* (pp. 128–159). Springfield, IL: Thomas.

Morris HL. (1973) Velopharyngeal competence and primary cleft palate surgery: 1960–1971: a critical review. *Cleft Palate Journal* 10, 62–71.

Nishio J, Matsuya T, Machida J, Miyazaki T. (1976a) The motor nerve supply of the velopharyngeal muscles. *Cleft Palate Journal* 13, 20–30.

Nishio J, Matsuya T, Ibuki K, Miyazaki T. (1976b) Roles of the facial, glossopharyngeal and vagus nerves in velopharyngeal movement. *Cleft Palate Journal* 13, 201–214.

Noll JD. (1982) Remediation of Impaired Resonance Among Patients with Neuropathologies of Speech. In NJ Lass, LV McReynolds, JL Northern, DE Yoder (eds), *Speech, Language, and Hearing. Volume II: Pathologies of Speech and Language* (pp. 556–571). Philadelphia: Saunders.

O'Gara MM, Logemann JA. (1988) Phonetic analyses of the speech development of babies with cleft palate. *Cleft Palate Journal* 25, 122–134.

O'Gara MM, Logemann JA. (1990) Early Speech Development in Cleft Palate Babies. In J Bardach, HL Morris (eds), *Multidisciplinary Management of Cleft Lip and Palate* (pp. 717–721). Philadelphia: Saunders.

Okazaki K, Satoh K, Kato M, et al. (1993) Speech and velopharyngeal function following maxillary advancement in patients with cleft lip and palate. *Annals of Plastic Surgery* 30, 304–311.

Peterson SJ. (1975) Nasal emission as a component of the misarticulation of sibilants and affricates. *Journal of Speech and Hearing Disorders* 40, 106–114.

Peterson-Falzone SJ. (November 1993) Speech Outcomes from the Furlow Double Opposing Z-Plasty. Presented before the Seventh International Congress on Cleft Palate and Related Craniofacial Anomalies, Broadbent, Australia.

Peterson-Falzone SJ. (1985) Velopharyngeal inadequacy in the absence of overt cleft. *Journal of Craniofacial Genetics and Developmental Biology* Supplement 1, 97–124.

Peterson-Falzone SJ. (1988) Speech Disorders Related to Craniofacial Structural Defects: Part 1. In NJ Lass, LV McReynolds, JL Northern, DE Yoder (eds), *Handbook of Speech-Language Pathology and Audiology* (pp. 442–476). Toronto: BC Decker.

Peterson-Falzone SJ, Graham MS. (1990) Phoneme-specific nasal emission in children with and without physical anomalies of the velopharyngeal mechanism. *Journal of Speech and Hearing Disorders* 55, 132–139.

Philips BJ, Kent RD. (1984) Acoustic-Phonetic Descriptions of Speech Production in Speakers with Cleft Palate and Other Velopharyngeal Disorders. In NJ Lass (ed), *Speech and Language: Advances in Basic Research and Practice* (pp. 113–168). New York: Academic Press.

Pigott RW. (1969) The nasoendoscopic appearance of the normal palato-pharyngeal valve. *Plastic and Reconstructive Surgery* 43, 19–24.

Powers MH. (1971) Functional Disorders of Articulation—Symptomatology and Etiology. In LE Travis (ed), *Handbook of Speech Pathology* (pp. 837–876). New York: Appleton-Century-Crofts.

Redenbaugh M, Reich A. (1985) Correspondence between an accelerometric nasal/voice amplitude ratio and listeners' direct magnitude estimations of hypernasality. *Journal of Speech and Hearing Research* 18, 273–281.

Reisberg D, Gold H, Dorf DS. (1985) A technique for obturating palatal fistulae. *Cleft Palate Journal* 22, 286–289.

Rosenbeck JC. (1985) Treating Apraxia of Speech. In DF Johns (ed), *Clinical Management of Neurogenic Communicative Disorders* (2nd ed) (pp. 267–312). Boston: Little, Brown.

Ruscello DM. (1989) Modifying Velopharyngeal Closure Through Training Procedures. In KR Bzoch (ed), *Communicative Disorders Related to Cleft Lip and Palate* (3rd ed) (pp. 338–349). Boston: College-Hill Press.

Schwartz MF, McCarthy JG, Coccaro PJ, et al. (1979) Velopharyngeal Function Following Maxillary Advancement. In JM Converse, JG McCarthy, D Wood-Smith (eds), *Symposium on Diagnosis and Treatment of Craniofacial Anomalies* (pp. 277–281). St. Louis: Mosby.

Schwarz C, Gruner E. (1976) Logopaedic findings following advancement of the maxilla. *Journal of Maxillofacial Surgery* 4, 40–55.

Shprintzen RJ. (1997) Nasopharyngoscopy. In KR Bzoch (ed), *Communicative Disorders Related to Cleft Lip and Palate* (4th ed) (pp. 387–409). Austin, TX: PRO-ED.

Shprintzen RJ. (1995a) Instrumental Assessment of Velopharyngeal Valving. In RJ Shprintzen, J Bardach (eds), *Management of Cleft Palate Speech* (pp. 221–256). St. Louis: Mosby.

Shprintzen RJ. (1995b) The Use of Information Obtained from Speech and Instrumental Evaluations in Treatment Planning for Velopharyngeal Insufficiency. In RJ Shprintzen, J Bardach (eds), *Management of Cleft Palate Speech* (pp. 257–276). St. Louis: Mosby.

Shprintzen RJ, Bardach J. (1995) *Management of Cleft Palate Speech*. St. Louis: Mosby.

Shprintzen RJ, Sher AE, Croft CB. (1987) Hypernasal speech caused by tonsillar hypertrophy. *International Journal of Pediatric Otorhinolaryngology* 14, 45–56.

Skolnick ML, Cohn ER. (1989) *Videofluoroscopic Studies of Speech in Patients with Cleft Palate*. New York: Springer-Verlag.

Skolnick ML, McCall GN, Barnes M. (1973) The sphincteric mechanism of velopharyngeal closure. *Cleft Palate Journal* 10, 286–304.

Starr CD. (1993) Behavioral Approaches to Treating Velopharyngeal Closure and Nasality. In KT Moller, CD Starr (eds), *Cleft Palate: Interdisciplinary Issues and Treatment* (pp. 337–356). Austin, TX; PRO-ED.

Stoel-Gammon C. (1988) Prelinguistic vocalizations of hearing impaired and normal hearing subjects: a comparison of consonantal inventories. *Journal of Speech and Hearing Disorders* 53, 302–315.

Sulter AM, Miller DG, Wolf RF, et al. (1992) On the relation between the dimensions and resonance characteristics of the vocal tract: a study with MRI. *Magnetic Resonance Imaging* 10, 365–373.

Taub S. (1966) The Taub oral panendoscope: a new technique. *Cleft Palate Journal* 3, 328–346.

Tomes L, Kuehn DP, Peterson-Falzone SJ. (1997) Behavioral Therapy for Speakers with Velopharyngeal Impairment. In KR Bzoch (ed), *Communicative Disorders Related to Cleft Lip and Palate* (4th ed) (pp. 529–562). Austin, TX: PRO-ED.

Trost JE. (1981a) Articulatory additions to the classical description of the speech of persons with cleft palate. *Cleft Palate Journal* 18, 193–203.

Trost JE. (1981b) Differential diagnosis of velopharyngeal disorders. *Communication Disorders: An Audio Journal of Continuing Education* 6.

Trost-Cardamone JE. (1987) Cleft Palate Misarticulations: A Teaching Tape. Videotape produced by the Instructional Media Center, California State University, Northridge, CA.

Trost-Cardamone JE, Bernthal JE. (1993) Articulation Assessment and Procedures and Treatment Decisions. In KT Moller, CD Starr (eds), *Cleft Palate: Interdisciplinary Issues and Treatment* (pp. 307–336). Austin, TX; PRO-ED.

Vallino LD. (1990) Speech, velopharyngeal function, and hearing before and after orthognathic surgery. *Journal of Oral and Maxillofacial Surgery* 48, 1274–1281.

Van Dantzig G. (1940) The nomenclature of certain forms of sigmatism. *Journal of Speech Disorders* 5, 209–210.

Van Riper CR. (1972) *Speech Correction: Principles and Methods* (5th ed). Englewood Cliffs, NJ: Prentice-Hall.

Warren DW. (1979) PERCI: a method for rating palatal efficiency. *Cleft Palate Journal* 16, 279–285.

Warren DW. (1986) The velopharyngeal sphincter: a control factor in the speech regulating system [abstract]. *Asha* 28, 103.

Warren DW. (1989) Aerodynamic Assessment of Velopharyngeal Performance. In KR Bzoch (ed), *Communicative Disorders Related to Cleft Lip and Palate* (3rd ed) (pp. 230–245). Boston: College-Hill Press.

Warren DW, Dubois AB. (1964) A pressure-flow technique for measuring velopharyngeal orifice area during continuous speech. *Cleft Palate Journal* 1, 52–71.

Warren DW, Bevin AG, Winslow RB. (1978) Posterior pillar webbing and palatopharyngeal displacement: possible causes of congenital palatal incompetence. *Cleft Palate Journal* 15, 68–72.

Weber JA, Chase RA. (1970) Stress velopharyngeal incompetence in an oboe player. *Cleft Palate Journal* 7, 858–861.

Weiss CE. (1971) Success of an obturator reduction program. *Cleft Palate Journal* 8, 291–297.

Weiss CE, Louis H. (1972) Toward a more objective approach to obturator reduction. *Cleft Palate Journal* 9, 157–160.

Weiss CE, Gordon ME, Lillywhite HS. (1987) *Clinical Management of Articulatory and Phonologic Disorders*. Baltimore: Williams & Wilkins.

West R, Ansberry M. (1968) *The Rehabilitation of Speech* (4th ed). New York: Harper & Row.

West R, Ansberry M, Carr A. (1957) *The Rehabilitation of Speech* (3rd ed). New York: Harper & Row.

West R, Kennedy L, Carr A. (1937) *The Rehabilitation of Speech*. New York: Harper & Row.

West R, Kennedy L, Carr A. (1947) *The Rehabilitation of Speech* (2nd ed). New York: Harper & Row.

Willis CR, Stutz ML. (1972) The clinical use of the Taub oral panendoscope in the observation of velopharyngeal function. *Journal of Speech and Hearing Disorders* 37, 495–502.

Witt PD, Marsh JL, Marty-Grames L, et al. (1995) Management of the hypodynamic velopharynx. *Cleft Palate–Craniofacial Journal* 32, 179–187.

Witzel MA, Munro IR. (1977) Velopharyngeal insufficiency after maxillary advancement. *Cleft Palate Journal* 14, 176–180.

Witzel MA, Stringer DA. (1990) Methods of Assessing Velopharyngeal Function. In J Bardach, HL Morris (eds), *Multidisciplinary Management of Cleft Lip and Palate* (pp. 763–776). Philadelphia: Saunders.

Witzel MA, Tobe J, Salyer KE. (1989) The use of videonasopharyngoscopy for biofeedback therapy in adults after pharyngeal flap surgery. *Cleft Palate Journal* 26, 129–134.

Worster-Drought C. (1956) Congenital suprabulbar paresis. *Journal of Laryngology and Otology* 70, 453–463.

Yoss KA, Darley FL. (1974) Developmental apraxia of speech in children with defective articulation. *Journal of Speech and Hearing Research* 17, 399–416.

Zemlin WR. (1988) *Speech and Hearing Science: Anatomy and Physiology* (3rd ed). Englewood Cliffs, NJ: Prentice-Hall.

Zwitman DH, Gyepes MT, Ward PH. (1976) Assessment of velar and lateral wall movement by oral telescope and radiographic examination in patients with velopharyngeal inadequacy and in normal subjects. *Journal of Speech and Hearing Disorders* 41, 381–389.

Zwitman DH, Sonderman JC, Ward PH. (1974) Variations in velopharyngeal closure assessed by endoscopy. *Journal of Speech and Hearing Disorders* 39, 366–372.

Appendix

CASE REPORTS

CASE 1: CONGENITAL MYOPATHY

EZ first presented to the Craniofacial Center at the age of 8 years, 11 months, with severely disordered speech and a puzzling medical history. His speech was characterized by a somewhat slowed rate; hypernasality; consistent use of glottal stops as either substitutions or simultaneous productions with oral stops; pharyngeal fricatives and affricates (affricates were actually a glottal stop followed by the glide /j/); nasal emission on attempted oral placements; severe hypernasal resonance; production of bilabial consonants as labiodental placements with simultaneous glottal stops for /p/ or /b/; and absence of lip rounding for /w/ with compensatory protrusion of the tongue. He could not approximate his lips for bilabials without using his finger to push his lower lip upward, a compensatory strategy taught to him in therapy. He could raise the tongue tip to the alveolar ridge for appropriate production of /n/ and /l/, but production of /t/ and /d/ consisted essentially of glottal stops. In addition, his laryngeal quality was breathy and weak, and he could only utter one or two syllables in a single-breath pulse. His referral diagnosis was Möbius' syndrome, but further work-up proved this to be erroneous, and the medical diagnosis proved to be congenital myopathy.

At the time of the initial visit, EZ was in second grade and enjoyed school but was acutely aware of his speech problems. He exhibited a constant mouth-open posture and a severe open bite, with the tongue resting between the teeth (Figure 8.6). The palatal vault was extremely narrow and high, and there was constant central grooving of the tongue. (These are common findings in someone who exhibits a constant open-mouth posture.) No movement of the velum was seen during speech. He had reportedly had a palatal lift appliance earlier, but neither he nor his parents could recall when this had been fitted or how long he had worn it. Arrangements were made for refitting of another lift, but the family disappeared from follow-up. Seven years later, they reappeared. The plans for another palatal lift were finally carried out, as was orthognathic surgery to lengthen the lower jaw, reducing the open bite and bringing the lips into better proximity (Figures 8.7 and 8.8). At the last team evaluation, he could produce four to five syllables on a breath pulse. He could produce anterior stop plosives and fricatives with-

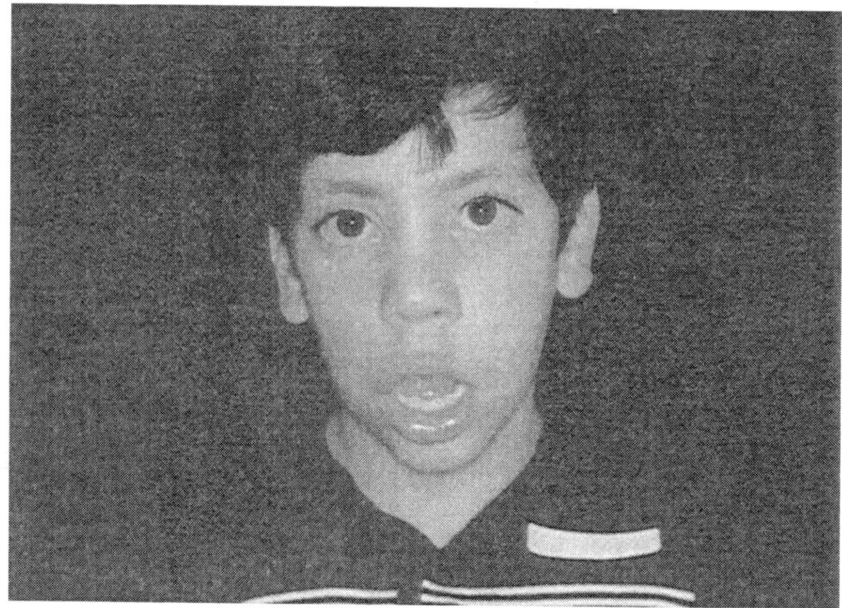

A

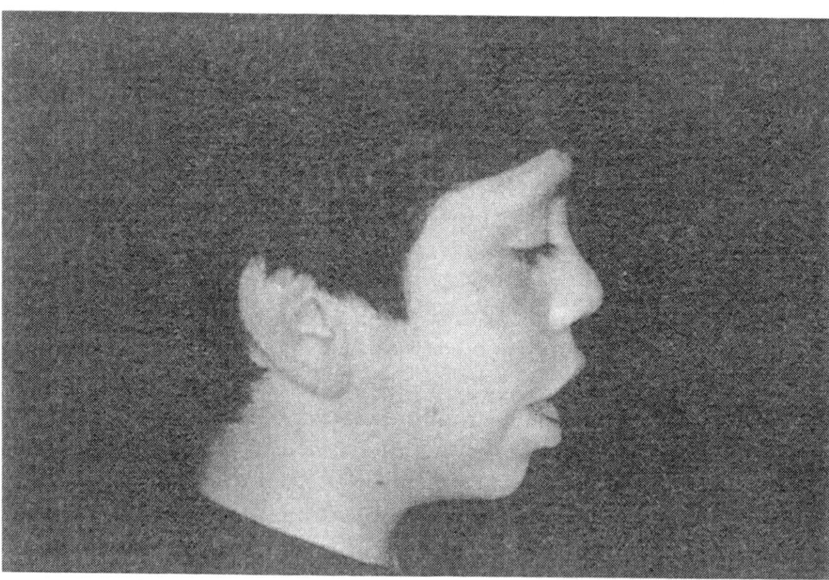

B

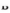

Figure 8.6 A. Full face of EZ at the age of 8 years, 11 months. B. Profile view of EZ.

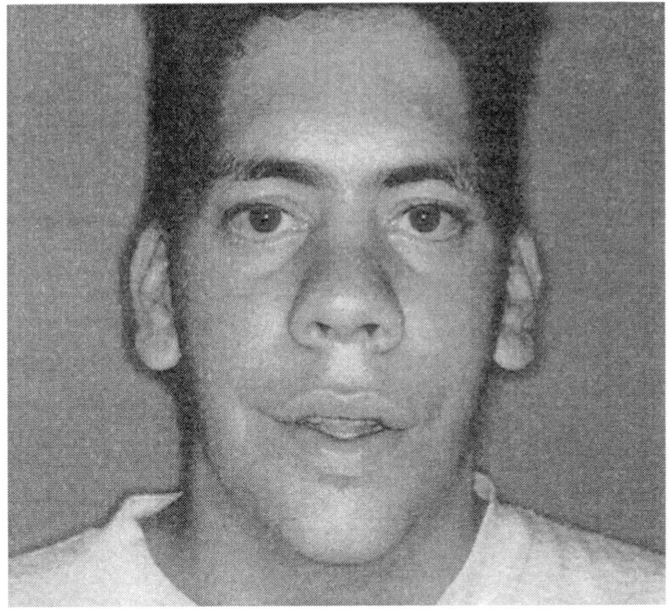

A

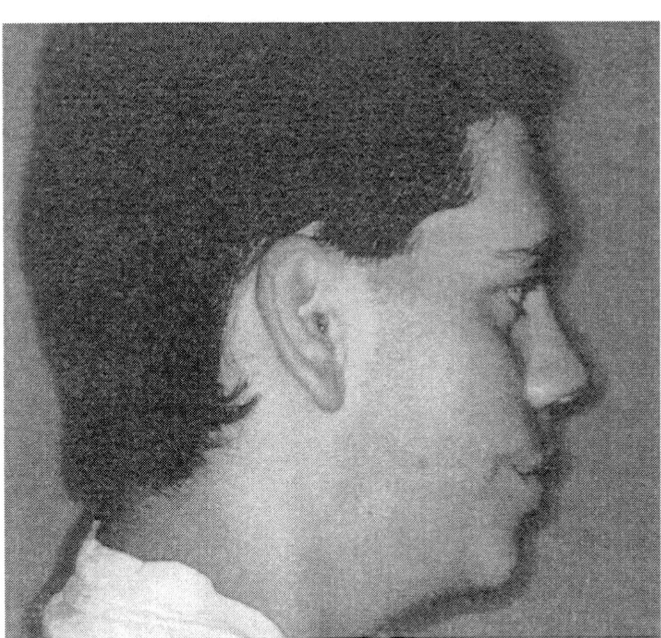

B

Figure 8.7 Full face (A) and profile view (B) of EZ at the age of 16 years.

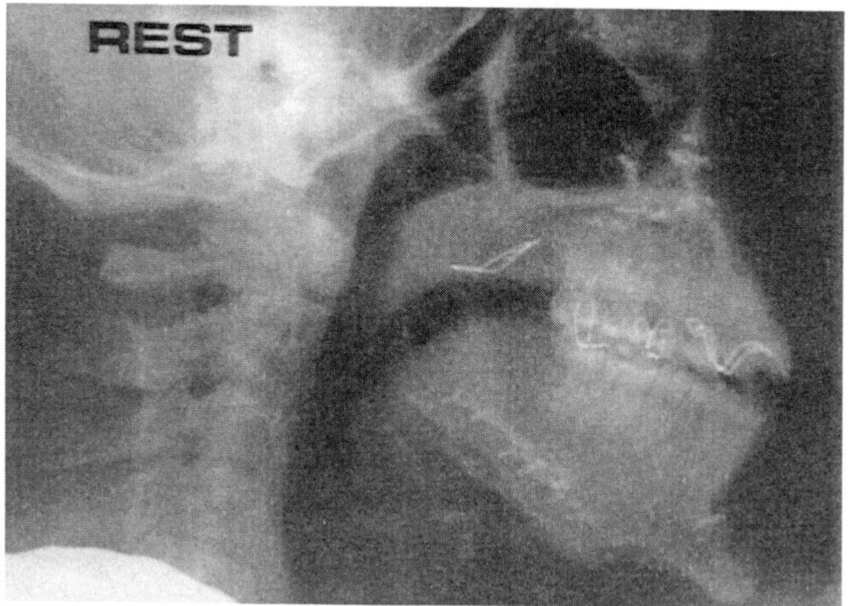

A

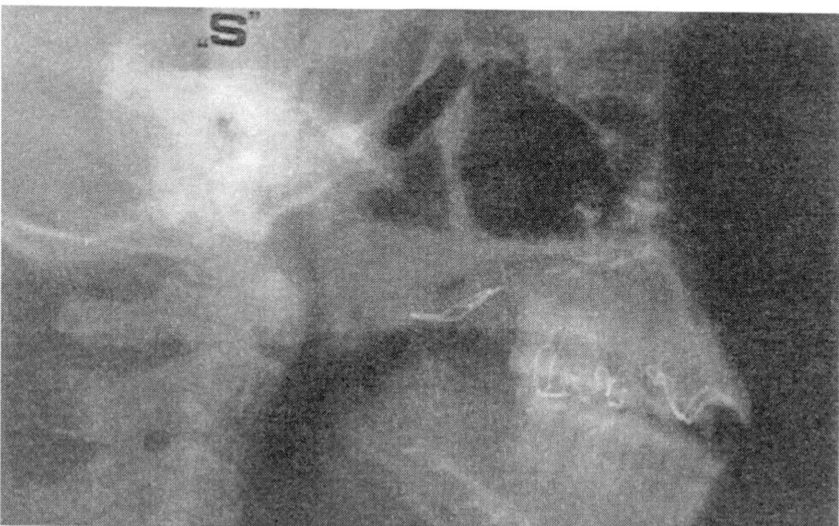

B

Figure 8.8 A. Lateral cephalometric film taken at rest of EZ at 16 years of age with his palatal lift in place. B. Lateral cephalometric film taken during sustained /s/ of EZ with his palatal lift in place. Note that with the support of the lift the velum is close enough to the posterior pharyngeal wall that the small amount of velar movement is enough to accomplish closure.

out nasal emission and could bring his lips together for bilabial consonants without using his finger. Glottal stops were still used as substitutions for velar stops and still occurred inconsistently as replacements for anterior stops in consonant clusters. Speech was still slow and dysarthric, although far more intelligible with the elimination of nasal air loss and the consequent increase in loudness and number of syllables produced per breath pulse. Intelligibility was estimated to be 70–75% to the casual listener, higher in short answers to questions or when the listener knew the context. EZ is doing well in high school, excelling in trigonometry and computer programming. He is planning on college and a career in engineering.

CASE 2: PHONEME-SPECIFIC NASAL EMISSION IN A NORMAL CHILD

SP was first referred to the center at the age of 10 years, 10 months, with a diagnosis of velopharyngeal inadequacy due to asymmetric movement of the velum. He had been seen by another cleft palate team because he had been in speech therapy for several years but still exhibited nasal emission. For reasons that were not clear, previous examiners had carried out lateral videofluorographic studies from both the left and right sides (lateral videofluorographic studies are focused in the midsagittal plane, meaning that two studies in the same plane were obtained). SP and his family brought a videotape of these studies to their first clinic visit, and the "two" views, not surprisingly, were exactly the same. Both showed good elevation of the velum and complete closure at the midsagittal plane throughout speech except in production of /s/, /z/, and /ʃ/. In production of the remaining sibilants, affricates, and stop plosives, closure was complete.

The intraoral examination was essentially negative. There were no visible or palpable stigmata or a submucous cleft, the palatal vault was normal in appearance, and there was consistent *and symmetric* upward movement of the velum on phonation.

The perceptual impression of SP's speech was exactly the same as one would expect from viewing the "two" videofluorographic samples. He showed no signs of nasal emission with the following exceptions: (1) /s/ was produced with a slightly fronted tongue placement and simultaneous nasal emission or posterior nasal frication; (2) for the targets /z/ and /ʃ/, he raised the dorsum of the tongue against the palate (the same tongue position that would normally be seen for production of /k/, /g/, or /ŋ/), completely precluding any oral emission of the air stream; (3) the sibilant /ʃ/ was appropriately produced except in the prevocalic position in his own name (Sean), in which he used his own pattern of nasal direction of the airstream for production of /s/ in *S*ean.

This boy was exhibiting a fairly classic pattern of phoneme-specific nasal emission (Peterson 1975; Peterson-Falzone and Graham 1990; Trost 1981a, b; Trost-Cardamone 1987). To demonstrate the nature of this speech

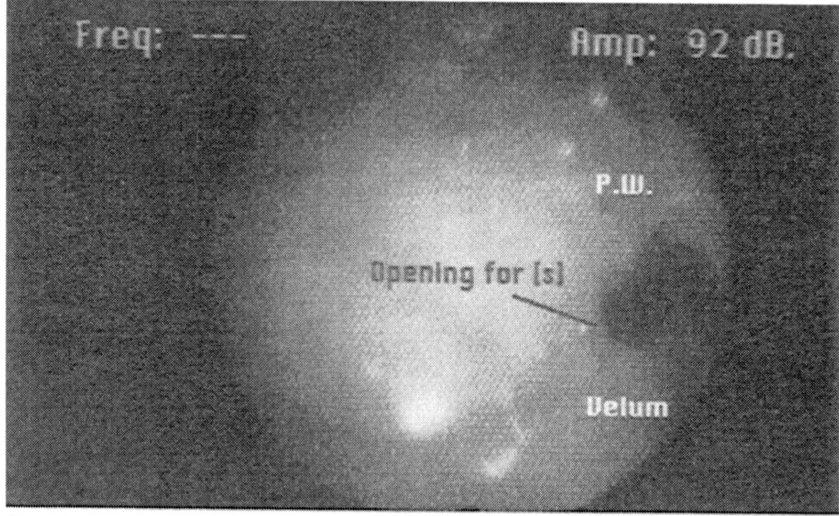

A

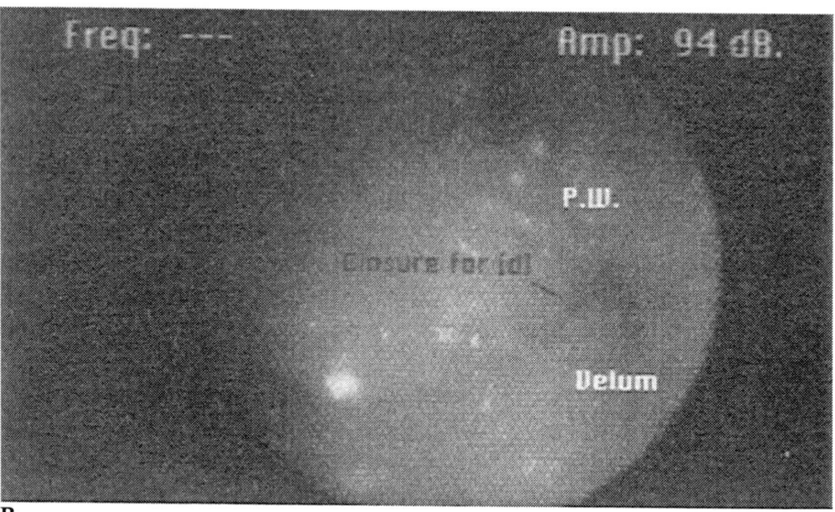

B

Figure 8.9 A. Nasopharyngoscopic view of the posterior pharyngeal wall (P.W.) and velum in SP during production of the posterior nasal fricative he habitually substituted for /s/. B. Nasopharyngoscopic view of the velopharyngeal closure in SP as seen during production of a nonsibilant pressure consonant. The posterior pharyngeal wall is contacted by the velum, providing closure of the nasopharyngeal port.

behavior to SP and to his parents, nasopharyngoscopy was performed on the first clinic visit (Figure 8.9). SP consistently showed velopharyngeal closure in speech in everything except the specific phonemes just described. He was easily stimulable (even without the nasopharyngoscopy) for correct oral production of all sibilants in all contexts. The nature of this speech behavior was explained to the patient and to his parents, and there were subsequent written and telephone communications with his speech pathologist. When he returned for re-evaluation 5 months later, he was free of any signs of nasal emission in his speech except for occasional relapse into the use of a posterior nasal fricative as a replacement for the prevocalic sibilant in his own first name. At his next visit, the residual problem had been eradicated.

9

Differential Diagnosis for Autism

Lynne E. Hewitt

Speech-language pathologists are key players in assessing individuals with autism, because lack of communicative competence is a hallmark of the syndrome. Although few speech-language pathologists take sole responsibility for assigning this diagnosis (opinion on the degree to which speech-language pathologists should participate in assigning the diagnosis varies), they, in any case, need to understand the implications of the diagnosis. This is not to say that familiarity with the meaning of labels such as autism, Asperger's syndrome, or Rett syndrome teaches clinicians what to do with clients who come to them with these diagnoses. Experts on autism urge caution: "no diagnostic number or label can mean any more than what is known about the condition represented by that label" (Schopler and Mesibov 1988, p. 4). Before the 1980s, the actual amount of what was known about autism was disturbingly small. Indeed, many myths and unfounded beliefs about autism have been put forward without research verification. Such myths have found their way into both clinical practice and popular imagination, complicating work with individuals with autism and their families. The echoes of these early mistakes reverberate even today.

Best practice in managing complex developmental disorders dictates use of a transdisciplinary assessment model. One goal of this chapter is to provide clinicians with basic information about diagnostic terms and what they mean. Another, broader goal is to prepare language clinicians for the possibility that they may be the first professional to suspect autism in a child (or even, rarely, an adult). This occurs because frequently the first concern of parents arises from the child's failure to acquire language. In such cases, the speech-language pathologist may be placed in a position in which detailed understanding of the characteristics of autism is crucial to making appropriate and timely referrals to other professionals. An even more difficult situation can arise for the experienced clinician who recognizes that a diagnosis given by another professional for an individual who has been referred for speech-language services is not appropriate. Opening a dialog with the professional who gave the prior diagnosis may not be possible. Although changing the record may be out of the question, the speech-language pathologist should proceed to carefully describe the results of the speech-language assessment using the most current terminology to meet the patient's needs when designing treatment recommendations. Taking a critical stance toward diagnoses provided by other professionals enables speech-language pathologists to consider alternative ideas about the nature of a client's problems and to develop an appropriate management program.

Even when a label is accurate, it can limit vision. A classic example of this in the literature on developmental language pathology is the case of echolalia. From the earliest description of autism (Kanner 1943), echolalia was thought of as a symptom of the abnormal language processes characteristic of the disorder. When thus viewed as a symptom, echolalia could not be seen as serving any purpose. Its presence was merely noted and used as diagnostic of autism (American Psychiatric Association 1980). Prizant and Duchan (1981), in contrast, entertained the hypothesis that echolalia was a means of communication. In fact, they were able to document a number of communicative functions served by it. In this new light, echolalia was no longer a disease symptom but a strategy for overcoming severe communication disability.

In the past, the label of autism entailed the notion that those so labeled had little or no interest in others, and, for this reason, communicative strategies were believed to be absent from all but a high-functioning few. The label of autism is particularly vulnerable to such mistakes, because it is based purely on behavioral observations. Many past inferences drawn from observations of "autistic behavior" have proved false, and there is no reason to believe that the process of improved understanding of this disorder has come to a halt.

The emphasis throughout this chapter is on in-depth, individualized assessment. Modern authorities on autism urge ongoing, detailed assessment of individuals and their significant others as the cornerstone of any intervention (Wetherby and Prizant 1992; Schopler and Mesibov 1988). The goal is to catalog the unique constellation of features that make up the communicative strengths and weaknesses of an individual with a severe communication disability such as autism. Assessment of language and communication on a microanalytic level provides the foundation for effective speech language intervention.

OVERVIEW OF DEFINITIONS AND THEORIES OF AUTISM

Biological Basis of Autism

After many years of struggle against assumptions made by Kanner and others (Bettelheim 1959; Kanner 1943), near-universal agreement on the biological nature of autism has been reached (see Tsai and Ghaziuddin 1992 for a review). Advances in this area point to the likelihood that autism is a disorder with multiple etiologies, and the list of medical problems associated with autism has lengthened (Gillberg 1990, 1992). Associated medical problems range from tuberous sclerosis to maternal rubella, to perinatal trauma, to fragile X chromosome abnormality. It has long been known that an increased prevalence of seizure disorders occurs in people who have autism, with sudden onset at or during puberty not uncommon (American Psychiatric Association 1994). These findings have put to rest previous notions of autism as a mysterious disorder in which otherwise normal children withdraw from the world.

Improved understanding of the organic nature of the disorder has helped in recognizing that the mental retardation often observed to accompany autism is not an artifact of poor test procedures. Rather, as Frith (1989) has outlined with particular lucidity, it is no surprise that an organic brain disorder having a pervasive effect on the course of development should in its severest forms co-occur with other cognitive problems. This fact has been obscured because there are individuals with autism who have average and even, in rare cases, superior intelligence. Debate continues on whether such cases represent the "purest" form of autism. Frith has argued that the "true" nature of the disorder is best revealed in individuals who have the least amount of diffuse brain damage, with one system only being impaired. Other authorities (Gillberg 1992) think that the notion of "pure" autism obscures more than it reveals. Instead, they advocate that the term can best be used as a description of a family of disabilities of diverse organic causes, ranging across a wide spectrum of ability.

As of this writing, autism is estimated to occur at rates of between 2 and 5 in 10,000; the ratio of males to females is approximately 4–5 to 1. Mental retardation is seen in 75–80% of the autistic population. Evidence from British, Swedish, Japanese, and New Zealand epidemiologic studies indicate similar, although not identical, figures (see Gillberg 1992 for review). Research suggests that autism occurs at similar rates in all social classes and in all cultures studied to date. However, Gillberg claimed lower incidence among native-born populations in Sweden than in immigrant populations and suggested that this difference may be linked to poor prenatal care and lack of maternal immunizations.

Defining Autism

To unravel some of the confusion surrounding the term *autism,* it is necessary to see how its use has evolved in the 50 years since it was first introduced. Originally, autism was classed with childhood schizophrenia. As understanding of the differences between schizophrenia and autism evolved, this early classification was abandoned. However, practitioners still encounter individuals who, in the past, were diagnosed as having childhood schizophrenia or a variant thereof and who would today likely be classified as autistic. (The term *childhood schizophrenia* is no longer used but may persist in old records.) To complicate matters further, in the *Diagnostic and Statistical Manual of Mental Disorders* (DSM) the definition of autism has changed in every one of its last three editions (American Psychiatric Association 1980, 1987, 1994). In DSM-IV, autism is defined as a subcategory of pervasive developmental disorders and is characterized by "severe and pervasive impairment in several areas of development: reciprocal social interaction skills, communication skills, or the presence of stereotyped behavior, interests, and activities" (American Psychiatric Association 1994, p. 65).

The social problems, language and communication disorders, and restricted repertoire of interests often remarked on as characteristic of autism are seen in DSM-IV as hallmarks of a group of disorders, of which autism is merely one type. The differential diagnosis of other pervasive developmental disorders in DSM-IV is further discussed in the following text. The diagnostic criteria for autism, in particular, involve the following:

- Delay or abnormal functioning in at least one of the core areas before 3 years of age
- At least two items from a checklist relating to qualitative impairment in social interaction
- At least one item from a checklist of qualitative impairments in communication
- At least one item from a list of restricted, repetitive, and stereotyped patterns of behavior; interests; and activities (an absence of pretend play is often the first sign of the presence of unusually restricted interests and activities)
- The disorder is not better accounted for by Rett syndrome or childhood disintegrative disorder

Associated, nondefinitional features include the following:

- Abnormal responses (hypo- and hypersensitivity) to sensory stimuli
- Abnormalities of mood and affect
- Self-injurious behaviors
- Prosodic abnormalities (including both unusually monotone vocal inflection and unusually "sing-song" or over-learned prosody)

Individuals with autism may display unusual patterns of ability and disability, such as so-called *hyperlexia,* in which the ability to decode the phoneme-grapheme correspondences of text is more advanced than the ability to integrate the meaning of the words read. Other types of unusual abilities have also been reported, including artistic (musical or drawing), mathematical, and mnemonic abilities. These so-called *idiot savant* abilities, which loom large in the popular imagination, are somewhat out of proportion to their actual incidence. They are more common in individuals whose adaptive functioning is in the normal or above-average range, but they have been seen in those who are severely impaired in all other domains. The degree to which perceptual features of autism are core characteristics is a matter of some debate (Bettison 1996; Grandin 1995), and the exact nature of perceptual differences and disturbances in people with autism is highly varied.

The DSM-IV definition provides examples of communication impairment in high-functioning individuals and emphasizes that the disorder can manifest itself quite differently at different ages. This is an important emphasis, because the lack of understanding of the developmental course of autism and autistic spectrum disorders has been second only to psychogenic theories in sowing confusion about this disability. In particular, many have been confused about whether social relatedness in autism is always absent, or whether it is at times present but manifested in unusual ways. In fact, an infant who apparently lacked awareness of and interest in close family members may in early childhood begin treating people as instruments to fulfill his or her wants and needs. In adolescence, this person may become very interested in friendships and relationships but uses idiosyncratic and nonreciprocal strategies in attempting to relate to others. Useful insight into the nature of the autistic experience across the lifespan may be gained by reading autobiographic accounts of very high-functioning individuals (Barron and Barron 1992; Grandin and Scariano 1986; Williams 1992). It is also important to be aware that, in rare instances, adults with a diagnosis of childhood autism may no longer exhibit any obvious signs of autism.

One challenge to diagnosticians involved with children with suspected autism is posed by cases in which intellectual functioning is limited. In such cases, all domains are likely to be impaired, including those thought of as associated with autism. Thus it may not be possible to differentiate autistic features caused by low overall potential from those linked to the specific disturbances seen in the autistic spectrum disorders in individuals with severe to profound mental retardation. Indeed, at the current level of knowledge, the impact of such a differential diagnosis on treatment approaches may be minimal.

Current Psychological Theories on Autism

There are a number of current theories of autism that can aid in clinical work. The first describes autism as primarily a social-affective disorder resulting in lifelong socioemotional impairment. This theory is primarily attributable to Hobson (see Hobson 1993 for an overview), who has investigated the ability of autistic individuals to recognize faces and facially expressed emotions and to use and understand vocabulary related to the emotions. Others take issue with Hobson, arguing that the social deficits in autism are secondary features not primary causes (e.g., Frith 1989).

An alternative to Hobson's view is the theory of mind or mind-blindness view of autism (Frith 1989; Happé 1995). In this theory, it is hypothesized that individuals with autism exhibit a specific cognitive deficit in the development of the ability to make inferences about mental states. Evidence exists that individuals with autism have special difficulty, when compared with Down syndrome controls, in succeeding at tasks involving understanding of deception and false belief. (See Frith 1989 and Happé 1995 for reviews.) Moreover, analyses of their language abilities have suggested that deficits are most pronounced in those areas requiring active tracking of the listener's mental state (Hewitt 1994; Tager-Flusberg 1994). For example, ability to make unambiguous and clear references is impaired (e.g., overuse of proper names unlikely to be known to the listener or excessive use of pronouns), while overall lexical and syntactic ability appears commensurate with IQ. This discrepancy occurs because referential communication involves making assumptions about the listener's knowledge state.

The theory of mind hypothesis has been challenged on a number of fronts. For example, it does not account for the stereotypes and routines exhibited by individuals with autism. Moreover, critics point out that some individuals with autism have the ability to make correct responses in tasks involving deception and false belief. If some do pass the tasks, then lack of theory of mind may be a common feature of autism but not an explanation for it. Ozonoff and colleagues (1991b) presented an alternative hypothesis that autism is caused by an "executive function deficit" similar to that seen in patients with frontal-lobe damage. They provided evidence that individuals with autism perform more poorly on assessment batteries designed to evaluate executive function than IQ-matched controls. From this view, many of the problems of autistic individuals stem from inability to plan and to inhibit prepotent responses. Theory of mind deficits may relate to executive function problems or possibly arise from some other, nonprimary source of difficulty.

Lifespan Perspectives on Autism

As noted above in the section *Defining Autism*, one of the least understood aspects of autism is that it is a disorder that shows changes across the lifespan. This has been documented by case studies (Windsor et al. 1994) and epidemiologic approaches (Wing and Gould 1979). For purposes of differential diagnosis, as well as long-range intervention planning, it is important to understand that a child's present level of functioning and style of behavior can change dramatically over the course of a lifetime. It is this aspect of autism that is responsible for causing much confusion about the true nature of the disability, because individuals who may use little or no language until their late preschool years and use primarily echolalia and routines to communicate may ultimately achieve some degree of conversational ability in adulthood.

CASE 1

Ben was nonverbal until 4 years of age. Until then, he appeared to have little interest in others, engaging in hand-flapping, spinning, and rocking for most of the time. He began speaking primarily via echolalia at the age of 4 years and then progressed slowly through the elementary years via a gradual process of increasing numbers of self-initiated utterances and decreasing echolalia. Ben was enrolled in a special school for children with language disabilities and received intensive pull-out as well as classroom-based language intervention. As he became older, he developed a strong interest in asking questions and would interact with anyone who would respond to his questions. These questions tended to revolve around restricted and unusual topic domains (e.g., which stores the listener shopped at, the color of the team jackets in the listener's high school). He was mainstreamed in a regular high school, where, with resource-room support, he was able to do grade-level work. Ben ultimately developed the ability to respond appropriately to many conversational overtures, to read for content, and to interact verbally, even when his special topics were not being discussed. Following his experience in high school, Ben began to express concerns about social interaction and how he "fit in" to his social environment.

Subclassifications of Autistic Spectrum Disorders

The degree to which autism can be subdivided into distinct categories is controversial. A number of related syndromes have been proposed, and there is controversy over which of these disorders represent types of autism and which are similar but unrelated entities (Table 9.1). See Provence and Dahl (1987) for presentation of a view of autism as a spectrum disorder.

Kanner's Syndrome

Classic autism is known as *Kanner's syndrome*, for the first to describe autism, Leo Kanner, and *early infantile autism* to distinguish it from adult-onset social withdrawal. These labels are often most closely associated with the features of autism linked to social difficulties and isolation. While social difficulties are indeed inherently a part of autism, the overemphasis on the self-involvement of autistic individuals has led to confusion. In particular, the notion that individuals with "pure" autism lack all interest in others has persisted. Given the knowledge that individual differences in autism can be extreme, the most cautious clinical approach would avoid emphasis on such notions as "classic" autism, since its differentiation from other categories on the autistic spectrum is unclear.

High-Functioning and Low-Functioning Autism

Two terms purporting to describe subcategories of autism have achieved popularity: *high functioning* and *low functioning*. The use of these terms relates to the wide range of intellectual ability and adaptive functioning seen in this disorder. It is a curious fact that two individuals of quite different ability can both be classified as autistic. Experienced practitioners recognize a cluster of characteristics (captured fairly well in the DSM-IV definition) even in widely diverse individuals. Those with less severe problems in the social, cognitive, and linguistic domains may function at considerably advanced levels in educational and even vocational contexts. There may also be a relationship between the level of ability to function in society and the degree to which perceptual and attention distortions and difficulty in achieving intentional control over motor acts affects the individual with autism (Duchan 1993). The labels *high* and *low functioning*

Table 9.1
Features of autistic spectrum disorders and related syndromes

Diagnosis	*Relationship to Autism*	*Differential Diagnostic Considerations*
Autism	—	Onset before 3 years of age Delay or disorder in language development Restricted repertoire of interests and activities Impairment in social cognition
Kanner's syndrome	Older, less-used label for autism	See Autism
Early infantile autism	Older, less-used label for autism	See Autism
Asperger's syndrome	Some authorities classify with high-functioning autism	No history of language delay Normal intelligence
PDDNOS	Some authorities include on autistic spectrum	Less severe social and linguistic impairments than seen with autism
Semantic-pragmatic disorder	Intended as language disorder classification for individuals not classified as autistic Unclear status vis-à-vis autism and PDDNOS	Similar to PDDNOS
Rett syndrome	Linguistic and behavioral features similar to autism	Only in females Head growth deceleration in infancy Marked loss of hand coordination and increasing gait impairment
Childhood disintegrative disorder	Linguistic and behavioral features similar to autism	Prolonged period of typical development (unclear how long)
Childhood schizophrenia	Not currently used for children meeting the criteria for autism	Not used in current practice. Childhood onset of schizophrenia differs from autism by hallucinations and delusions and periodic recovery and acute episodes Very rare in preschool years Onset usually during adolescence

Table 9.1
Continued

Diagnosis	*Relationship to Autism*	*Differential Diagnostic Considerations*
Profound mental retardation	Can co-occur with autism	Differential diagnosis difficult because of overall low function
Obsessive-compulsive disorder	Obsessions and compulsions sometimes exhibited by individuals with autism	Awareness by the individual of unusual nature of or lack of factual basis for obsession Absence of other features of autism
Tourette's syndrome	Repetitive verbal behaviors sometimes exhibited by individuals with autism	Awareness by the individual of the unwanted nature of tics Absence of other features of autism
Elective mutism	Reluctance to communicate orally by some autistic individuals	Otherwise normal development in speech and language Social impairments less marked Usually able to communicate normally in certain situations

PDDNOS = pervasive developmental disorder not otherwise specified.

can be considered useful clinical shorthand, although their scientific status is unclear.

Asperger's Syndrome

At almost the same time Kanner (1943) was publishing the first description of autism in English, Asperger was publishing his findings about a similar group of individuals in German (Asperger tr. Frith 1995). The differences and similarities between Kanner's and Asperger's ideas make an interesting historical study (Frith 1995). Because Asperger's work was not previously available in English, there has been uncertainty whether the two populations are identical. Many authorities have considered Asperger's syndrome (called in DSM-IV, APA 1994, *Asperger's disorder*) to refer to autistic people who are high functioning and who do not exhibit a language delay or obvious language disorder (although their social problems may result in conversational difficulty). Others have argued for distinguishing between autism and Asperger's (Ozonoff et al. 1991a; Frith 1995). For speech-language pathologists, perhaps the most important aspect of this controversy is that evidence is emerging that there may be many individuals with Asperger-type difficulties in social interaction who have not been formally diagnosed. Such individuals are at risk for undiagnosed pragmatic language impairment, with possibly serious consequences for their social and vocational functioning. Patients with Asperger's syndrome, very high-functioning individuals with autism, or both may perform fairly well in educational contexts, even with their social differences. The structured nature of expectations in school settings may enable them to achieve success with their high intelligence alone. However, in the world of work, more flexibility in adapting to the expectations of others, general social awareness, and skill are necessary to succeed. Individual differences are less likely to be tolerated when they impact economic productivity. These factors suggest that use of the term *Asperger's syndrome* may be helpful in delivering much-needed language services to individuals who do not entirely fit the usual definition of autism.

Pervasive Developmental Disorder Not Otherwise Specified

The diagnosis of a pervasive developmental disorder not otherwise specified (PDDNOS) was first put forward in DSM-III (American Psychiatric Association 1980). It refers to the clinical impression that there are children who fit some, but not all, of the characteristics listed in the definition of autism. This diagnosis is probably one of the more challenging for parents, because its meaning is unclear. It suggests a milder impairment than autism but recognizes that somehow development is proceeding abnormally. It probably has a connection with the frustrating term *autistic-like*. There has been a history of reluctance on the part of some medical and psychological professionals to give the diagnosis of autism, especially if there are prognostic indicators that the developmental course may be tending toward a better outcome than that traditionally foreseen in autism. The use of this diagnostic term can be beneficial, in that some children with special needs who would not have been identified as autistic can begin receiving the intervention services they need. Speech-language pathologists should note unusual social patterns, restricted repertoires of interests, or both in children who exhibit signs of conversational impairment. Referral for psychological assessment may be appropriate even when actual autism is not suspected.

Semantic-Pragmatic Disorder

Semantic-pragmatic disorder is a term coined by specialists in communication disorders (Bishop and Rosenbloom 1987; Rapin and Allen 1983). Semantic-pragmatic disorder may relate historically to the period when most clinicians believed individuals with true autism must be socially withdrawn. Some authorities now argue that semantic-pragmatic disorder does not represent a true subcategory but rather a point on the high-functioning, more social end of the autistic continuum (Brook and Bowler 1992; Happé 1995). Others continue the use of this descriptor for children whose primary problems seem to lie in pragmatic language but not in other domains traditionally linked to autism (e.g., social relatedness). As it is a diagnostic category squarely within the purview of speech-language pathology, it is useful to retain this term for individuals who do not have a specific diagnosis but show signs of the types of pragmatic impairment seen in individuals with autistic spectrum disorders. If circumstances, such as parental reluctance, prohibit a closer look at the possibility of autism, use of the term *semantic-pragmatic disorder* allows the speech-language pathologist to tackle the language problems while setting aside the thornier issues of etiology and psychological classification. It also has the advantage of carrying less catastrophic overtones than autism for family members.

Use of the Term **Autistic-Like**

The term *autistic-like* has little clinical use and no real scientific basis (Happé 1995). If the term is seen in diagnostic reports, it may have a particularly insidious effect in coloring the speech-language pathologist's clinical vision, such that he or she perceives all observed behaviors to perhaps be caused by autism. At times, *autistic-like* may be comforting to parents who are not prepared to accept a definitive diagnosis for their child. However, in such cases it would be better to provide no diagnosis at all, since this noncategory has the potential drawback of a label without conveying any of its benefits. It is perhaps for this reason that the term *PDDNOS* has been instituted. The use of *autistic-like* may decline in favor of PDDNOS. In addition, increased understanding of the wide variety of autistic spectrum disorders and possible outcomes may help increase acceptance of the term *autism* itself.

In the interests of dispelling the confusion brought about by the term *autistic-like*, speech-language pathologists should not perpetuate its use. If autism is suspected, referral to a specialist or team experienced in the evaluation of autism and similar disorders is indicated. The speech-language pathologist's report should avoid uncertain and vague diagnostic terms that are misleading in favor of descriptions of observed behaviors and caregiver reports. Careful documentation of difficulties in language areas often impaired in autism will be most useful to psychological professionals charged with evaluating an individual for autism.

Syndromes Sometimes Confused with Autism

Rett Syndrome

Rett syndrome is a developmental disorder exclusively seen in females, with onset following a period of normal development. DSM-IV (American Psychiatric Association 1994) reports a characteristic pattern of head growth deceleration, which may be observed as early as 5 months of age. Onset is before 4 years of age and usually occurs by 2 years of age. People with Rett syndrome regress (it also has been described as arrested development), losing hand coordination (ultimately resulting in stereotyped hand movements) and developing impairments in gait, social interaction, receptive and expressive language, and intellectual functioning. Rett syndrome is differentiated from autism by its gender specificity, the characteristic head growth deceleration, and the severe motor problems observed. Language disorders and social interaction patterns are similar to those seen in autism. As with autism, individuals with Rett syndrome may develop increased interest in social interaction in adolescence. In terms of language intervention, similarities between Rett syndrome and autism suggest similar approaches. However, clinicians working with very young individuals with Rett syndrome need to consider the future effect of years of developmental regression (or arrest), followed by limited recovery, on long-term intervention planning.

Childhood Disintegrative Disorder

Childhood disintegrative disorder is differentiated from autism by a prolonged period of typical development. Differential diagnosis is complicated by the fact that in DSM-IV (American Psychiatric Association 1994) it is reported that, in rare cases, autistic individuals may also exhibit a period of normal development for 1–2 years. Childhood disintegrative disorder may be diagnosed following a period of normal development as short as 2 years (although typically it is much longer). Thus, there is an overlap in the definitions of these disorders that allows the possibility for borderline cases. This is particularly confusing in that children with childhood disintegrative disorder are described as exhibiting the social and communicative deficits seen in autism. To add to the confusion, in a minority of cases, regression in language use has been reported in autism. Unlike Rett syndrome, there are no physical differentiating features or associated medical conditions (other than those also associated with autism) between autism and childhood disintegrative disorder. As with Rett syndrome, this diagnosis is associated with a language and communication profile very similar to autism. However, clinicians should be aware that childhood disintegrative disorder is usually associated with severe mental retardation.

Childhood Schizophrenia

As discussed under *Defining Autism,* childhood schizophrenia is a diagnosis that was for a number of years given to children who would today meet the DSM-IV criteria for autism (American Psychiatric Association 1994). For this reason, occasionally adults with a history that reports childhood schizophrenia who consult a speech-language pathologist exhibit the signs of Asperger's syndrome or autism. As of this writing, schizophrenia is not diagnosed in childhood unless it truly resembles adult- or adolescent-onset schizophrenia. The following features differentiate schizophrenia from autism: (1) people who are schizophrenic display periodic episodes of illness with recovery, while those with autism appear consistent in their behavior over time (except for slow developmental change over the lifespan); (2) schizophrenic individuals have hallucinations and delusions, while autistic individuals do not; and (3) schizophrenia rarely develops before adolescence and only a very few cases develop during the preschool years, unlike autism, the onset of which occurs by 3 years of age. Cases of autistic individuals developing true adolescent-onset schizophrenia have been reported, but it is rare.

CASE 2

Thomas, a 21-year-old man, came to a university speech and hearing clinic seeking help with his communicative style. He had a diagnosis of schizophrenia but did not suffer from delusions or hallucinations and had remained fairly constant in his demeanor and functioning over many years. Psychological testing provided evidence of mental ability in the superior range. A speech and language evaluation revealed that he exhibited prosodic anomalies (e.g., a "robotic" quality of speech caused by a monotone quality of intonation) and showed conversational disability in responding to other-initiated topics, lack of information-seeking questions, and difficulty in topic-shifting and topic-shading. Thomas was enrolled in the clinic for speech and language intervention to address these needs. He showed strong motivation to attend therapy and evidence of responsiveness to clinical direction. It was informally determined that it would be clinically useful to design intervention with features of autism or Asperger's syndrome in mind.

Profound Mental Retardation

Individuals with profound mental retardation may exhibit depressed abilities in language and social cognition that parallel those seen in lower-functioning autistic individuals. When an individual's profile of adaptive functioning is severely limited in all domains, it is difficult to make a useful distinction between overall low intelligence and true autism. Again, the clinical importance of this distinction may be minimal. However, it may be necessary to consider that a person with profound mental retardation may have a poorer prognosis for change across the lifespan and for ultimate development of language and communication than one with autism.

CASE 3

Joseph was enrolled in a self-contained classroom for students with autism. He used no verbal communication. Nonverbally, he communicated by means of eye contact, showing objects, and distress signals such as moaning and crying. He had several years of instruction in sign but did not use any signs expressively. He responded to his name and to physical prompts such as a touch on the elbow to indicate that he should stand up. Various approaches to augmentative communication had been tried with him without success. Joe had a pleasant demeanor and seemed happy to be with people and also happy when left alone. He enjoyed mouthing objects and vocalizing. The staff interacting with him suspected that the diagnosis of autism was mistaken, and that Joe was actually functioning in the profound range of mental retardation. Differential signs included the signs of interest in activities at an infantile level of development (mouthing objects) and good eye contact.

Tourette's Syndrome and Obsessive-Compulsive Disorder

Tourette's syndrome and obsessive-compulsive disorder are distinguished from autism by the patients' awareness of the unusual nature of their tics and compulsions and normal social and linguistic development, aside from the verbal tics sometimes associated with Tourette's syndrome. It is interesting to note, however, that some of the same medications used to control the symptoms of these disorders have shown benefit for individuals with autism. Some individuals with autism exhibit ritualistic and compulsive behavior similar to behavior seen in obsessive-compulsive disorder and Tourette's syndrome; however, in autism this co-occurs with unusual social-affective development.

Elective Mutism

In general, the diagnosis of elective mutism is not given unless an individual has previously exhibited a language system that is presumed to be intact. Such individuals display normal language ability in certain contexts, implying that the individual chooses not to speak rather than lacks the ability to express himself or herself. The opposite situation occurs in autism, in which at least the pragmatics of language are impaired, by definition. However, there are two scenarios in which elective mutism can be confused with autism. In some individuals with true autism, the lack of social responsiveness or interest in socializing results in a passive verbal style with very limited output. In such individuals, adequate receptive ability may be paired with little or no verbal expression. This situation is similar to elective mutism, although the latter cannot be diagnosed in the presence of a neurologic difference such as those seen in autism (Harris 1996). A somewhat different situation occurs when a toddler or preschool child who has mastered some language suddenly stops talking. This scenario is occasionally associated with autism, and careful clinical observation is needed to ensure that a timely referral is made.

CASE 4

When Mr. and Mrs. Jones first brought their son, John, into the clinic for a speech and language evaluation, he was 24 months of age. Their primary concern was that he had stopped talking. He had begun to say a few words when he was a little older than 1 year. When his baby sister was born, when he was 24 months of age, he stopped verbalizing. The speech-language pathologist administered a standardized inventory via parent report, and John scored within normal limits for his reported functioning before the birth of his sister. No formal receptive or expressive language testing could be completed with John because of his lack of attention to testing materials. Informal observation confirmed his parents' report of lack of spontaneous verbalization and lack of response to language addressed to him. A program of informal language stimulation was recommended, to be followed by a re-evaluation within 3 months. It was speculated that the birth of his sibling had caused a temporary regression. On re-evaluation, John exhibited no progress from the previous diagnostic.

He had been seen in two separate facilities in the interim, as the parents sought other professional opinions. In one of these settings, formal language therapy had been attempted, but Mr. and Mrs. Jones reported no progress. The staff at the other facility recommended a psychological evaluation and stated that they were not able to provide further assistance for John. During the diagnostic re-evaluation, it was noted that John exhibited a marked lack of eye contact, as well as a tendency to play with toys in unusual ways (sorting by color and size and lining them up). A referral for psychological evaluation was made, and John ultimately received the diagnosis of autism. He was enrolled in a school specializing in intervention for children with autism.

An important feature of this case study is the clinician's optimism regarding the possibility of some type of elective mutism following the birth of a sibling. As Harris (1996) noted, such "reactive" mutism is rare. Parental concern coupled with such a severe regression should have been taken more seriously from the beginning.

ROLE OF THE SPEECH-LANGUAGE PATHOLOGIST IN DIAGNOSING AUTISM

Careful consideration of Case 4 leads to certain conclusions about the speech-language pathologist's role as communication disorders specialist in diagnosing a disorder that is so closely related with his or her specialty. First, it is important to recognize that the speech-language pathologist is likely to be the first professional to see young children who are ultimately diagnosed as autistic, since the first signal to parents of something wrong is often absence of language development. Second, close monitoring of unusual cases is vital, especially if the following are present:

- Language regression
- Suspected receptive language delay
- Impairment of nonverbal communication
- Lack of development of pretend play
- Unusually restricted interests and activities
- Unusual patterns of eye gaze and eye contact
- Report of unusual reactions to sensory stimuli
- In older individuals, conversational disability with marked lack of ability to succeed in listener-focused domains (referencing, spontaneous requests for information, maintenance of other-initiated topics)

Third, speech-language pathologists must carefully evaluate their role in offering information to parents at a difficult time in their lives. Although autism is a diagnosis that depends on psychological evaluation, the use of the word is not forbidden. It is likely that the speech-language pathologist who offered no information to Mr. and Mrs. Jones thought it inappropriate to suggest a possible diagnosis and wanted to avoid infringement on the psychologist. It is difficult to imagine what could be more alarming to parents than to be told by a speech-language pathologist that there is very limited help for their nonspeaking child and that they must seek unspecified psychological help. Given that, following diagnosis, it was likely that a speech-language pathologist would be involved in a transdisciplinary treatment team, and clear communication and mutual understanding should be established from the beginning. Speech-language pathologists who do not have access to team support can at a minimum suggest further evaluation to assist in determining the possible diagnosis of autism. Negative situations will become less likely with the increasing availability of transdisciplinary teams composed of people experienced in working with children who have developmental disorders.

CASE 5

Mrs. Johnson brought Jim to a speech and hearing center because he was not yet speaking at 3 years of age. The speech-language pathologist observed that Jim stood for a long period in front of the coat rack in the waiting room, making unusual hand gestures and moving his body rhythmically. He did not make eye contact during the evaluation, and no verbal or nonverbal communicative attempts were observed. Formal testing was abandoned following lack of success on training plates. When she was questioned about Jim's behavior with the coat rack, his mother became agitated and related how difficult it was even to walk down the street with Jim because of his apparent need to stop and perform this ritual with all tall thin objects (e.g., parking meters, telephone poles). His mother stated: "I have two other children, and lots of cousins, nieces and nephews, and he is not like any other child I've ever seen. Have you ever seen a child like this?" The clinician decided that in the face of clear-cut evidence of autism (i.e., marked language delay, impairment of nonverbal communication, unusual and restricted repertoire of interests and activities), it was important to reassure Mrs. Johnson that indeed there are other children like this and to mention the existence of the condition autism. The speech-language pathologist stated that the psychologist should be consulted in seeking a definitive diagnosis, but that Jim demonstrated some of the same characteristics of children with a known disorder.

DIFFERENTIAL DIAGNOSIS IN AUTISM: FOCUS ON LANGUAGE AND COMMUNICATION

Transdisciplinary Team

A speech-language pathologist who participates in a diagnostic evaluation of an individual with suspected autism has a dual role. He or she must conduct an in-depth analysis of language and communication, documenting strengths and weaknesses, for purposes of intervention programming. In addition, the speech-language pathologist is the person who has the expertise and responsibility to provide the information, opinions, and recommendations about the client's communicative functioning to the psychological, medical, and educational professionals who are involved. Ideally, the speech-language pathologist is a member of a transdisciplinary team. Other members of the team for evaluation of childhood developmental disorders are likely to include medical and allied health professionals (e.g., a pediatrician, geneticist, neurologist psychologist, occupational therapist, special educator, and audiologist). The ideal situation does not always exist, and, when it does not, the services must be arranged by referrals to and consultations with other professionals.

Consulting with Other Professionals

It is important that the speech-language pathologist provide information to fellow professionals on the exact characteristics of a client's competence in receptive and expressive domains. To this end, report summaries should include specific opinions about the client's ability to operate in these domains. However, few outside the profession of speech-language pathology are aware of the existence of pragmatic language problems. Even when some awareness of conversational disability exists, it typically does not extend to awareness of the complex interaction of form and function that takes place in successful comprehension. This may result in failure to consult a speech-language pathologist when people with borderline abilities are first seen by psychologists, who may diagnose broad-based "comprehension deficits" that in fact may have a basis not in typical problems with vocabulary and syntax but rather arise from special pragmatic problems experienced by people with autism. Obviously, the team approach helps to avoid such problems.

Purpose of Formal Language Testing

An assessment battery for an individual suspected of having autism may include some formal tests. These tests may be useful in establishing areas of competence, such as vocabulary knowledge. However, poor performance on formal language assessment batteries does not differentiate autistic from nonautistic individuals. To successfully document the presence of a communicative profile consistent with an autistic spectrum disorder, informal analysis is imperative. As previously noted, the individual differences that can be seen in individuals with autism are extreme, and clients may range from nonverbal toddlers to adults who have jobs and college degrees. For this reason, a prescribed approach to assessment is inappropriate. Rather, the structural-analytic approach advocated by Lund and Duchan (1993) is recommended. In structural analysis, the clinician collects samples of communicative performance in a variety of contexts and seeks to establish observed regularities. The goal is to be able to infer the nature of the underlying system.

In addition to direct observation, the insights of caregivers should be sought in attempting to establish a diagnosis of autism. Parents have the most ample opportunities to observe patterns of social interaction, communicative behavior, and other clues that may point to autism (e.g., routines, motor stereotypes). Careful interviewing in a sensitive manner can reveal unexpected competencies not observed in the clinical setting, as well as providing the parents' insights into the sources of their child's greatest difficulties.

As with any complex language disorder, assessment in a range of contexts is important for establishing the parameters of ability displayed by an individual. In autism, the restricted range of interests and difficulty in dealing with unfamiliar persons and environments can contribute to an unnecessarily negative impression of a client seen only in a typical clinical setting. For differential diagnostic purposes in uncertain cases, a range of contexts is also necessary. These contexts allow for adequate sampling of the range of behaviors necessary for documenting a suspicion of autism. By the same token, use of dynamic assessment can be helpful in probing for hidden abilities. (See Olswang and Bain 1991 for a discussion of dynamic assessment techniques.) Dynamic assessment actually allows for and encourages modifications of standard assessment tools. It is therefore ideal for assessing clients who may be autistic, in that modifications to a task to make it fit in with the client's world view can reveal cues as to what leads to success and failure in a given communication domain.

Assessment of Expressive Communication

Systems that should be considered for an assessment of expressive communication include the following:

1. Unintentional behavior patterns correlating with nonverbal communication, including unusual behavior patterns (e.g., signs of extreme distress resulting from apparently ordinary situations), body posture and movements that indicate emotional status, patterns of self-stimulatory behavior as they correlate with external situations (for their potential unintentional communicative value), change of affect within and across situations, and interactants.

2. Intentional nonverbal communicative behaviors, including gesture, eye-gaze patterns, vocalizations indicative of pleasure or distress, and possible vocables or protowords. Nonverbal communication needs careful attention in suspected autism, as both verbal and nonverbal communication are typically affected in this population. In addition, documenting lack of nonverbal gestural communication is important for differentiating autism from other language disorders of childhood. There is evidence that children with autism show deficits in gestural joint attention (e.g., failing to follow a communicative partner's point with their gaze) even when matched for IQ and language with controls (Mundy et al. 1990).

3. Linguistic vocalizations. Linguistic vocalizations can be intentional or unintentional; however, this determination may be impossible for the observer to make. Observation should instead focus on documenting the form of utterances and correlating forms with inferred purposes. Analysis of echolalic utterances is particularly important as research has shown that individuals with autism may use echolalia for communicative purposes (Prizant and Duchan 1981; Prizant and Rydell 1984). Even noncommunicative echoes need to be inventoried, and their role in the client's speech repertoire examined, for possible cues to intervention strategies.

In terms of differential diagnosis, the clinician is strongly cautioned against considering echolalia alone to be a sufficient basis for the diagnosis of autism. Even normal children can go through a stage of echoing, especially when very young. People with visual impairments or other sensory problems may echo as a means of confirming what was said, or because they don't have the ability to generate language spontaneously in a given situation. Brain insults of various kinds can also leave patients with some tendency to rely on echolalia.

Pronominal reversal in speakers with autism has received much attention, but caution is needed here as well. Speakers with other disorders and young, normally developing children may say *I* for *you* and vice versa. Mastery of these deictic shifts in discourse is a slow process, and the mere presence of pronominal reversal in the absence of other indicators is an inadequate basis for the diagnosis of autism.

In general, the language used by individuals with autism tends to exhibit the inflexible, routinized nature that characterizes much of their interactions with the world. However, the exact nature of a person's routines and patterns is highly individual. In very high-functioning individuals, even the detection of routines can be problematic. This is because they can, at times, incorporate routines into discourse in a manner that appears on the surface to be natural, at least the first time the listener hears it. The input of individuals familiar with the autistic person is essential for discovering the existence of these patterns.

CASE 6

Luke was a 20-year-old man with autism. He conversed readily with both familiar and unfamiliar individuals and sought out peer interactions. An inexperienced clinician was conversing with Luke one day, and, during the course of the conversation, Luke happened to mention that he had a sunburn and described himself as "red as a lobster" with great verve and appropriate intonation. Later, he mentioned an episode in which he had a cold and fever, during the course of which illness he sweated and was given an aspirin. Still later, the clinician observed him spontaneously questioning a peer during group conversation-based therapy. Luke inquired about what the student had for dinner at a restaurant, what he had to drink, whether it was diet or regular, and whether it had ice. These observations suggested to the novice speech-language pathologist that Luke had some of the strongest and most appropriate conversational abilities among the more linguistically advanced students. However, during the course of the next year, the clinician had the opportunity to hear Luke, at plausible points in the conversation, repeat these same series of utterances (and other routines as well), almost verbatim. Luke's interest in preservation of sameness and dwelling on certain topics had blossomed into a highly skilled ability to intertwine his interests with the ongoing conversation in a manner which, to an untutored observer, seemed spontaneous.

Assessment of Receptive Abilities

There are no receptive language disorders uniquely associated with autism. In general, receptive vocabulary and syntactic ability appear to be commensurate with intellectual functioning (as measured by nonverbal testing) in autistic individuals. However, problems can arise for pragmatic reasons. These are difficult to assess, since most formal testing is not designed to discover problems in areas such as drawing inferences in conversation. Research by Paul and Cohen (1985) suggests that individuals with autism may have special difficulty in understanding indirect requests. My own research (Hewitt 1994) found that individuals with autism were less able to respond in naturalistic contexts to questions requiring drawing of inferences and taking the perspective of the listener. These data indicate that informal assessment of ability to respond to direct (e.g., Give me the salt, Open the window) versus indirect (e.g., Can you pass me the salt? Gee, it's cold in here) requests may help pinpoint comprehension problems arising from an autistic spectrum disorder. Observation of a pattern of success and failure in questions requiring more and less inferencing may also be helpful.

There is one specific aspect of receptive ability that can, in fact, differentiate autism from other problems in some cases. A frequent early sign of autism troubling to parents is that toddlers with autism appear not to attend to human voices. It is for this reason that hearing impairment is sometimes suspected before autism is diagnosed. If a baby or toddler clearly startles at environmental noise, while appearing not to attend to caregivers' speech, the possibility of autism should be explored carefully.

Impairment in central auditory processing abilities has been suspected in some individuals with autism. This may impact receptive and expressive language ability, especially in noisy or distracting environments.

Assessment for Other Speech and Hearing Disorders

Standard batteries routinely carried out in a comprehensive speech, language, and hearing assessment are of course necessary. Other than ruling out hearing loss as a cause of autistic-seeming behaviors, the primary speech-related domain that is helpful in differential diagnosis is an assessment of prosody. Prosodic disturbances are a sign of autism according to DSM-IV (American Psychiatric Association 1994), and while not alone sufficient to establish the diagnosis, their presence may fit into a larger overall pattern. Phonologic or vocal patterns may be unusual in certain individuals, but they are not diagnostic indicators of autism per se. Some high-functioning people who are particularly uncomfortable in social situations may border on elective mutism, and autism should be considered as one possible reason for reluctance to use known communication abilities.

Other Behavioral Aspects to Consider

Perceptual Factors

Abnormal perceptual processes resulting in hyper- and hyposensitivity to certain types of sensory stimuli can frequently co-occur with autism. Indeed, Grandin (1995) argued that perceptual disturbances, in fact, cause autism by preventing affected individuals from attending to social and other important stimuli in infancy. Parent report and self-report of such problems should be a factor in considering a referral for assessment of suspected autism in the presence of other factors indicating the diagnosis to be a possibility. Some high-functioning people with autism report that they are unable to listen at all in the presence of background noise or to function when multiple speakers address them (Grandin 1995; Williams 1992). Grandin (1995) advocated central auditory testing for people with autism although such evaluations are not yet standard.

Gait and Motor Stereotypes

Stiff and unusual gait patterns, as well as the often reported motor stereotypes involving flapping and spinning of self or objects, rocking, and other self-stimulatory behaviors, are indicators of possible autism. However, care is needed, as other types of problems can result in some of these behaviors, especially unusual gait patterns (e.g., some children with cerebral palsy exhibit stiff gait patterns at times similar to those seen in certain individuals with autism). Marked presence of self-stimulatory behaviors is an important sign of autism, but it should be considered in light of all factors.

Routines and Preservation of Sameness

Unusual and marked distress at changes in routine and preference for limited activities is not unusual in autism. Examples of unusual hobbies and repetitive verbal routines include a young man primarily interested in studying his high school algebra text, a young adult who spent his leisure time writing letters requesting celebrities to send him a copy of a *TV Guide* they had used, a person who gathered information on the addresses of juvenile courts in the British Isles (Frith 1989), a young man who enjoyed reciting from memory routines from the television show *Sesame Street*, and a boy who asked everyone he met the location of a store chain where they shopped (saying, "What K-Mart do you shop at?"). As previously noted, routines can be verbal (e.g., repetitive questioning) or may more closely resemble narrowly focused hobbies in high-functioning individuals. Indeed, in some individuals, narrowness of interests can fade off the end of the autistic spectrum out of the domain of clearly clinically significant behavior. Some of the more bizarre manifestations of autistic individuals may seem highly unusual; however, obsessive interest in a hobby is not far from behavior that falls within normal limits. In borderline cases such as these, whether the client is actually autistic or has Asperger's syndrome is not as important as what type of communication disorder he or she presents.

CASE 7

Mrs. Gold was referred for an evaluation for a possible communication disorder and autism by her husband. She was an articulate and intelligent individual holding a doctorate in a highly specialized scientific technical field. However, she had trouble finding employment in her field and reported difficulties in successfully negotiating the social requirements of the interview process. She had been evaluated by an audiologist for reported hypersensitivity to noise, with a lack of clear-cut findings. In her self-report, she mentioned avoiding almost all social situations, stores, and restaurants, as the background noise of talking and music was physically painful to her and caused her terrible distress. Mrs. Gold had excellent eye contact and, while discussing her auditory and communication problems, was very articulate and thoughtful. She exhibited excellent nonverbal communication skills and evidenced a very fast rate of speech with no prosodic anomalies. However, the clinician interviewing her found that she had difficulty discussing subjects that she had not introduced and also exhibited a loquacity that made it difficult to terminate the conversation. A referral for psychological evaluation was suggested. A feature of this case worth noting is that Mrs. Gold exhibited a number of signs of an autistic spectrum disorder such as Asperger's syndrome. These included a somewhat restricted range of interests and activities, perceptual abnormalities, and mild conversational difficulties. Nonetheless, her adaptive functioning was at a level that placed her at or beyond the top end of the autistic spectrum.

In addition to routines and restricted interests, many individuals with autism show marked distress in new environments or sometimes over household routines of which they disapprove. Mothers have reported infants who would not eat unless the caregiver wore a particular flowered dress, children who would not sleep and become hysterically destructive if a certain pattern of sheets was not on the bed, and a boy who screamed if the car he was riding in turned left. In this boy's world, if the car went right, everything was fine, but if it went left and he hadn't predicted it, chaos and misery would result (Barron and Barron 1992). Reports of this type of behavior should be examined carefully if autism is suspected.

Social Factors

Social withdrawal as a hallmark of the syndrome of autism is the single most familiar aspect of the syndrome to the general public. The notion of the autistic person who needs no one, does not differentiate between close relatives and strangers, and is completely happy in isolation from social contact is far from being the typical case. In fact, as several of the case studies illustrate, while virtually all individuals who receive a diagnosis of autism do, in fact, demonstrate unusual social relatedness, they do not necessarily demonstrate social withdrawal. (See

Mundy and Sigman 1989 for a discussion of social relatedness in autism.) For practical clinical purposes, speech-language pathologists need to be looking for those unusual patterns in social relations. Autism cannot be eliminated as a possibility merely because the speech-language pathologist is aware that a child relates to peers at times or, perhaps, has an attachment to a certain caregiver.

Cases of near-total social avoidance in individuals with autism do exist. There are, for example, infants or toddlers who become rigid when held and are only relaxed and happy when left alone. Many individuals with autism report a need to spend significant amounts of time alone. But the speech-language pathologist must also consider cases like that of Ben (Case 1), who, when mainstreamed in a regular high school, began to ask his mother questions about what being a friend meant and to seek out interactions with peers. Some type of difficulty in social relatedness is virtually always present in individuals with autism. But difficulty in handling a given domain is far from total absence of interest or ability in that domain.

ADDITIONAL RESOURCES FOR DESIGNING ASSESSMENT FOR INDIVIDUALS WITH AUTISM

There are a number of resources offering clinicians direction in the design of informal assessment for individuals with autism. Lund and Duchan (1993) published a general guide to language assessment in naturalistic contexts. For more specific suggestions relevant to autism, Wetherby and Prizant (1992) provided a brief but relatively comprehensive chapter listing important considerations and offering specific suggestions. Wetherby and Prutting's (1984) research protocol can also serve as a guide to the analysis of communicative and social abilities in autistic children. The TEACCH program (Watson et al. 1989) gave detailed, step-by-step assessment suggestions, including obtaining a communication sample, interviewing caregivers, and determining goals held by teachers and caregivers for improving communication. A comprehensive overview of the "state of the art," according to many working in the area of autism, is found in the April 1996 issue of the *Journal of Autism and Developmental Disorders* (Plenum Publishing Corporation 1996). In addition, Internet searches of World Wide Web sites and listserves on autism and related disorders can turn up an interesting range of information and opinion. Of course, caution is needed, as always, in using Internet resources, since most are not refereed and quality varies widely.

CONCLUSION

The role of the speech-language pathologist in identifying and working with people with autism is not clearly defined. Reports of tentativeness and uncertainty in such situations are not uncommon. For example, at a recent presentation on autism, an audience member asked me, "Who should diagnose autism?" She came up later and explained that there was a child in her preschool program whom she suspected had autism, and she was not sure how to proceed. A further anecdote is an example of how *not* to proceed in such a situation. The father of a child with autism described how he received the news his child was autistic. A psychologist came for a home visit, left without saying anything specific, and said a speech-language pathologist would schedule a follow-up. The speech-language pathologist then conducted a home-based assessment. As she was leaving, she said something to the effect of, "The psychologist mentioned he saw signs of autism, and what I have seen confirms this. I'm very sorry. Have a nice day." The fact that reactions by the clinicians placed in this situation varied from "we can't tell you anything, go see a psychologist," to dropping a bombshell and leaving suggests a high level of professional discomfort with this domain.

Many speech-language pathologists, as well as other professionals, are also very uncomfortable when planning for appropriate management. The speech-language pathologist is the person who needs to provide the leadership in the planning for assistance in the development of communication skills. Obviously, understanding of the diagnosis is necessary for effective planning. The diagnostic process extends into the treatment phase of a management program. Changes that occur with maturation and those occurring in response to treatment require continued assessment. The management program also requires revisions in response to these changes. One avenue for increased competency in the domain of autism is the approach to differential diagnosis outlined in this chapter, in which the emphasis is placed on understanding autism as a spectrum disorder marked by extreme individual differences. Moreover, as understanding of the complexity and range of problems associated with autism improves, hope increases for improved outcomes. With increased early identification, intervention and a lifespan approach will be key components in achieving those outcomes. Perhaps as the gloom and confusion surrounding autism begin to lift, more speech-language pathologists will take a positive and confident approach.

After all, the training of speech-language pathologists provides unique qualifications to allow the most insight into a key component of autism, communicative impairment. Speech-language pathologists have an important place as key players on assessment teams. As practice shifts to true transdisciplinary teams with porous disciplinary boundaries, service delivery to persons with autism will achieve a new level of excellence.

REFERENCES

American Psychiatric Association. (1980) *Diagnostic and Statistical Manual of Mental Disorders* (3rd ed). Washington, DC: American Psychiatric Association.

American Psychiatric Association. (1987) *Diagnostic and Statistical Manual of Mental Disorders* (3rd ed). Washington, DC: American Psychiatric Association.

American Psychiatric Association. (1994) *Diagnostic and Statistical Manual of Mental Disorders* (4th ed). Washington, DC: American Psychiatric Association.

Asperger H. (1995) Autistic Psychopathy in Childhood (U Frith, trans.). In U Frith (ed), *Autism and Asperger Syndrome* (pp. 37–92). New York: Cambridge University Press. (Original work published in 1944.)

Barron J, Barron S. (1992) *There's a Boy in Here.* New York: Simon & Schuster.

Bettelheim B. (1959) Joey: a "mechanical boy." *Scientific American* 200, 116–127.

Bettison S. (1996) The long-term effects of auditory training on children with autism. *Journal of Autism and Developmental Disorders* 26, 361–374.

Bishop D, Rosenbloom L. (1987) Classification of Childhood Language Disorders. In W Yule, M Rutter (eds), *Language Development and Disorders. Clinics in Developmental Medicine,* nos. 101–102. London: MacKeith Press.

Brook S, Bowler D. (1992) Autism by another name? Semantic and pragmatic impairments in children. *Journal of Autism and Developmental Disorders* 22, 61–81.

Duchan J. (1993) Issues raised by facilitated communication for theorizing and research on autism. *Journal of Speech and Hearing Research* 36, 1108–1119.

Frith U. (1989) *Autism: Explaining the Enigma.* Oxford, England: Basil Blackwell.

Frith U. (1995) Asperger and His Syndrome. In U Frith (ed), *Autism and Asperger Syndrome* (pp. 1–36). New York: Cambridge University Press.

Gillberg C. (1990) Autism and pervasive developmental disorders. *Journal of Child Psychology* 31, 99–119.

Gillberg C. (1992) Autism and autistic-like conditions: subclasses among disorders of empathy. *Journal of Child Psychology* 33, 813–842.

Grandin T. (1995) *Thinking in Pictures and Other Reports from My Life with Autism.* New York: Doubleday.

Grandin T, Scariano MM. (1986) *Emergence Labeled Autistic.* Novato, CA: Arena Press.

Happé F. (1995) *Autism: An Introduction to Psychological Theory.* Cambridge, MA: Harvard University Press.

Harris HF. (1996) Elective mutism: a tutorial. *Language, Speech, and Hearing Services in Schools* 27, 10–15.

Hewitt L. (1994) Communicative competence of young adults with autism: ability to meet listener's needs, Ph.D. diss., State University of New York at Buffalo, 1994. *Dissertation Abstracts International.*

Hobson P. (1993) *Autism and the Development of Mind.* Hillsdale, NJ: Erlbaum.

Kanner L. (1943) Autistic disturbances of affective contact. *Nervous Child* 2, 217–250.

Lund N, Duchan J. (1993) *Assessing Children's Language in Naturalistic Contexts* (3rd ed). Englewood Cliffs, NJ: Prentice-Hall.

Mundy P, Sigman M. (1989) Specifying the Nature of the Social Impairment in Autism. In G Dawson (ed), *Autism: Nature, Diagnosis, and Treatment* (pp. 3–21). New York: Guilford Press.

Mundy P, Sigman M, Kasari C. (1990) A longitudinal study of joint attention and language development in autistic children. *Journal of Autism and Developmental Disorders* 20, 115–128.

Olswang L, Bain B. (1991) When to recommend intervention. *Language, Speech, and Hearing Services in Schools* 22, 255–263.

Ozonoff S, Rogers S, Pennington B. (1991a) Asperger's syndrome: evidence of an empirical distinction from high-functioning autism. *Journal of Child Psychology* 32, 1107–1122.

Ozonoff S, Rogers S, Pennington B. (1991b) Executive function deficits in high-functioning autistic individuals: relationship to theory of mind. *Journal of Child Psychology* 32, 1081–1105.

Paul R, Cohen D. (1985) Comprehension of indirect requests in adults with autistic disorders and mental retardation. *Journal of Speech and Hearing Research* 28, 475–479.

Prizant B, Duchan J. (1981) The functions of immediate echolalia in autistic children. *Journal of Speech and Hearing Disorders* 46, 241–249.

Prizant B, Rydell P. (1984) Analysis of functions of delayed echolalia in autistic children. *Journal of Speech and Hearing Research* 27, 183–192.

Provence S, Dahl K. (1987) Disorders of Atypical Development: Diagnostic Issues Raised by a Spectrum Disorder. In D Cohen, A Donnellan, R Paul (eds) *Handbook of Autism and Pervasive Developmental Disorders* (pp. 677–689). New York: Wiley.

Rapin I, Allen D. (1983) Developmental Language Disorders: Nosologic Considerations. In U Kirk (ed), *Neuropsychology of Language, Reading and Spelling* (pp. 155–184). New York: Academic Press.

Schopler E, Mesibov G. (1988) Introduction to Diagnosis and Assessment of Autism. In E Schopler, G Mesibov (eds), *Diagnosis and Assessment in Autism* (pp. 3–14). New York: Plenum.

Tager-Flusberg H. (1994) Dissociations in Form and Function in the Acquisition of Language by Autistic Children. In H Tager-Flusberg (ed), *Constraints on Language Acquisition: Studies of Atypical Children* (pp. 175–194). Hillsdale, NJ: Erlbaum.

Tsai L, Ghaziuddin M. (1992) Biomedical Research in Autism. In D Berkell (ed), *Autism: Identification, Education, and Treatment* (pp. 53–76). Hillsdale, NJ: Erlbaum.

Watson L, Lord C, Schaffer B, Schopler E. (1989) *Teaching Spontaneous Communication to Autistic and Developmentally Handicapped Children.* Austin, TX: PRO-ED.

Wetherby A, Prizant B. (1992) Facilitating Language and Communication Development in Autism: Assessment and Intervention Guidelines. In D Berkell (ed), *Autism: Identification, Education, and Treatment* (pp. 107–134). Hillsdale, NJ: Erlbaum.

Wetherby A, Prutting C. (1984) Profiles of communicative and cognitive-social abilities in autistic children. *Journal of Speech and Hearing Research* 27, 364–377.

Williams D. (1992) *Nobody, Nowhere*. New York: Doubleday.

Windsor J, Doyle S, Siegel G. (1994) Language acquisition after mutism: a longitudinal case study of autism. *Journal of Speech and Hearing Research* 37, 96–105.

Wing L, Gould J. (1979). Severe impairments of social interaction and associated abnormalities in children: epidemiology and classification. *Journal of Autism and Developmental Disorders* 9, 11–29.

10

Differential Diagnosis for Aphasia

Richard K. Peach

For some, differential diagnosis for aphasia is assumed to involve simply the assignment of patients to one of the nine or so traditional categories or types of aphasia. Indeed, the teaching of these diagnostic algorithms usually proceeds from the assumption that the language disorder with which a patient presents is, in fact, aphasia. But the differential diagnosis of aphasia in daily clinical practice has more to do with identifying whether the neurologic communication disorder that a patient presents is truly one of aphasia versus another clinical entity that shares symptoms to warrant consideration of a diagnosis of aphasia. For example, among the "aphasic" patients seen on a given day in any large medical center, there may be individuals who actually present with communication problems from such diverse disorders as conversion reaction, dementia, anoxic encephalopathy, epilepsy, confusional state, apraxia, psychiatric disturbance, or lacunar syndrome, to name a few. So, while a portion of this chapter is given necessarily to identifying the characteristics of the different varieties of aphasia, substantial discussion is also devoted to describing the signs and symptoms that aid in discriminating among aphasic versus nonaphasic language disorders.

Perhaps the most appropriate way to begin this discussion is with a clear description of what is meant by the term *aphasia*, at least insofar as it is used in this chapter. Darley (1967, p. 236) recognized that "not everything called aphasia by someone is, indeed, aphasia" and framed the nosologic significance of this exercise by pointing out that the treatment of patients with nonaphasic language disorders is quite different from those who are aphasic. Comprehensive reviews of the historical use of the term *aphasia* are provided by Chapey (1994), Davis (1993), and Rosenbek and colleagues (1989). The key issues addressed in these reviews concern (1) whether aphasia produces a general impairment to all language input-output modalities simultaneously (Darley 1982;

Schuell et al. 1964) or can selectively involve particular modalities (Damasio 1981; Goodglass and Kaplan 1983); (2) whether it damages the components of language symmetrically (i.e., to a similar degree) (Darley 1982; Schuell et al. 1964) or differentially, yielding novel combinations that result in various types (Benson 1979; Benson and Ardila 1996; Goodglass and Kaplan 1983); (3) whether aphasia consists of a primary loss in language competence for producing propositions (Jackson 1864) or an inefficiency for performing language computations secondary to physiologic deficits (McNeil 1988); and (4) whether it affects language representations without impairing the cognitive processes acting on those representations or involves the entire cognitive system necessary for processing linguistic information (Chapey 1994; Davis 1993).

In this chapter, aphasia refers to the broad range of linguistic processes underlying language activities in both input (listening, reading) and output (speaking, writing) modalities. Deficits that are selective with regard to a single input or output modality involve different neuropsychological impairments from those observed in aphasia and are described respectively as agnosic or apraxic in nature. The distributed character of the neural systems underlying language behavior (Mesulam 1990) supports the notion of crossmodal rather than unimodal impairment following cerebral damage. These networks nonetheless engage cortical centers that are predominately lexical-semantic and posteriorly located on the one hand and articulatory-syntactic and anteriorly related on the other hand, giving rise to differential effects in the severity of the impairments within modalities following brain damage. Aphasia, then, is a general impairment that involves all language activities (i.e., speaking, listening, reading, writing), most frequently to disproportionate degrees. Aphasia is also less likely the result of a loss of language competence (i.e., knowledge of representations) as it is an impairment in the real-time processes that act on such representations (Caplan 1987; McNeil et al. 1991; Zurif 1990). More than just a circumscribed language impairment then, aphasia is a disorder that involves information-processing disturbances at the attentional, memorial, linguistic, and executive levels of the cognitive system used for processing language (Beeson et al. 1993; Margolin 1991; Tseng et al. 1993).

Historically, views such as these have been developed following investigations of individuals with chronic aphasia secondary to focal brain lesions. The most common etiologies for these aphasia-producing lesions have been cerebrovascular accidents (CVA) and open-head injuries (e.g., gunshot wounds). From a differential diagnostic perspective, the belief that aphasia produces a general, simultaneous impairment to all language modalities allows the examiner to rule out a diagnosis of aphasia when the deficits impair as a single modality, as

Table 10.1
Traditional criteria for aphasia diagnosis

Parameter	*Criterion*
Onset	Paroxysmal versus insidious
Number of affected modalities	Multiple versus single
Localization of underlying brain damage	Cortical versus subcortical
Extent of brain damage	Focal versus diffuse versus mixed
Mental status	Alert and aware versus lethargic and obtunded
Mental competence	Preserved versus impaired thought
Specificity of cognitive impairment	Primarily linguistic versus linguistic and nonlinguistic
Personality characteristics	Normal versus muted or bizarre

in the case of agnosia or apraxia. But these notions do not provide clinical guidance for distinguishing aphasia from the larger group of general language impairments that result from a variety of neurologic conditions. To do this, additional criteria have been applied in aphasia diagnosis that concern the onset of the condition (paroxysmal versus insidious), the localization of the underlying brain damage (cortical versus subcortical), the extent of the brain damage (focal, diffuse, or mixed), the mental status of the patient (alert and aware versus lethargic or obtunded), the mental competence of the patient (preserved versus impaired thought), the specificity of cognitive impairment (primarily verbal versus verbal and nonverbal), and the personality characteristics of the patient (normal versus muted versus bizarre) (Table 10.1). Using these criteria, aphasia has been described traditionally as a language impairment of sudden onset resulting from focal, unilateral neurologic damage involving the cortex of the dominant hemisphere, not attributable to sensorimotor deficits, decreased mentation, or altered thought processes, and coexisting with relatively preserved nonverbal cognitive abilities.

Yet these guidelines have been blurred when the term *aphasia* is used to describe the language impairments associated with other diverse conditions such as Alzheimer's disease (Croisile et al. 1991; Yesavage et al. 1993), Pick's disease and aspecific gliosis (Croisile et al. 1991), chronic subdural hematoma (Kaminski et al. 1992), closed-head injury (Peach 1992), epilepsy (Abou-Khalil et al. 1994), multiple sclerosis (Spatt et al. 1994), progressive supranuclear palsy (Capitani et al. 1993), mental retardation (Gordon 1993), herpes simplex encephalitis (Benson 1991; Caselli et al. 1991), and schizophrenia (Sambunaris and Hyde 1994). Most of these conditions have been associated with diffuse, cognitive decline and organic brain syndrome, so that the resulting language deficits have been described otherwise as a product of confusion or generalized intellectual impairment rather than aphasia (Wertz 1985).

Does the frequent description of these language impairments as aphasia suggest an acceptance of the alternative, broader use of the term (i.e., any language impairment following brain damage) (Benson 1979; Benson and Ardila 1996)? Or do their characteristics conform closely enough to the aphasias observed following CVA or open-head injury that they meet the essential definition just suggested, thereby requiring only modification based on improved understanding of the medical circumstances that may produce these aphasias? These questions address the issue of when the language disorder associated with at least some of these conditions should be considered an aphasia and when it should not. To be sure, the issue is not a new one (see, for example, the series of papers presented by Holland, Wertz, and Rosenbek at the 1982 Clinical Aphasiology Conference [Brookshire 1982]); it merely has been placed in the updated context of medical practice.

In this chapter, aphasia diagnosis is described in terms of an orderly process of data collection that allows the clinician to converge on whether an acquired language impairment is aphasic or nonaphasic, and, if aphasic, what the nature of the aphasia is. The process is characterized by a series of judgments at selected junctures that bring in or rule out various alternative diagnoses that explain the language disorder, until the full complement of evidence delimits the choices to just one but no more than a few. Data collection to diagnose aphasia is organized around the patient's (1) medical history, (2) mental status, (3) speech fluency and speech patterns, (4) oral and visual language capabilities, (5) nonverbal cognitive abilities, and (6) pragmatic abilities. The diagnosis provides the basis on which a prognosis is developed for the patient's future communication abilities and the direction for management of the patient's language disorder.

MEDICAL HISTORY

Request for Consultation and Review of the Medical Record

The first "contact" with a patient is through the request for consultation services. Frequently, the only information contained in the consult is the need for speech evaluation or speech therapy. However, on other occasions, the presenting problem is described in terms of broad diagnoses (e.g., CVA, intractable seizures) that nonetheless allow the clinician to delimit the range of possible communication disorders. That is, given an admitting diagnosis that suggests a paroxysmal (versus an insidious) event, the clinician can bring disorders into his or her differential diagnosis that have a greater probability of being associated with such illnesses and assign secondary status to those that do not. Based on these expectations, the clinician can consider, well before the bedside examination, modifications that may need to be made to the diagnostic battery to answer specific questions raised by the disorders receiving primary consideration.

The review of the patient's medical record provides focus to the primary communication disorders that may be encountered during examination. This is usually accomplished by obtaining a thorough picture of the patient's medical history and relating this to possible diagnoses, by comparing this information to the descriptions of the patient's speech and language symptoms appearing in the progress notes section of the chart and by considering the speech-language diagnoses provided by physicians or other health care professionals before the point of speech-language pathology contact. Important information to be considered in the medical history includes the patient's reason for hospital admission, the patient's medical history before the current admission, the results of neuroradiologic procedures (e.g., computed tomography [CT], magnetic resonance imaging [MRI], angiography, positron emission tomography [PET], transcranial Doppler sonography), Wada test results (as appropriate), consultation reports from other clinical services, operative information, the medication record, and the progress notes. The description of the patient's speech-language symptoms provides both a timeline for the evolution of speech-language changes, if applicable, and a snapshot of the patient's communication status just before examination, the interpretation of which may be heavily dependent on the former observations. Any prior speech-language diagnoses, if accurate, provide essential background for interpreting the behaviors observed during speech-language evaluation but should be acknowledged with caution due to the terminologic differences described regarding aphasic behavior and the variable expertise of the individuals making these diagnoses.

Admitting Diagnoses

As mentioned, the patient's admitting diagnosis should be interpreted with regard to whether it signals a paroxysmal (sudden onset of symp-

Table 10.2
Admitting diagnoses: the neuropathology of aphasia

Paroxysmal etiologies (sudden onset of symptoms or disease)
Cerebrovascular disease
Trauma
Infectious disease
Tumors
Epilepsy
Toxins
Insidious etiologies (progressive onset of symptoms or disease)
Diseases of cerebral cortex
Alzheimer's disease
Pick's disease
Creutzfeldt-Jakob disease
Disease of basal ganglia
Corticobasal degeneration

toms or disease) or insidious (progressive onset of symptoms or disease) event (Table 10.2). This information is important because generally focal cerebral damage is associated more often with paroxysmal events, and diffuse cerebral damage is identified more with insidious events. Since the aphasias are commonly a manifestation of focal cerebral damage, the clinician's initial hypotheses should entertain a diagnosis of aphasia more strongly when the neurologic event is paroxysmal versus when the event is found to be of insidious onset. On the other hand, early focal cortical degeneration and resulting aphasia have been associated increasingly with a number of well-recognized progressive diseases. In this section, the neuropathologic underpinnings of aphasia are described with regard to the rapidity of their onset.

Paroxysmal Etiologies

Cerebrovascular Disease

Spontaneous vascular events (i.e., CVAs, or strokes) resulting from cerebrovascular disease are a frequent paroxysmal cause of cortical and subcortical aphasias and their related disorders. These events include both ischemic and hemorrhagic insults to the brain. Ischemic strokes result from obstruction of the cerebral blood supply, which deprives the brain of oxygen and produces cerebral infarction (i.e., tissue destruction). The major causes of ischemic strokes are thrombosis and embolism in the cerebral artery or venous systems, the internal carotid arteries, and the vertebral arteries. Cerebral ischemia can also result from traumatic occlusion of the cervical segment of the internal carotid artery.

Thrombosis is clotting within a blood vessel and is most often the result of atherosclerotic plaques (Gilroy 1990). The factors that contribute to accelerated atherosclerosis include hypertension, diabetes mellitus, obesity, hyperuricemia, hyperlipidemia, and smoking. Other causes of thrombosis include hypertrophic arteriosclerosis (hardening of the arteries) associated with chronic hypertension, cerebral arteritis (vasculitis) (e.g., systemic lupus erythematosus), fibromuscular dysplasia producing stenosis of the carotid arteries, abnormalities of the blood, and critical reductions in cerebral perfusion (blood flow). Cerebral thrombosis affects both the large and small, perforating arteries of the cerebral tissues (lacunar syndrome).

In young adults, thrombosis can result from nonpenetrating trauma to the carotid artery and arterial dissections. Nonpenetrating trauma is a common risk factor for ischemia in young adults and is associated with motor vehicle accidents, falls, strangulation, and other causes (Caplan LR 1993; Saver et al. 1992). Arterial dissections result from intense physical exertion or trivial trauma to the cervical and intracranial carotid and middle cerebral arteries. Dissections occur when blood hemorrhages into the wall of an artery forming a hematoma. As the hematoma enlarges, it reduces the arterial lumen (space) and produces a pseudoaneurysm. The hematoma eventually ruptures through the wall of the artery and into the lumen of the artery forming a thrombus that, in turn, produces cerebral ischemia.

Thrombosis of the cerebral venous system also produces infarction of brain tissue nourished by cerebral arteries farther away. Cerebral venous thrombosis can be caused by infection (e.g., infection of face, otitis media, mastoiditis, acute sinusitis). It is also associated with head trauma, sickle cell disease, neoplasms, and the immediate postpartum period.

Cerebral embolism is the occlusion of a vessel by a transported blood clot or other material. The most common source of blood clotting is the heart. Cardiac emboli result from atherosclerotic disease; aneurysms of the ascending aorta; and such valvular diseases as rheumatic heart disease, prolapsed mitral valve, and endocarditis. Others result from fragments of thrombi, due to myocardial infarction, cardiac arrhythmias (e.g., atrial fibrillation), and heart surgery, that have broken free and lodged in the bloodstream at more narrow vessels. Emboli of cardiac origin have a greater likelihood of entering the common carotid arteries than the vertebral arteries and tend to enter the middle cerebral artery via the internal carotid artery (Gilroy 1990).

Traumatic sources of emboli include bleeding due to injury or arterial dissection and thrombosis of the neck vessels, fat emboli from fracture of long bones, and air emboli subsequent to arterial catheterization or surgeries for the heart, the thorax, or vascularized tumors. Septic emboli from systemic infections arise in the lungs as well as other areas.

When the focal deficits resulting from ischemic episodes last 24 hours or less, the patient is said to have experienced a transient ischemic attack. Some patients, however, demonstrate symptoms that persist more than 24 hours but appear to resolve totally within 3 weeks. Although this condition is referred to as *reversible ischemic neurologic deficit,* Kelley (1989) suggested that such scenarios are indicative of a completed stroke and, therefore, at least subtle, and probably permanent, neurologic impairment.

Hemorrhagic strokes include primary intracerebral hemorrhage and subarachnoid hemorrhage. Primary intracerebral hemorrhage is characterized by bleeding into the substance of the brain. The most frequent causes of intracerebral hemorrhage are hypertension and head trauma. A high incidence of intracerebral hemorrhage is also found in patients with leukemia, and a hemorrhagic stroke can be the initial manifestation of the disorder (Garcia et al. 1992).

Chronic hypertension produces arteriosclerotic weakening of blood vessels particularly involving the lenticulostriate branches of the middle cerebral artery. These changes eventually result in the formation and rupture of small aneurysms. The most frequent sites for hypertensive intracerebral hemorrhage are the basal ganglia, the thalamus, and the internal capsule (Bhatnagar and Andy 1995; Gilroy 1990; Kelley 1989). Intracerebral hemorrhages also are observed in the white matter of each of the cerebral lobes (Toole 1990). Blood released from the ruptured blood vessels can accumulate to form a hematoma that then acts as a mass lesion. Intracerebral hemorrhages cause direct destruction of tissue and compression of the surrounding brain parenchyma (the essential internal tissue) that can impinge on important cortical centers. Aphasia resulting from spontaneous-hypertensive posterior temporal lobe hemorrhages in the left hemisphere has been associated with a good outcome due to spontaneous resolution of the causative hematomas (Weisberg et al. 1991).

Subarachnoid hemorrhage is characterized by bleeding into the subarachnoid space. The most common nontraumatic causes of primary subarachnoid hemorrhage are rupture of an intracranial aneurysm due to hypertension and bleeding from an arteriovenous malformation (AVM). Aphasia has been found to be the predominate complaint associated with chronic subdural hematomas resulting from subarachnoid hemorrhage (Kamiski et al. 1992). Secondary subarachnoid hemorrhage occurs when an intracerebral hemorrhage ruptures through the brain parenchyma into the subarachnoid space or the ventricles (Toole 1990).

Aneurysms manifest themselves as dilatations, or pouching, in the arterial wall that assume a simple spherical form. Ninety percent of cerebral aneurysms are berry or saccular aneurysms and occur most often at points of bifurcation along the large arteries of the cerebrovasculature (Hademenos 1995). The most common sites of berry aneurysms are the junction of the internal carotid and the posterior communicating arteries and the junction of the anterior cerebral and anterior communicating arteries and the origin of the middle cerebral artery (Gilroy 1990; Kelley 1989). Neurologic symptoms can result either from compression of surrounding areas due to arterial dilation or from the irritating effects of blood released into the brain or onto its surface (Bhatnagar and Andy 1995). Vasospasm (contraction of the coats of the blood vessels) with delayed cerebral ischemia develops within the first week of a ruptured aneurysm in approximately one-third of the cases of subarachnoid hemorrhage.

CASE 1

CG, a 36-year-old African American woman, was admitted to Rush-Presbyterian-St. Luke's Medical Center with a diagnosis of subarachnoid hemorrhage. A cerebral angiogram revealed a left posterior communicating artery aneurysm without other aneurysms or arteriovenous malformations. She underwent partial craniotomy with a wrap of the cerebral aneurysm. Three days later, she was noted to have a change in mental status that included decreased responsiveness, speech-language disturbances, left facial droop, and right hemiparesis. Transcranial Dopplers revealed severe vasospasm in the distribution of the left internal carotid artery and left middle cerebral artery, with diffuse vasospasm extending over the vessels in the vertebrobasilar system as well. A CT scan demonstrated a diffuse lucency to the left hemisphere suggestive of a sizable infarct or area of ischemia in the territory of the left middle cerebral artery. Results of speech-language evaluation performed approximately 7 weeks later revealed a moderate-to-marked conduction aphasia.

AVMs, or angiomas, are congenital tangles of abnormal vessels composed of arteries and veins of varying size without intervening capillaries. Hemorrhage from an AVM is not strictly limited to the subarachnoid space but can contain a large parenchymatous component (Caplan LR 1993). The majority of AVMs occur in the parietal or frontoparietal regions, but they can occur anywhere in the brain, including the brain stem and cerebellum (Gilroy 1990; Mohr et al. 1992). The surrounding brain shows numerous small hemorrhages and disruption of neurons that can cause loss of brain substance as clot and necrotic tissue are reabsorbed (Caplan LR 1993).

Trauma

Traumatic brain injury is the second most common cause of sudden-onset aphasia (Helm-Estabrooks and Albert 1991). Both the open-head (penetrating) and closed-head (nonpenetrating) types are included under this category and are essentially differentiated by whether the integrity of the meninges has been maintained. Open-head injuries result from gunshot or stabbing wounds and produce more localized cerebral damage. Closed-head injuries can result from motor vehicle accidents, assaults, and accidental falls and produce more diffuse brain damage. Of the two types, nonpenetrating forces are the more common cause of traumatic brain injury.

Traumatic impacts to the head often produce sudden horizontal and rotational movements of the head. Horizontal movements result in focal effects such as cerebral contusions, lacerations, intracranial and intracerebral hematomas, and skull fractures. Rotational movements are associated with loss of consciousness and shear strains (separation of axons and disruption to cell bodies) within the gray and white matter of the brain (Ommaya and Gennarelli 1974). The response to this trauma is a variable mixture of focal and cerebral concussion (i.e., restricted, as well as diffuse, disruption of function) accompanied by primary brain lesions. The clinical picture is frequently complicated by secondary cerebral processes. These processes include edema; increased intracranial pressure; and ischemia due to hypoxia or anoxia, pulmonary insufficiency, hypotension following shock, or fat emboli from long-bone fractures.

The locus of lesion and the type of aphasia in closed-head injury are consistent with the clinicopathologic correlations observed in focal injuries due to cerebrovascular origin. The full range of classical aphasia syndromes following closed-head injury, with few exceptions, has been reported in the literature (Kertesz 1979). It also appears that aphasia in individuals with nonpenetrating head injuries does not necessarily result from discrete focal brain lesions (Peach 1992). Even mild aphasic disturbances can appear as severe language disorders after head injury, due to complications from the presence of confusion. More rapid language recovery is associated with closed-head injury than with CVA, although persistent speech-language deficits are associated with severe closed-head injury.

Infectious Disease

Bacterial and viral infections of the central nervous system produce numerous conditions that can be associated with communicative impairment. Noteworthy among these are bacterial meningitis, viral meningitis, and encephalitis. Acute bacterial meningitis develops over the course of hours to days from a variety of microorganisms and produces an inflammatory response in the pia and arachnoid membranes. The inflammation extends into the first two layers of the cortex and cortical veins. Cortical thrombophlebitis results, followed by thrombosis and infarction (Gilroy 1990). Neuropsychological impairment is common and is characterized by generalized mental status changes (Gade et al. 1992). Focal neurologic deficits can become evident during the chronic stage of the disease (Harris and Benson 1989), and the cerebral lesions causing them can be identified effectively by CT scanning and MRI.

CASE 2

AM, a 47-year-old African American woman, was hospitalized status post bacterial meningitis. CT scan with contrast performed 9 days after admission demonstrated multiple areas of decreased attenuation in the left parietal lobe and the right frontoparietal junction involving the subcortical white matter and extending out toward the cortex. Repeat contrast CT scan performed 18 days after admission demonstrated increased enhancement in the right frontoparietal and left parietal cortices and a new area of abnormal density with cortical enhancement in the left frontal region. Results of a language evaluation performed at approximately 6 months after onset demonstrated moderate-to-marked cognitive-communicative disturbances characterized by impaired lexical-semantic abilities with relatively preserved syntactic and phonologic processing; disruption of higher-order abilities, including the recall, organization, and production of verbal information; and impaired functional communication.

Viral infections confined to the meninges result in aseptic meningitis, which is difficult to distinguish clinically from bacterial meningitis (Gilroy 1990; Harris and Benson 1989). Viral meningitis is frequently associated with polio virus, measles, mumps, herpes virus, and human immunodeficiency virus (HIV). Additionally, tuberculosis can occasionally produce an acute viral meningitis.

Viral infections that invade the brain parenchyma produce viral encephalitis. Acute viral encephalitis causes inflammation and damage to the central nervous system gray matter. The most common infection resulting in aphasia is herpes simplex I encephalitis. Caused by the same virus that causes herpes labialis (i.e., cold sores), herpes simplex I encephalitis invades the temporal and orbitofrontal areas of the brain (Damasio and Van Hoesen 1985; Davis et al. 1978), producing disorientation, hallucinations, and memory disturbances. Aphasia and other focal neurologic signs appear following these broader cognitive changes (Benson 1979; Benson and Ardila 1996; Caselli et al. 1991; De Renzi and Lucchelli 1994; Gilroy 1990; Goetz and Wilson 1989; Pietrini et al. 1988; Warrington and Shallice 1984).

Progressive intellectual and cognitive deterioration also results from the subacute encephalitis associated with HIV and acquired immunodeficiency syndrome (AIDS). Language, as well as attention, concentration, and most visuospatial construction abilities, remains essentially preserved during the early phases of the disease (Van Gorp et al. 1989). In the later stages of the disease, however, an AIDS dementia complex develops that can ultimately result in mutism (Lezak 1995). Unlike the cortical effects produced by herpes simplex encephalitis, HIV infection generally spares the cortex, while producing diffuse lesions within the white matter and subcortical structures.

CASE 3

MJ, a 69-year-old white man, was admitted to the hospital with a diagnosis of pneumonia of the lower lobe of the left lung and herpes simplex encephalitis. MRI performed 3 days after admission indicated a left hemisphere insult in the temporoparietal region, including the insula. Results of bedside and videofluoroscopic swallow studies performed 11 and 13 days after admission, respectively, demonstrated mild-to-moderate oral dysphagia and moderate-to-severe pharyngeal dysphagia. At the time of speech-language evaluation 15 days after admission, the patient was lethargic but cooperative and mildly to moderately confused. Initial language results suggested moderate anomic aphasia. Performance on follow-up testing 19 days after admission was characterized by severe lethargy and decreased attention more suggestive of confusion at this time than aphasia. MJ continued to demonstrate severe mental status changes over the next 8 days and received treatment to improve attention and orientation. On the twenty-seventh day post admission, the patient returned to an alert and fully oriented state. Repeat language testing performed on the thirty-second day post admission demonstrated severe anomic aphasia. He was transferred 2 days later for continued speech-language treatment and other rehabilitation services.

Tumors

Tumors are spontaneous new and abnormal growths of tissue. Although anomia is a common outcome of the mass effects produced by tumors in their early stages, the presence and characteristics of any of the classic aphasia syndromes in association with a tumor generally is dependent on the location of that tumor (e.g., Broca's area, superior temporal gyrus). In some cases, aphasia arises only as a consequence of surgery to resect the tumor.

Gliomas arising from neuroectodermal glial cells compose the majority of intracranial tumors. The most common type of glioma in adults is the astrocytoma. Astrocytomas are rapidly growing neoplasms with extensive cerebral invasion. They develop along a spectrum of differentiation from a benign, well-differentiated astrocytoma (grade I), to the less malignant anaplastic astrocytoma (grade II), to the more malignant glioblastoma multiforme (grades III and IV). The most common sites for astrocytomas are the frontal lobes, followed by the temporal lobes, the parietal lobes, the basal ganglia, and the occipital lobes. Glioblastomas are frequently found in one frontal lobe and spread to the other side through the corpus callosum. They are also found in the temporal, parietal, and occipital lobes, as well as in the basal ganglia and the thalamus (Gilroy 1990).

Oligodendrogliomas are relatively slow-growing and moderately well-differentiated tumors. They constitute a small percentage of all gliomas (approximately 5%) and usually occur in the frontal lobes (Gilroy 1990). Given their predilection for bleeding, they sometimes present with stroke characteristics (Levin 1989).

Ependymomas are derived from the ependymal cells (inner layer of neuroectodermal cells) lining the ventricles and the central canal of the spinal cord. They are found more often in children and arise from the fourth ventricle in the posterior fossa. Supratentorial ependymomas are more aggressive than those of the posterior fossa and can have features similar to those of glioblastoma multiforme. They usually involve the parieto-occipital area and can grow for a considerable amount of time before being detected.

CASE 4

JK, a 64-year-old white woman, presented with a diagnosis of glioblastoma multiforme, verified by pathology, in the temporoparieto-occipital junction of the dominant left hemisphere. The tumor was debulked and shrunk from 7 mm to 3 mm, after which the patient was treated with dexamethasone (Decadron) and chemotherapy. The patient subsequently underwent neurosurgery for total resection of tumor. The mass was found to be well differentiated and identified as an ependymoma. Following surgery, the patient presented with a transcortical sensory aphasia and was treated with radiation therapy.

Epilepsy

Epileptogenic aphasia is observed commonly in both children and adults. In children, acquired epileptiform aphasia (i.e., Landau-Kleffner syndrome) arises between the ages of 2.5 and 6 years for unknown reasons and is characterized by severe, bilateral encephalographic abnormalities and disruption of language generally following a normal developmental schedule. Moderate-to-severe aphasia can continue to be evident in these patients many years after onset, even after the seizure activity has been controlled (Mantovani and Landau 1980; Paquier et al. 1992; Peter and Assal 1992; Zardini et al. 1995).

In adults, ictal and postictal aphasias are a frequent sequel to partial and complex focal seizures. In parietal-lobe epilepsy, aphasia can comprise the aura preceding the seizure (Salanova et al. 1995). Aphasic seizures have been described following focal seizure activity confined to the speech (eloquent) cortex of the dominant hemisphere (Gilroy 1990; Spatt et al. 1994). In temporal lobe epilepsy, global (total) or nonfluent aphasia has been reported exclusively after simple and complex partial seizures of the dominant left hemisphere (Abou-Khalil et al. 1994; Chiba et al. 1991; Devinsky et al. 1994), while fluent aphasia with comprehension impairment has been observed following complex partial seizures of either hemisphere (Devinsky et al. 1994; Fakhoury et al. 1994). Postictal aphasia, on the average, generally lasts between 3 and 5 minutes before a correct verbal response is produced (Devinsky et al. 1994). Frank aphasic deficits, however, may be observed during the interictal period due to the irritative effects of chronic epilepsy. Patients with long-standing epilepsy frequently demonstrate low or below-normal functioning on selected language tasks during formal testing.

CASE 5

ML, a 47-year-old white woman, presented with a history of nocturnal epilepsy and grand mal seizures of approximately 19 years duration. According to the patient, she had been diagnosed with scar tissue in the left cerebral hemisphere. She began having word-finding difficulty approximately 3 years before the evaluation, with progressive worsening over the previous 6–8 months. She described her problem as having difficulty thinking of and saying words. She stated that she produces "unrecognizable" words that are backwards or sound completely different. She also complained that her reading was much slower, that she does not understand well sometimes, and that she has significant memory difficulties. Presurgical language evaluation demonstrated general language skills within the normal to low-normal range of performance. Occasional failure in word retrieval and paraphasia was observed in spontaneous speech production. Mild auditory processing difficulty was observed for sentence- and paragraph-length material, possibly related to the reported memory difficulties. Electroencephalogram (EEG) demonstrated left anterior and midtemporal sharp waves, sometimes more posteriorly, with an additional focus in the motor strip. The ictal EEG focus occurred in a fairly widespread area of the temporal lobe. ML underwent resection of the anterior temporal lobe and multiple subpial transection of the motor strip for treatment of her intractable epilepsy. Results of postsurgical speech-language evaluation demonstrated marked-to-severe mixed nonfluent aphasia with mild-to-moderate oral apraxia and apraxia of speech.

TOXINS

Neurotoxic compounds include metals (e.g., lead, mercury, arsenic), industrial toxins (e.g., organic solvents, gases, pesticides, other environmental toxins), biologic toxins (e.g., bacterial exotoxins, animal poisons, venoms, botanical poisons), and prescription drugs (e.g., antibiotics, cardiac drugs, psychiatric drugs, anti-inflammatory agents) (Goetz 1989). Aphasia is a somewhat uncommon outcome of toxic encephalopathy, suggesting that neurotoxins probably affect subcortical and mesial temporal structures more than cortical gray matter (White et al. 1993). Nonetheless, several reports have documented acute aphasia of toxic origin. For example, mild, transient aphasia has been observed following injection of high doses of botulinum toxin type A for the treatment of spastic torticollis (Mezaki et al. 1995). Infusion of ifosfamide, a chemotherapeutic agent used in a variety of gynecologic tumors, can produce severe neurotoxicity with resulting aphasia in the context of significant mental status changes (Curtin et al. 1991). Delayed mixed aphasia has been reported from poisoning by organophosphorous pesticides (Zhang 1991). Carbon-monoxide poisoning is associated with subcortical aphasia (Sovilla et al. 1988). These studies demonstrate that toxins having an affinity for the central nervous system have the potential to cause aphasic deficits.

Insidious Etiologies

DISEASES OF THE CEREBRAL CORTEX

Conditions, including Alzheimer's disease, Pick's disease, and Creutzfeldt-Jakob disease, are associated with language impairment in a context of global cognitive decline. Some authors have suggested that the accompanying "aphasia" in Alzheimer's disease may even be a predictor of more rapid decline than that observed in patients not developing these signs (Yesavage et al. 1993). However, as indicated in the introduction to this chapter, the progressive onset of these dementing diseases, the diffuse nature of the cortical involvement, and the coexistence of both linguistic and nonlinguistic cognitive impairments often coalesce against the description of such language impairment as aphasic.

A growing number of cases have been reported in which the aphasia accompanying these diseases conforms to the pattern expected in aphasias resulting from conditions with paroxysmal onsets. Classified as a primary progressive aphasia (PPA), the syndrome has been described as one of four behaviorally focal dementia syndromes (Weintraub and Mesulam 1993). In PPA, the insidious onset and gradual exacerbation of the language deficits constitute the only detectable abnormality for at least the first 2 years after the symptoms appear. Nonlanguage cognitive activities during this period remain relatively preserved.

Neuropathologic studies of PPA demonstrate predominantly focal atrophy with nonspecific neuronal loss, gliosis, and spongiform changes with or without findings associated with Alzheimer's disease (e.g., neurofibrillary tangles, senile plaques), Pick's disease (e.g., argentophilic inclusions [Pick's cells]) or Creutzfeldt-Jakob disease (e.g., accompanying myoclonus, rigidity, dystonia) (Croisile et al. 1991; Gilroy 1990; Karbe et al. 1993; Kirk and Ang 1994; Weintraub and Mesulam 1993). Eleven of the 19 patients with PPA reviewed by Weintraub and Mesulam (1993) had focal atrophy with nonspecific neuronal loss; three had features of Pick's disease; and five had findings of Alzheimer's disease. The PPA patients described by Scheltens and colleagues (1993) and Ikejiri and colleagues (1993) were diagnosed with Pick's disease. The patient described by Pantel (1991) was diagnosed with Alzheimer's disease. Habib and colleagues (1993) and Kertesz and colleagues (1994) argued that the neuropathologic pattern in the majority of PPA patients is nearer to Pick's disease and devoid of the characteristic features of Alzheimer's disease.

To resolve these differences, Weintraub and Mesulam (1993) suggested that PPA, as well as other focal dementing syndromes, is the result of the distribution of the causative lesions rather than the nature of the underlying disease (e.g., Alzheimer tangles or plaques, Pick's inclusions). Structural (i.e., CT, MRI) and functional (i.e., PET, single photon emission CT) imaging in patients with primary progressive aphasia shows the most severe pathology in the left frontoperisylvian regions, areas consistent with the localization of the cortical language network (Croisile et al. 1991; Habib et al. 1993; McDaniel et al. 1991; Parkin 1993; Weintraub and Mesulam 1993). In contrast, the neuropathology associated with Alzheimer's disease initially appears in the limbic structures and then spreads into language cortex as the disease progresses.

The language characteristics in PPA are diverse. In their review, Duffy and Peterson (1992) found that many of the reported cases of PPA had predominantly fluent, anomic, or Wernicke's-like verbal output, but there was substantial variability in this clinical picture. Weintraub and Mesulam (1993) found that nearly half the cases of PPA demonstrated a nonfluent aphasia. Karbe and colleagues (1993) found expressive language disabilities in their PPA patients typically characterized by reduced speech fluency and anomia with preserved language comprehension. Spontaneous speech was significantly more impaired in PPA patients in comparison with patients with aphasia due to left-hemisphere stroke. Croisile and colleagues (1991) reported one PPA case with Broca's aphasia, but two others that demonstrated anomia in one instance and pure-word deafness in the other. Parkin's (1993) case presented anomia, surface dyslexia, and surface dysgraphia, along with a mild grammatical disturbance and deficits in both visual and auditory word comprehension. The most important outcome associated with this variability is that PPA patients with nonfluent or Broca's-like characteristics seem to be more likely to demonstrate longer durations of isolated language difficulties and more stable nonlanguage cognitive functions than patients demonstrating fluent language characteristics (Duffy and Petersen 1992; Weintraub and Mesulam 1993).

CASE 6

DK, a 54-year-old white man, presented with a history of aphasia and a slow and progressive decline of approximately 2 years duration. MRI performed approximately 6 months before language evaluation revealed mild-to-moderate atrophy, more prominent in the frontal and temporal lobes, accompanied by mild generalized cerebral atrophy. Single photon emission CT scan demonstrated a small area of hypoconcentration at the periphery of the left temporal lobe. Two neuropsychological examinations also performed 6 months after language evaluation demonstrated a moderate aphasia syndrome with above average and well preserved performance on nonlanguage-based tests. Speech-language evaluation performed 3 months before presentation at the medical center suggested a moderately severe aphasia with mixed fluency characteristics but predominately fluent and anomic output. A subtle apraxia of speech and an equivocal oral apraxia were also found. DK progress was followed at the medical center to document the severity and rate of progression of his aphasia and to provide counseling regarding strategies to enhance communication consistent with his level of functioning. On examination, DK presented with moderate aphasia characterized by reduced but fluent speech and some telegraphic output accompanied by at least mild cognitive deficits in higher-order reasoning skills and thinking. Follow-up language examination was performed 8 months later. DK presented moderate nonfluent aphasia similar to transcortical motor aphasia, suggesting increasing frontal-lobe involvement. The findings indicated substantial decline in DK's verbal skills with perhaps only mild diminution of nonverbal, intellectual skills during the same period. A third language evaluation was performed 6 months later, 14 months after the initial evaluation at the medical center and approximately 3.5 years after the onset of the disorder. DK presented marked nonfluent aphasia similar to Broca's aphasia, consistent with the previous suggestions of increasing frontal-lobe involvement. In addition, the findings suggested significant decline in both verbal and nonverbal intellectual skills during the intervening period, indicating that the disorder had evolved to a full dementia syndrome.

Disease of the Basal Ganglia

The presence of aphasia has been cited as a possible basis for distinguishing two other degenerative diseases—progressive supranuclear palsy (PSP) and corticobasal degeneration. PSP is a chronic degenerative condition of the central nervous system characterized by early paralysis of eye movements accompanied by parkinsonian features and generalized spasticity. The pathology is associated with decreased pigment in the substantia nigra and locus ceruleus and loss of neurons in the basal ganglia, brain stem, and cerebellum (Gilroy 1990). Capitani and colleagues (1993) reported a case of a patient with a clinical syndrome closely resembling PSP but accompanied by progressive aphasia and apraxia not consistent with the usual profile of PSP. The authors concluded that these findings are more suggestive of an alternative diagnosis of corticobasal degeneration and that the presence of these neuropsychological deficits are critical to establishing a correct diagnosis.

MENTAL STATUS

The assessment of a patient's mental status before subsequent formal or informal language evaluation is one of the most important steps in establishing a differential diagnosis for aphasia. Information obtained from the mental status examination is basic to determining whether language deficiencies are more reflective of impairments to the patient's language system (i.e., linguistic competence or the processes acting on that competence) or to cognitive functions responsible for orienting to language inputs, sustaining attention for those inputs, and evaluating the meaningfulness or relevance of language. That is, the patient's mental status must be determined and significant mental status deficits ruled out before the validity of the language examination results can be assumed and a diagnosis of aphasia confirmed.

The goal of the mental status examination is to assess the patient's general cerebral functioning before language evaluation. Orientation, attention, perception, and memory are evaluated to exclude confusion as a primary factor for observed language deficits. Confusion, characterized by inappropriate reactions to environmental stimuli, is a common sequel to strokes and head injuries (especially during the early stages of recovery), drugs, toxins, and metabolic imbalances. It is often accompanied by disorientation, difficulty in concentration, poor memory and recall, and a range of behavioral abnormalities (e.g., fatigue, irritability, agitation, lability) (Goetz and Wilson 1989; Lezak 1995). The verbal deficits associated with confusion are easily mistaken for aphasic disturbances (e.g., misnamings, perseveration, dysgraphia, confabulation, bizarreness) (Chedru and Geschwind 1972; DeLuca and Cicerone 1991; Geschwind 1967; Wallesch and Hundsalz 1994). On the other hand, it is not uncommon for some aphasic patients, especially those with Wernicke's aphasia, to be diagnosed as confused (Goetz and Wilson 1989).

Since the majority of items used to test the cognitive functions assessed in the mental status examination load heavily on verbal skills, it is essential that the examiner recognize that aphasic patients who demonstrate impairments on such tasks are not necessarily confused. Alternatively, the examiner should not assume that the presence of confusion contraindicates the need for further, in-depth language testing in aphasic or other language-impaired patients. Indeed, such testing, when a patient is capable of withstanding such procedures, provides a baseline against which to measure the patient's recovery or regression with regard to the onset of the neurologic event. The important point is to use the information from the mental status examination to further support, clarify, or rule out a diagnosis of aphasia.

The mental status examination can be performed informally through the presentation of series of questions, commands, and paper and pencil tasks, or it can be accomplished through any one of a large number of formal tests (e.g., Mini-Mental State) (Folstein et al. 1975) (Table 10.3). Assessment of orientation usually investigates the patient's awareness of time, place, personal information, reason for hospitalization, and current events. Attention and concentration are tested by having the patient perform phoneme-monitoring or letter-cancellation tasks, repeat digits or sentences, count or spell backward, and serial subtractions. Perceptual tasks can include phoneme discrimination; object, picture or color matching; line marking and bisection; and sound, object, picture, or facial recognition. At a minimum, memory testing can include tasks for immediate recall and verbal retention by having the patient repeat a series of words and then repeating those words when requested after several minutes of continued testing.

The mental-status examination can also include assessment of a patient's conceptual functioning and reasoning (Lezak 1995), although

Table 10.3
Mental status examination

Variable	*Test*
Orientation	Awareness of time, place, personal information, reason for hospitalization, current events
Attention and concentration	Phoneme monitoring, letter cancellation, repeating digits and sentences, counting and spelling backwards, serial subtractions
Perceptual	Phoneme discrimination; object, picture, and color matching; line marking and bisection
	Presence of illusions, delusions, hallucinations
Memory	Immediate recall and verbal retention of word series

generally not for the purpose of assisting in the interpretation of results from basic language testing as suggested earlier in this section. Rather, such additional information can be worthwhile in diagnosing the language disturbance when it appears to be more related to confusion or intellectual impairment than to aphasia. Tasks that can be used for these purposes usually include interpretations of proverbs or idioms and descriptions of similarities or absurdities.

The examiner's impressions regarding the patient's mental state provide the basis for responding to some of the basic questions that need to be considered when assessing patients with language disorders of neurologic origin. For example, is the patient's level of alertness and responsiveness sufficient to support a level of sustained attention that will result in reliable responses to language testing? Is the patient oriented to himself or herself and to his or her surroundings to the degree that the patient understands the reasons for language testing, is motivated to participate in testing, and provides valid responses to the tasks required? Can the patient sustain the concentration (attention) necessary for adequately retaining the response requirements for a given task, focusing on and processing the test stimuli (especially for lengthier or syntactically complex stimuli), and maintaining his or her mental set for the completion of a subtest or battery? In patients seeming to have the requisite attention and concentration, is their verbal retention sufficient to support a full analysis of and response to stimuli of lengths comparable to sentences or greater? Does the patient perform better on visual versus auditory tasks, suggesting some benefit from continuous exposure to visual stimuli (i.e., decreased demands on auditory retention)?

CASE 7

MZ, an 86-year-old white woman, was admitted to the medical center with a history of a rapidly growing neck mass over the previous 5 months. Previous medical history included hypertension and atrial fibrillation. She was diagnosed with undifferentiated carcinoma of the thyroid and underwent excision of the left common carotid artery with interposition of a segment of the left greater saphenous vein. She presented with new onset of right-sided weakness and speech disturbances 1 day after surgery. Impressions derived from neurologic consultation suggested cerebral infarction of the area supplied by the left middle cerebral artery secondary to cardiac embolus versus carotid surgery. Speech-language pathology consultation was requested, wherein the patient was described as demonstrating expressive aphasia status post CVA. On examination, the patient was lethargic but responsive with apparently functional hearing for conversation. Mental status could not be assessed further. Language evaluation demonstrated aphonic, nonfluent speech with occasional echolalia, unintelligible utterances, and frequent failure to respond. She showed moderate impairment for comprehension of simple yes and no questions and did not condition to word-recognition tasks. She did not follow commands spontaneously but did perform such tasks to imitation. Her repetition was disproportionately preserved for words and sentences and her naming to confrontation was generally accurate following tactile or phonemic cues. Impressions derived from these results suggested nonfluent aphasia versus communication disturbances secondary to altered mental status. One week later, MZ remained lethargic but responsive to verbal input and demonstrated reduced attention to the right hemifield. Her speech and language were characterized by frequent hesitations but with increased fluency, grammatical completeness, and informational content. Responses to simple yes and no questions were mildly impaired. Impressions at that time attributed the patient's moderate reductions in communication to her altered mental status more so than to aphasia. On return the next day for treatment, the patient needed to be awoken, remained lethargic but responsive to verbal input, then subsequently became somnolent. After an additional week (2 weeks post onset), MZ was lethargic but responsive with a flat affect, continued to demonstrate inattention to the right side, and was oriented to person and the reason for her hospitalization but not to time or place. Speech was reduced in initiation but grammatically complete and with good informational content. She continued to show mild-to-moderate impairment for simple yes and no questions but could name three items within specified categories with a high degree of success. Improvements in language functioning were generally commensurate with increases in the patient's mental status. MZ was discharged from the medical center and transferred to another facility closer to her home for further rehabilitation services.

SPEECH FLUENCY AND SPEECH PATTERNS

During the initial interview with a patient, as well as throughout the mental status examination, the clinician forms an impression of the patient's speech fluency (i.e., the ease with which speech is produced) (Table 10.4). The purpose of this exercise is to categorize the patient into a fluent versus a nonfluent syndrome. If the patient demonstrates fluent speech characteristics, the differential diagnosis at this point considers whether the patient exhibits fluent aphasia versus another neurogenic language condition with fluent symptomatology (e.g., confusion, dementia, schizophrenia, depression, alexia with or without agraphia, auditory verbal agnosia, regression associated with aging). The differential diagnosis for patients with nonfluent characteristics attempts to distinguish nonfluent aphasia from apraxia of speech, anarthria, mutism, frontal-lobe syndrome, decreased arousal associated with diffuse cortical dysfunction, or psychotic disturbances. As described in the introduction to this chapter, the etiology and onset of the disorder, the localization and extent of any possible brain damage, the mental status and competence of the patient, the specificity of the cognitive impairment, and the patient's personality characteristics are considered in addition to the speech and language profile to determine whether the language impairment is of aphasic or nonaphasic origin. Once it has been determined that the disorder is aphasic in nature using data collected from these sources, the assessment of the patient's speech fluency comprises the first step in establishing an aphasia diagnosis.

Measures of phrase length provide the primary means for categorizing aphasic patients as fluent or nonfluent. Goodglass and colleagues (1964) demonstrated that aphasic patients distribute themselves naturally into long-phrase dominant (five or more words) and short-phrase dominant (one or two words) types, and that clinicians could make this distinction reliably by evaluating the maximum length of word groups produced by a patient. Benson (1979) and Benson and Ardila (1996) associated these output characteristics with speech rates of 100–150 words per minute (normal), up to more than 200 words per minute (super-normal) for fluent patients, and with less than 50 words per minute for nonfluent aphasia. Fluent patients tend to produce utterances that are grammatically complete or "paragrammatic" (containing errors of syntactic usage) and containing a dearth of substantive words, while nonfluent patients produce utterances that are grammatically sparse or "agrammatic" (errors of syntactic omission or simplification) and lacking in functor words. Goodglass and colleagues (1993) demonstrated that nonfluent, agrammatic aphasic subjects were

Table 10.4
Differential diagnoses based on speech fluency

Fluent speech characteristics
Fluent aphasia
Confusion
Dementia
Schizophrenia
Depression
Alexia with or without agraphia
Auditory verbal agnosia
Normal aging
Nonfluent speech characteristics
Nonfluent aphasia
Apraxia of speech
Anarthria
Mutism
Frontal-lobe syndrome
Decreased arousal
Psychotic disturbances

inferior to fluent aphasic subjects in the use of auxiliaries, verb inflection, and passive word order. In addition, only agrammatic subjects omitted articles or main verbs. The use of noun plurals and possessives did not discriminate between the groups.

Other factors that are considered in assessing speech fluency include the occurrence and prevalence of paraphasias, perseveration, effort, the rate of speaking, pauses, speech prosody, and articulatory agility (Davis 1983; Helm-Estabrooks and Albert 1991). Using these parameters, Rosenbek and colleagues (1989, p. 43) summarized the distinctions between the two aphasia types in the following manner:

> The nonfluent patient should be characterized by sparse, effortful, sometimes perseverative speech; many pauses; disturbances in prosody; abnormal pronunciation; single word utterances or short phrases; and, sometimes, word substitutions. Conversely, the fluent patient produces a great deal of speech; few pauses; normal prosody; few, if any, perseverations; a lack of abnormal pronunciation; and normal phrase length.

It is important to note the role of articulatory errors in distinguishing fluent from nonfluent speech. Generally, the phonologic errors associated with these aphasias are either literal paraphasic or apraxic in nature and represent impairments at two distinct levels of motor speech programming. The literal paraphasic errors observed with fluent speech result from deficient sensory guidance for motor programming (impaired phonologic representations or disrupted auditory association networks). Apraxia of speech in nonfluent patients results from impairment to the motor association mechanisms that transduce sensory information into motor impulses for phoneme production (Tonkovich and Peach 1989). Literal paraphasic errors arise from either posterior temporoparietal or subcortical damage and are characterized by generally unpredictable phoneme substitutions or sequencing errors. Apraxia of speech is found with anterior, inferior cortical, or subcortical damage; is characterized by rather predictable phoneme substitutions and distortions; and is accompanied by difficult speech initiation and articulatory transition (Canter et al. 1985; Odell et al. 1990). Rather than consider all surface articulatory errors as representative of a unitary problem, an inventory of these speech patterns assists in categorizing the aphasia as fluent or nonfluent and assists in hypothesizing with regard to the nature of the articulation deficits.

Despite the range of factors that should be considered when making such judgments, establishing whether a patient presents fluent or nonfluent speech is a relatively easy perceptual task, even to the untrained listener. In some instances, however, the distinction may not be so straightforward, as, for example, when patients with nonfluent characteristics are evolving to fluent syndromes, or when frequent paraphasic errors in some fluent aphasias combine to substantially disrupt fluency (a "nonfluent" fluent aphasia!). Formal rating scales have been included in several aphasia batteries to assist in determining a patient's speech fluency, including the Boston Diagnostic Aphasia Examination (Goodglass and Kaplan 1983), the Western Aphasia Battery (Kertesz 1982), and Aphasia Diagnostic Profiles (Helm-Estabrooks 1992).

Once a patient has been assigned to a fluent or nonfluent group, the clinician focuses on the diagnoses that fit with the patient's speech characteristics and rules out those aphasia syndromes that do not (Table 10.5). The fluent aphasias include Wernicke's aphasia, transcortical sensory aphasia, conduction aphasia, and anomic aphasia; the nonfluent aphasias include global aphasia, Broca's aphasia, nonfluent mixed aphasia, transcortical motor aphasia, and transcortical mixed aphasia (isolation syndrome). At this juncture, however, the relevant syndromes enter the differential diagnosis only tentatively, since these traditional aphasia classifications have been estimated to account for less than half of all cases within this population and may therefore be insufficient for identifying the unique language impairments in a given case (Goodglass 1981; Schwartz 1984). Also, while some have claimed that the aphasic deficits arising from subcortical lesions can be described

Table 10.5
Classification of aphasia syndromes

Cortical aphasias
Fluent
Anomic aphasia
Conduction aphasia
Transcortical sensory aphasia
Wernicke's aphasia
Nonfluent
Broca's aphasia
Global aphasia
Mixed nonfluent aphasia
Mixed transcortical aphasia (isolation syndrome)
Transcortical motor aphasia
Subcortical aphasias
Striatal aphasias with or without white matter extension
Thalamic aphasia
Progressive aphasia

using the same traditional categories developed for cortical aphasias (Kirk and Kertesz 1994), others suggest that the subcortical aphasia syndromes often share features found within different cortical aphasia syndromes and cannot be described in traditional terms (Helm-Estabrooks and Albert 1991). Whether the syndrome conforms to one of the traditional classifications or not, describing the language impairment as a fluent or nonfluent aphasia remains preferable to such popular terminology as *receptive* or *expressive aphasia*, because (1) such descriptors do not convey the impression that the language impairment is limited to the receptive or expressive domain, and (2) such an approach does not attempt to maintain the input-output dichotomies of previous approaches (e.g., sensory versus motor aphasia, receptive versus expressive aphasia, posterior versus anterior aphasia) that underspecify the nature of the deficits found across aphasia types (Peach 1995).

ORAL AND VISUAL LANGUAGE CAPABILITIES

Fluent and nonfluent aphasia syndromes are distinguished further within each category and differentiated from related disorders, such as apraxia of speech or the agnosias, by assessment of the patient's performance on tasks involving auditory and visual comprehension, oral repetition and reading, naming, and written expression. Assessment should be performed using a formal aphasia test battery (1) to control the stimuli used across tasks, (2) to assure comprehensive evaluation of all input-output modalities, (3) to allow examination of the similarities and differences among responses to the same stimuli processed through different modalities, and (4) to improve the reliability of test results. Clinicians who choose to assess performance informally or to administer only selected portions of these batteries (a common but unfortunate practice!) are certain to lose the above advantages, as well as other important information necessary to making an appropriate diagnosis.

Differential diagnosis of the fluent and nonfluent aphasias is delineated further by determining whether a patient's auditory comprehension and repetition abilities are more or less preserved, whether the observed pattern maintains when the same or similar stimuli are processed through alternate input-output modalities (i.e., visual comprehension and oral reading), and whether the language impairments can be observed across all language modalities or are restricted to single input or output modalities (e.g., speech and writing versus speech or writing only). Here the term *more preserved* can be subjectively defined as clinically normal to mildly impaired abilities, while *less preserved* suggests moderately to severely impaired abilities. Kertesz (1982) provided a more operational definition for these terms using cutoff scores derived from administration of the Western Aphasia Battery. Fluent patients demonstrating more impaired auditory comprehension may be presenting either Wernicke's or transcortical sensory aphasia, while those demonstrating relatively less comprehension impairment may have conduction or anomic aphasia. Nonfluent patients with more impaired auditory comprehension are likely to have either global aphasia, mixed nonfluent aphasia, or transcortical mixed aphasia (isolation syndrome), while those with less comprehension impairment are likely to have either Broca's aphasia or transcortical motor aphasia.

Having assigned the patient to either a fluent or nonfluent aphasia type with relatively impaired or preserved auditory comprehension, the patient's repetition abilities are assessed to determine whether he or she fits into one of the traditional categories of aphasia. Here, repetition is evaluated relative to the patient's spontaneous speech production. For example, patients who demonstrate minimal to no paraphasic errors in their spontaneous speech, but who show increased paraphasia in their speech when repeating words and sentences, regardless of how mild, are said to demonstrate a repetition impairment that is *disproportionate to their level of spontaneous speech*. The same would be true for patients having markedly paraphasic speech that breaks down even more substantially than that observed spontaneously. Conversely, patients having repetition difficulties that are equivalent to, or even less severe than, those observed in spontaneous speech (e.g., marked deficits in phoneme initiation, selection, transitionalization, or sequencing; grammatical impairments; lexical-semantic problems) are not said to have a special repetition impairment.

Fluent aphasic patients with more impaired auditory comprehension are classified as having Wernicke's aphasia, if they have disproportionately impaired repetition, or as having transcortical sensory aphasia, if they have disproportionately preserved repetition. Fluent aphasic patients who have more preserved auditory comprehension demonstrate conduction aphasia, if they have disproportionately impaired repetition, or anomic aphasia, if they have relatively preserved repetition. Nonfluent aphasic patients with more impaired auditory comprehension and repetition impairment commensurate with their spontaneous speech are classified as having either global aphasia or mixed nonfluent aphasia, depending on the severity of their comprehension deficits. When nonfluent aphasic patients with more impaired auditory comprehension demonstrate disproportionately preserved repetition, they are classified as having transcortical mixed aphasia (isolation of the speech-zone syndrome). Finally, nonfluent aphasic patients with relatively preserved auditory comprehension and repetition impairment equivalent to their spontaneous speech are classified as having Broca's aphasia, while nonfluent aphasic patients with relatively preserved auditory comprehension and disproportionately preserved repetition are classified as having transcortical motor aphasia.

The oral language assessment concludes with an evaluation of the patient's naming abilities. Since all aphasic patients have naming problems, the information is obtained not so much for the purposes of classification as it is for qualifying the nature and severity of the errors and the underlying mechanisms responsible for the patient's anomia. Linebaugh (1990) described three such mechanisms associated with the fluent aphasias: (1) damage to the neuronal representations of lexical entries resulting in word omissions, partial responses, semantic paraphasias, and neologisms; (2) delay or failure to activate substantially intact neuronal networks resulting in increased response latencies, partially accurate responses, circumlocutions, word omissions, and production of unrelated words; and (3) failure to inhibit lexical entries sharing a substantial number of common features resulting in semantic paraphasia. Alternately, naming failures in nonfluent aphasia can be related to the initiation difficulties, restrictions in vocabulary, or perseverative responses that are pathognomonic of these aphasia types.

CASE 8

MB, an 84-year-old white woman, was seen for speech-language evaluation after hitting her head during an accidental fall that was caused by stepping in a pothole. She did not lose consciousness but observed significant changes in speech immediately following the incident. She was taken by ambulance to a local hospital, where she presented with a laceration of the right eyebrow, subconjunctival hemorrhage, and contusion of the right scalp and knee. She received three sutures to her right eyebrow and was discharged to her home with instruction for follow-up in 1–2 days. No further neurologic work-up was undertaken.

On examination, MB described her speech as "terrible" and said that she "couldn't talk for nothing" since her accident. She denied weakness of the upper or lower extremities, difficulty walking, visual disturbances, or swallowing problems. She did not pass a hearing screening bilaterally at 40 dB HL; hearing status for conversational speech was functional. The Mini-Mental State Examination was administered to assess general cognitive status. She achieved a raw score of 27 of 30, placing her within the normal range of functioning. Administration of the Western Aphasia Battery yielded an aphasia quotient of 81.5 (cutoff for normal performance is 93.8) and a cortical quotient of 84.6 (cutoff for normal performance is 90.0). Spontaneous speech was characterized by reduced fluency with good grammatical organization and information content. Frequent literal paraphasic errors were observed consisting of sound substitutions and deletions. Articulation was distorted but easily produced. Speech rate was rapid. Auditory verbal comprehension was preserved generally (19.5 of 20.0). Word and sentence repetition was moderately impaired (7.5 of 10.0) and characterized by phonemic errors and word omissions. Naming was mildly impaired (8.5 of 10.0) and characterized by occasional phonemic errors and decreased word fluency. Reading comprehension and writing were mildly impaired (17.2 of 20.0). Writing was performed cursively with her preferred right hand. Facial and limb praxis were generally preserved (9.2 of 10.0) for performance of instrumental and noninstrumental commands. Constructional, visuospatial, and simple calculation tasks were mildly to moderately impaired (7.7 of 10.0). Performance on the Ravens Coloured Progressive Matrices (RCPM) (Raven 1965) placed her at the seventy-fifth percentile for individuals of her age, which was consistent with above-average intellectual functioning. Speech-language impressions following evaluation indicated a mild-to-moderate conduction aphasia and relatively preserved nonverbal cognitive skills. Functional communication was adequate for activities of daily living but moderately reduced in intelligibility. MB was referred for medical and neuroradiologic follow-up to determine the cause of her significant speech disturbance. Speech-language treatment and a complete audiologic examination were recommended pending the outcome of this work-up. MB was seen for CT scan of the brain the next day. Results obtained at that time demonstrated regions of ischemic change in the periventricular white matter, a left parietal convexity infarct, and a right frontal lobe infarct of indeterminate age. There was no evidence of intracranial hemorrhage.

CASE 9

JO, a 62-year-old white man with a past history of hypertension, was hospitalized after a transient episode of inability to talk and right arm weakness. CT scan was normal, but angiogram demonstrated a high degree of bilateral extracranial occlusive disease. Emergency carotid endarterectomy was performed, after which JO did well; however, several hours later he became aphasic and was unable to move his right side. CT scan performed the next day showed an area of wedge-shaped density in the midfrontal lobe extending to the high convexity and no evidence of hemorrhage. Speech-language evaluation performed 3 days later found the patient to be lethargic and echolalic. Conversational and expository speech production were nonfluent and characterized by phrase lengths of one to two words, no grammatical form, and good articulatory agility. Word finding was restricted to simple automatisms, and paraphasia was absent. JO provided undifferentiated responses to yes and no questions and did not respond to other auditory comprehension tasks. His repetition of words and phrases was superior to his conversational speech but was marked by frequent perseveration. Word reading was relatively intact but responsive, and confrontation naming was characterized by perseveration. Speech-language impressions at that time were to rule out transcortical motor aphasia versus frontal-lobe syndrome characterized by reduced attention, initiation, and perseveration of response. JO was seen for speech-language treatment and was transferred for rehabilitation 10 days later. His speech-language diagnosis at the time of discharge was transcortical motor aphasia.

The aphasia diagnosis is confirmed or ruled out on the basis of results obtained from visual language testing. Recalling that aphasia is a general impairment that involves all language activities but to disproportionate degrees, the clinician should expect the patient's reading and writing to be impaired in a manner proportional to, or perhaps somewhat in excess of, his or her speaking and listening. To assess visual language, then, the examination should include tasks evaluating the patient's comprehension of printed words, sentences, and paragraphs; his or her ability to read words or sentences aloud; his or her ability to write such nonpropositional sequences as numbers or the alphabet; his or her ability to copy sentences or write them to dictation; and his or her ability to write words, sentences, or paragraphs propositionally (Davis 1983). If the combined oral and visual language test results reveal a selective impairment for only one input-output modality, then a diagnosis of aphasia must be questioned. For example, patients who demonstrate significant errors in spontaneous speech, repetition, and oral reading, yet produce normal writing with preserved auditory and visual comprehension, are probably apraxic rather than aphasic. Patients who have substantial auditory comprehension and repetition difficulties but generally preserved spontaneous speech, oral reading, visual comprehension, and writing likely demonstrate auditory-verbal agnosia (pure word deafness) instead of aphasia. The patient who speaks, understands, and writes normally but cannot read may be exhibiting alexia without agraphia, while the patient who reads but cannot write may have pure agraphia. These single-modality impairments are best understood as apraxic or agnosic rather than aphasic, and their diagnosis is dependent on collection of both oral and visual language responses.

A substantial body of literature has developed during the past two decades describing aphasic patients who do not fit any of the traditional aphasia syndromes. One reason for these developments is the recognition of aphasic deficits arising from subcortical versus cortical lesions, a trend obviously fueled by the evolution of noninvasive neuroimaging techniques to study aphasic patients. Helm-Estabrooks and Albert (1991) developed an algorithm for classifying three types of subcortical aphasia: (1) anterior capsular-putaminal aphasia, a syndrome sharing features of transcortical motor and Broca's aphasia; (2) posterior capsular-putaminal aphasia, a syndrome sharing features of Broca's and Wernicke's aphasia; and (3) thalamic aphasia, a syndrome sharing features of transcortical motor and transcortical sensory aphasia. In their scheme, the patient's speech fluency, auditory comprehension, and repetition; the patient's verbal and nonverbal agility; and the presence or absence of hemiplegia, hypophonia, or both comprise the judgment parameters necessary to distinguish among the variety of cortical versus subcortical aphasia syndromes. Although the literature has not supported the specificity of the language impairments reported to result from lesions to each of these sites (Bruyn 1989; Damasio et al. 1982; Kennedy and Murdoch 1993, 1994; Kirk and Kertesz 1994; Naeser et al. 1982; Robin and Schienberg 1990), there appears to be agreement that the location of the subcortical lesion, and not the size or extent of the lesion, is the primary determinant as to whether such infarcts yield an aphasia (Alexander et al. 1987; Kirk and Kertesz 1994; Naeser et al. 1982). Helm-Estabrooks and Albert's (1991) identification of the consistencies and discrepancies found between nonverbal and verbal agility in these groups may be an important diagnostic indicator awaiting further validation.

CASE 10

ES, a 79-year-old African American woman with a past medical history of hypertension, myocardial infarction, and hypercholesteremia, was hospitalized following sudden onset of mild right hemiparesis and speech disturbances. CT scan performed 2 days after admission revealed an infarct of the lenticulostriate arteries of the left middle cerebral artery involving the periventricular white matter deep to Broca's area and the basal ganglia. Administration of the Boston Diagnostic Aphasia Examination (Goodglass and Kaplan 1983) 3 days after onset revealed fluent spontaneous speech of normal phrase length and grammatical form with mildly reduced articulatory agility and melodic line. Frequent literal and semantic paraphasic errors, as well as speech perseveration, were observed. Verbal (7 of 14) and nonverbal (6 of 12) agility were moderately reduced. Vocal loudness was normal. Oral and visual language results were as follows: auditory comprehension in the forty-eighth percentile; repetition in the seventy-eighth percentile; naming in the thirty-seventh percentile; and reading in the fiftieth percentile. The patient was seen for speech-language treatment, where she demonstrated pronounced lexical-semantic deficits consisting of poor semantic categorization and minimal responsiveness to semantic prestimulation and hierarchical cues for naming to confrontation. Four days later, she was discharged to her home, where she was scheduled to receive continued speech-language treatment.

Recent applications of neuropsychological language models for aphasia diagnosis have also demonstrated that the criteria used for classifying patients into the traditional aphasia syndromes (i.e., entire language functions) are insufficient for identifying the unique language impairments in some cases (Caplan D 1993; Hillis 1994). This may be due to the reliance of the traditional approach on the classical model of language, a model that postulates only corticocortical connectivity among the major association areas of the cortex. Information-processing models specifying the types and sequences of language-related components and operations that underlie the performance of a given language task increasingly are replacing the traditional approach as a framework for better describing the selective language deficits of aphasic patients (Margolin 1991). The components of model-driven analyses include those that analyze auditory and visual inputs and those that activate spoken and written outputs for simple and morphologically complex words and sentences (Caplan D 1993). These finer analyses of aphasic patient's deficits provide more specific information regarding the nature of the language breakdown. For example, in the case reported by Peach (1996), the patient's word production deficits were localized to impairments associated with phonologic planning. Three sources of evidence were used to develop this conclusion: (1) the subject demonstrated not only marked literal paraphasia but also neologistic errors well after she had recovered aural comprehension that was only mildly impaired; (2) her writing exceeded her oral output at initial evaluation and at the time of a subsequent pre-experimental evaluation; and (3) her phonologic production was approximately equally impaired for repetition and naming but substantially improved for oral reading, thereby suggesting the use of a lexical strategy for the latter tasks. This type of information is more aligned with contemporary notions regarding the neuroanatomy of language in which the contributions of multiple cortical areas (e.g., heteromodal, paralimbic, limbic) and the distributed form of language representations are emphasized (Mesulam 1990, 1994). Although no formal test battery is available as of this writing to perform such a systematic analysis of these cognitive components, numerous informal test batteries have been described in reports using this approach to the assessment and treatment of aphasic patients (e.g., Caplan LR 1993).

NONVERBAL COGNITIVE ABILITIES

An important criterion for defining aphasia, as described in the introduction, is the relative preservation of nonverbal versus verbal cognitive abilities. Eisenson (1973, p. 61) defined cognitive, nonverbal tasks as "any activity which involves thinking in contrast to tasks which are of a more specific sensory or perceptual nature such as sensory discrimination, e.g., size or weight judgments, maze problems, etc. Presumably, such tasks can be performed without language mediation." Kertesz (1979) equated cognition with intelligence and viewed them as being independent from language. For Kertesz, intelligence included attention, retention, memory, discrimination, abstraction, recall, knowledge, motor skills, integration, problem solving, logic, and planning. Davis (1993) described cognition as consisting of specific subsystems with dedicated knowledge bases and processes specialized for different complex abilities, thereby including language, as well as, for example, visuospatial and musical skills. Although different in some respects, these three approaches recognize and identify common cognitive activities that are believed not to rely on linguistic mediation and have provided the focus for investigations of the nonverbal cognitive abilities of aphasic patients. Inferences regarding the integrity of a patient's nonverbal cognition, for the purposes of differentially diagnosing aphasia, are dependent on the conclusions that have been drawn from these studies.

Kertesz and McCabe (1975) analyzed the performances of aphasic patients on the RCPM (Raven 1965), a test of analogic reasoning, to assess nonverbal cognition in aphasia. Aphasic subjects with poor comprehension (patients with global, Wernicke's, transcortical sensory, and transcortical mixed aphasias) performed more poorly than either aphasic subjects without comprehension impairment or other brain-damaged subjects without aphasia, even though the test does not require any verbal instruction. The RCPM scores also correlated highly with those obtained from a drawing task. The authors concluded that there may be a visuospatial-nonverbal intelligence factor that is bilaterally distributed and may be impaired along with verbal cognitive functions following left-hemisphere damage. Gainotti et al. (1986), using a new version of the RCPM to minimize the influence of unilateral spatial neglect on test performance, found no differences between right- and left-brain–damaged subjects on this task; however, they found greater impairment in aphasic subjects when compared to nonaphasic left-hemisphere–damaged subjects. Similar to Kertesz and McCabe (1975), Gainotti et al. (1986) also found greater impairment in aphasic subjects with severe language comprehension deficits than in patients classified with less severe comprehension deficits.

Prescott and colleagues (Prescott et al. 1984, 1987) and Wolfe et al. (1987) investigated aphasic subjects' performances on a nonverbal problem-solving task called the Tower of Hanoi puzzle. The puzzle consists of a board with three pegs (A, B, and C), and three disks of progressively smaller sizes on Peg A that must be moved to Peg C. Only one disk can be moved at a time and no disk can be place on top of a disk smaller than itself. The solution to the puzzle requires at least seven moves and requires a degree of planning in selecting moves and generating subgoals that bring the problem closer to solution. Whether actual wooden stimuli or microcomputer simulations were used, aphasic subjects required a greater number of moves to complete the puzzle than normal subjects. The aphasic subjects also required the longest times to complete the puzzle relative to normal subjects and other brain-damaged groups (i.e., right hemisphere, bilateral). Aphasic subjects achieved fewer solutions and attempted more illegal moves than normal subjects. The authors concluded, like Kertesz and McCabe (1975) and Gainotti and colleagues (1986), that nonverbal problem-solving tasks may have equal potential for either hemisphere.

Della Sala (1987) constructed and administered a nonverbal Figure-Object Matching Test to a large group of focal brain-damaged subjects and found that a left-hemisphere lesion was more relevant to the outcome than a right-hemisphere lesion. Both the presence and severity of aphasia played roles in the poor outcome on the Figure-Object Matching Test, while the type of aphasia, degree of intellectual impairment (as assessed by the Wechsler-Bellevue Adult Intelligence Performance Scale [Wechsler 1944]), and presence of visual field defect did not. The results were interpreted as evidence for a basic nonverbal defect in aphasia that is linked in some way to language impairment.

Collectively, these studies demonstrate that aphasic subjects show impaired nonverbal cognitive abilities. What these studies do not address, however, is whether a single, unitary nonverbal defect accounts for all of these results. Basso and colleagues (1985) investigated this issue and found a clear-cut dissociation in the types of nonverbal impairments demonstrated by subjects with Broca's and Wernicke's aphasia. The authors concluded, therefore, that the breakdown of nonverbal resources varies with the different types of aphasia and that the nature of the nonverbal defect in aphasia is multidimensional rather than unitary.

How, then, can the criterion suggesting "preserved" nonverbal abilities for aphasia be interpreted in light of these results? The answer appears to be that the relationship between verbal and nonverbal cognitive abilities in aphasia is a relative one, with impairments to verbal cognition always exceeding those to nonverbal cognition. In this way, the defects to the more widely distributed intellectual functions that accompany most forms of brain damage should be expected, but the language impairment of the aphasia remains the primary, or most salient, cognitive impairment. A simple way to quantify these relationships is to administer the Western Aphasia Battery (Kertesz 1982), an aphasia test that includes such nonverbal tasks as block design, calculation, and RCPM, in addition to the expected tasks assessing oral and visual language capabilities. As impairments to nonverbal cognition become equivalent to, or exceed, that within the verbal sphere, evidence exists to suggest that language impairment is probably of nonaphasic origin.

PRAGMATIC ABILITIES

The final consideration for diagnosing whether a patient's language impairment is aphasic or otherwise does not involve notions of loss or impairment, as in preceding areas, but rather the integrity of the patient's communicative intent. The latter area falls within the rubric of pragmatics, which, of course, concern the rules that govern the use of language in context. A sizable literature describing the pragmatic skills of aphasic patients has appeared since the 1980s (see Davis 1993; Hough and Pierce 1994; Newhoff and Apel 1990 for reviews), and the results emerging from this body of information all converge on the simple observation that aphasic patients communicate better than they talk. In more formal terms, aphasic patients abide by Grice's (1975) conversational maxims that presuppose a willingness on the part of speakers to be informative, truthful, relevant, and concise.

Aphasic patients, even those with Wernicke's aphasia, can be distinguished from patients with other neurogenic language disorders (e.g., dementia) because their communicative intent remains discernible even in the face of substantial semantic and syntactic deficits (Albert 1981). Aphasic patients, as a group, are motivated to convey messages to their listeners, whereas confused or demented patients become communicatively "disconnected" from their environment by virtue of the disorientation and other cognitive deficits accompanying these and related conditions. The clinician's subjective impression of the patient's pragmatic adequacy, when considered with the data from the formal portions of the language evaluation, is an important factor contributing to the differential diagnosis of the language impairment. To paraphrase Holland (1982), if the patient's language problems do not look like aphasia, sound like aphasia, or act like aphasia, then they are not aphasia.

CASE 11

AK, a 78-year-old white woman residing in a skilled nursing facility, was hospitalized following a sudden change in mental status and new onset of right upper-extremity weakness that was preceded by an accidental fall from her bed. Previous medical history included a diagnosis of probable Alzheimer's disease with the ability to converse intelligibly. Speech-language consultation was requested for "testing of (the patient's) comprehension, etc." and to determine whether the patient demonstrated Wernicke's aphasia. On examination, AK was found to be awake, alert, and disoriented to person, place, and time. Administration of the oral language portions of the Western Aphasia Battery yielded fluent, grammatical speech production characterized by complete but often irrelevant sentences, frequent semantic jargon, and primarily verbal paraphasia. Auditory comprehension assessment revealed moderate auditory comprehension impairment with responses that were frequently off task. Repetition was relatively preserved for words and single sentences but characterized by verbal and literal paraphasic errors for more complex (lengthier) responses. Naming was moderately impaired with primarily verbal paraphasic errors. Narrative writing was characterized by sentences of two to three words, preserved orthography, and visuospatial disorganization. Impressions derived from the speech-language evaluation were consistent with moderate generalized intellectual deterioration. The language profile was distinguished from one of Wernicke's aphasia by the patient's irrelevant responses produced with relatively preserved phonology and syntax, affective changes, reduced intention to communicate, and fluctuating auditory comprehension that suggested an attentional versus associative basis for her listening deficits.

CONCLUSION

Classifying neurologic language disorders into their appropriate categories is not simply a diagnostic exercise but instead is an integral first step in the intervention process. The information derived from the differential diagnosis contributes to intervention in at least two important ways. First, classification relates the patient's language deficits to established hypotheses regarding the processing components that have been affected, thereby identifying the targets for language treatment. In essence, the diagnosis dictates whether the targets for language treatment reside outside the language system, as in the case of nonaphasic language disorders, or within the language system when treating deficits of aphasic origin. For example, apart from the gross auditory comprehension disturbance distinguishing Wernicke's and conduction aphasia, these two forms of fluent aphasia share the common characteristic of paraphasic errors in their language output. Although similar in many of their surface manifestations, the source of these two deficits in the two syndromes is thought to be quite different. The errors in Wernicke's aphasia can be attributed to disturbances in the representations for the sound patterns of words, while those in conduction aphasia can be attributed to disconnection between relatively preserved sound patterns and the speech-production mechanism. With this background, treatment to reduce paraphasic errors in the patient with Wernicke's aphasia is directed toward reestablishing the sound structure of words, while that for conduction aphasia focuses on stimulating the selection and sequencing of speech sounds. Numerous other examples can be found within aphasia symptomatology where the aphasia syndrome guides treatment approaches for seemingly similar deficits with rather disparate bases.

Second, the aphasia syndrome provides one factor for developing prognostic statements regarding the course of the aphasia. Although developing a prognosis for each of the aphasias remains an inexact undertaking, evidence has accumulated for estimating recovery using the patient's type of aphasia (Kertesz and McCabe 1977). Prognosis in aphasia impacts treatment during the acute recovery period because it influences the clinician to choose among restorative, compensatory, or combined approaches to the language impairment.

REFERENCES

Abou-Khalil B, Welch L, Blumenkopf B, et al. (1994) Global aphasia with seizure onset in the dominant basal temporal region. *Epilepsia* 35, 1079–1084.

Albert ML. (1981) Changes in language with aging. *Seminars in Neurology* 1, 43–46.

Alexander MP, Naeser MA, Palumbo CL. (1987) Correlations of subcortical lesion sites and aphasia profiles. *Brain* 110, 961–991.

Basso A, Capitani E, Luzzatti C, et al. (1985) Different basic components in the performance of Broca's and Wernicke's aphasics on the Colour-Figure Matching Test. *Neuropsychologia* 23, 51–59.

Beeson PM, Bayles KA, Rubens AB, Kazniak AW. (1993) Memory impairment and executive control in individuals with stroke-induced aphasia. *Brain and Language* 45, 253–275.

Benson DF. (1979) *Aphasia, Alexia, and Agraphia*. New York: Churchill Livingstone.

Benson DF. (1991) What's in a name? *Mayo Clinic Proceedings* 66, 865–867.

Benson DF, Ardila A. (1996) *Aphasia: A Clinical Perspective*. New York: Oxford University Press.

Bhatnagar SC, Andy OJ. (1995) *Neuroscience for the Study of Communicative Disorders*. Baltimore: Williams & Wilkins.

Brookshire RH. (1982) *Clinical Aphasiology: Conference Proceedings*. Minneapolis, MN: BRK Publishers.

Bruyn RPM. (1989) Thalamic aphasia: a conceptual critique. *Journal of Neurology* 236, 21–25.

Canter GJ, Trost JE, Burns MS. (1985) Contrasting speech patterns in apraxia of speech and phonemic paraphasia. *Brain and Language* 24, 204–222.

Capitani E, Laiacona M, Barbarotto R. (1993) Progressive neuropsychological and extrapyramidal deterioration resembling progressive supranuclear palsy: is aphasia relevant for correct diagnosis? *European Archives of Psychiatry and Clinical Neuroscience* 242, 347–351.

Caplan D. (1987) *Neurolinguistics and Linguistic Aphasiology: An Introduction*. New York: Cambridge University Press.

Caplan D. (1993) Toward a psycholinguistic approach to acquired neurogenic language disorders. *American Journal of Speech-Language Pathology* 2, 59–83.

Caplan LR. (1993) *Stroke: A Clinical Approach* (2nd ed). Boston: Butterworth–Heinemann.

Caselli RJ, Ivnik RJ, Duffy JR. (1991) Associative anomia: dissociating words and their definitions. *Mayo Clinic Proceedings* 66, 783–791.

Chapey R. (1994) Introduction to Language Intervention Strategies in Adult Aphasia. In R Chapey (ed), *Language Intervention Strategies in Adult Aphasia* (3rd ed) (pp. 3–26). Baltimore: Williams & Wilkins.

Chedru F, Geschwind N. (1972) Disorders of higher cortical function in acute confusional states. *Cortex* 8, 395–411.

Chiba S, Muneoka Y, Miyagashi T, Tanaka T. (1991) [A case of temporal lobe epilepsy with recurrent dysphasic seizures]. *No to Shinkei—Brain and Nerve* 43, 869–873.

Croisile B, Laurent B, Michel D, et al. (1991) Differentes modalites cliniques des aphasies degeneratives [Different clinical types of degenerative aphasia]. *Revue Neurologique* 147, 192–199.

Curtin JP, Koonings PP, Gutierrez M, et al. (1991). Ifosfamide-induced neurotoxicity. *Gynecologic Oncology* 42, 193–196.

Damasio A. (1981) The Nature of Aphasia: Signs and Syndromes. In MT Sarno (ed), *Acquired Aphasia* (pp. 51–65). New York: Academic Press.

Damasio AR, Van Hoesen GW. (1985) The limbic system and the localisation of herpes simplex encephalitis. *Journal of Neurology, Neurosurgery, and Psychiatry* 48, 297–301.

Damasio AR, Damasio H, Rizzo M, et al. (1982) Aphasia with nonhemorrhagic lesions in the basal ganglia and internal capsule. *Archives of Neurology* 39, 15–20.

Darley FL. (1967) Lacunae and Research Approaches to Them. IV. In CH Millikan, FL Darley (eds), *Brain Mechanisms Underlying Speech and Language* (pp. 236–240). New York: Grune & Stratton.

Darley FL. (1982) *Aphasia*. Philadelphia: Saunders.

Davis GA. (1983) *A Survey of Adult Aphasia*. Englewood Cliffs, NJ: Prentice-Hall.

Davis GA. (1993) *A Survey of Adult Aphasia and Related Language Disorders* (2nd ed). Englewood Cliffs, NJ: Prentice-Hall.

Davis JM, Davis KR, Kleinman GM, et al. (1978) Computed tomography of herpes simplex encephalitis, with clinicopathological correlation. *Radiology* 129, 409–417.

Della Sala S. (1987) Figure-object matching: another frequent nonverbal impairment of aphasics. *Italian Journal of Neurological Sciences* 8, 43–49.

DeLuca J, Cicerone KD. (1991) Confabulation following aneurysm of the anterior communicating artery. *Cortex* 27, 417–423.

De Renzi E, Lucchelli F. (1994). Are semantic systems separately represented in the brain? The case of living category impairment. *Cortex* 30, 3–25.

Devinsky O, Kelley K, Yacubian EM, et al. (1994) Postictal behavior: a clinical and subdural electroencephalographic study. *Archives of Neurology* 51, 254–259.

Duffy JR, Petersen RC. (1992) Primary progressive aphasia. *Aphasiology* 6, 1–15.

Eisenson J. (1973) *Adult Aphasia: Assessment and Treatment*. Englewood Cliffs, NJ: Prentice-Hall.

Fakhoury T, Abou-Khalil B, Peguero E. (1994) Differentiating clinical features of right and left temporal lobe seizures. *Epilepsia* 35, 1038–1044.

Folstein MF, Folstein SE, McHugh PR. (1975) "Mini-mental state": a practical method for grading the mental state of patients for the clinician. *Journal of Psychiatric Research* 12, 189–198.

Gade A, Bohr V, Bjerrum J, et al. (1992) Neuropsychological sequelae in 91 cases of pneumococcal meningitis. *Developmental Neuropsychology* 8, 447–457.

Gainotti G, D'Erme P, Villa G, Caltagirone C. (1986) Focal brain lesions and intelligence: a study with a new version of Raven's Colored Matrices. *Journal of Clinical and Experimental Neuropsychology* 8, 37–50.

Garcia JH, Ho K, Caccamo DV. (1992) Pathology of Stroke. In HJM Barnett, JP Mohr, BM Stein, FM Yatsu (eds), *Stroke: Pathophysiology, Diagnosis, and Management* (2nd ed) (pp. 125–146). New York: Churchill Livingstone.

Geschwind N. (1967) The varieties of naming errors. *Cortex* 3, 97–112.

Gilroy J. (1990) *Basic Neurology* (2nd ed). New York: Pergamon Press.

Goetz CG. (1989) Neurotoxic Effects of Drugs Prescribed by Non-Neurologists. In WJ Weiner, CG Goetz (eds), *Neurology for the Non-Neurologist* (2nd ed) (pp. 207–218). Philadelphia: Lippincott.

Goetz CG, Wilson RS. (1989) Behavioral Neurology. In WJ Weiner, CG Goetz (eds), *Neurology for the Non-Neurologist* (2nd ed) (pp. 187–197). Philadelphia: Lippincott.

Goodglass H. (1981) The syndromes of aphasia: similarities and differences in neurolinguistic features. *Topics in Language Disorders* 1, 1–15.

Goodglass H, Kaplan E. (1983) *The Assessment of Aphasia and Related Disorders* (2nd ed). Philadelphia: Lea & Febiger.

Goodglass H, Christiansen JA, Gallagher R. (1993) Comparison of morphology and syntax in free narrative and structured tests: fluent vs. nonfluent aphasics. *Cortex* 29, 377–407.

Goodglass H, Quadfasel FA, Timberlake WH. (1964) Phrase length and the type and severity of aphasia. *Cortex* 1, 133–153.

Gordon AG. (1993) Aphasia, deafness, or mental retardation. *Journal of Medical Genetics* 30, 262.

Grice LP. (1975) Logic and Conversation. In P Cole, JL Morgan (eds), *Syntax and Semantics: Speech Acts* (Vol. 3) (pp. 41–58). New York: Academic Press.

Habib M, Pelletier J, Khalil R. (1993) Aphasie progressive primaire (syndrome de Mesulam) [Primary progressive aphasia (Mesulam syndrome)]. *Presse Medicale*, 22, 757–764.

Hademenos GJ. (February 1995) The physics of cerebral aneurysms. *Physics Today* 24–30.

Harris AA, Benson CA. (1989) Central Nervous System Infection. In WJ Weiner, CG Goetz (eds), *Neurology for the Non-Neurologist* (2nd ed) (pp. 338–345). Philadelphia: Lippincott.

Helm-Estabrooks N. (1992). *Aphasia Diagnostic Profiles*. Chicago: Riverside.

Helm-Estabrooks N, Albert ML. (1991) *Manual of Aphasia Therapy*. Austin, TX: PRO-ED.

Hillis AE. (1994) Contributions from Cognitive Analyses. In R Chapey (ed), *Language Intervention Strategies in Adult Aphasia* (3rd ed) (pp. 207–219). Baltimore: Williams & Wilkins.

Holland AL. (1982) When Is Aphasia Aphasia? The Problem of Closed Head Injury. In RH Brookshire (ed), *Clinical Aphasiology: Conference Proceedings* (pp. 345–349). Minneapolis, MN: BRK Publishers.

Hough MS, Pierce RS. (1994) Pragmatic and Treatment. In R Chapey (ed), *Language Intervention Strategies in Adult Aphasia* (3rd ed) (pp. 246–268). Baltimore: Williams & Wilkins.

Ikejiri Y, Tanabe H, Nakagawa Y, et al. (1993) [Two cases of primary progressive non-fluent aphasia]. *No to Shinkei—Brain and Nerve* 45, 370–376.

Jackson JH. (1864) Loss of speech: its association with valvular disease of the heart and with hemiplegia on the right side. *Brain* 38, 28–42.

Kaminski HJ, Hlavin ML, Likavec MJ, Schmidley JW. (1992) Transient neurological deficit caused by chronic subdural hematoma. *American Journal of Medicine* 92, 698–700.

Karbe H, Kertesz A, Polk M. (1993) Profiles of language impairment in primary progressive aphasia. *Archives of Neurology* 50, 193–201.

Kelley RE. (1989) Cerebrovascular Disease. In WJ Weiner, CG Goetz (eds), *Neurology for the Non-Neurologist* (2nd ed) (pp. 52–66). Philadelphia: Lippincott.

Kennedy M, Murdoch B. (1993) Chronic aphasia subsequent to striato-capsular and thalamic lesions in the left hemisphere. *Brain and Language* 44, 284–295.

Kennedy M, Murdoch B. (1994) Thalamic aphasia and striato-capsular aphasia as independent aphasic syndromes: a review. *Aphasiology* 8, 303–313.

Kertesz A. (1979) *Aphasia and Associated Disorders: Taxonomy, Localization, and Recovery*. Orlando, FL: Grune & Stratton.

Kertesz A. (1982) *Western Aphasia Battery*. New York: Grune & Stratton.

Kertesz A, Hudson L, Mackenzie IR, Munoz DG. (1994) The pathology and nosology of primary progressive aphasia. *Neurology* 44, 2065–2072.

Kertesz A, McCabe P. (1975) Intelligence and aphasia: performance of aphasics on Raven's Coloured Progressive Matrices (RCPM). *Brain and Language* 2, 387–395.

Kertesz A, McCabe P. (1977) Recovery patterns and prognosis in aphasia. *Brain* 100, 1–18.

Kirk A, Ang LC. (1994) Unilateral Creutzfeldt-Jakob disease presenting as rapidly progressive aphasia. *Canadian Journal of Neurological Sciences* 21, 350–352.

Kirk A, Kertesz A. (1994) Cortical and subcortical aphasias compared. *Aphasiology* 8, 65–82

Levin IH. (1989) Neurological Aspects of Cancer. In WJ Weiner, CG Goetz (eds), *Neurology for the Non-Neurologist* (2nd ed) (pp. 247–259). Philadelphia: Lippincott.

Lezak MD. (1995) *Neuropsychological Assessment* (3rd ed). New York: Oxford University Press.

Linebaugh CW. (1990) Lexical Retrieval Problems: Anomia. In LL LaPointe (ed), *Aphasia and Related Neurogenic Language Disorders* (pp. 96–112). New York: Thieme.

Mantovani JF, Landau WM. (1980) Acquired aphasia with convulsive disorder: course and prognosis. *Neurology* 30, 524–529.

Margolin DI. (1991) Cognitive neuropsychology. Resolving enigmas about Wernicke's aphasia and other higher cortical disorders. *Archives of Neurology* 48, 751–765.

McDaniel KD, Wagner MT, Greenspan BS. (1991) The role of brain single photon emission computed tomography in the diagnosis of primary progressive aphasia. *Archives of Neurology* 48, 1257–1260.

McNeil MR. (1988) Aphasia in the Adult. In NJ Lass, LV McReynolds, JL Northern, DE Yoder (eds), *Handbook of Speech-Language Pathology and Audiology* (pp. 738–786). Toronto: BC Decker.

McNeil MR, Odell K, Tseng CH. (1991) Toward the integration of resource allocation into a general theory of aphasia. *Clinical Aphasiology* 20, 21–39.

Mesulam MM. (1990) Large-scale neurocognitive networks and distributed processing for attention, language, and memory. *Annals of Neurology* 28, 597–613.

Mesulam M. (1994) Neurocognitive networks and selectively distributed processing. *Revue Neurologique* 150, 564–569.

Mezaki T, Kanji R, Chimera J, Manned T. (1995) [Dose-response relationship in the treatment of cervical dystonia with botulinum toxin type A (AGN 191622) — A phase II study]. *No to Shinkei—Brain and Nerve* 47, 857–862.

Mohr JP, Hilal SK, Stein BM. (1992) Arteriovenous Malformations and Other Vascular Anomalies. In HJM Barnett, JP Mohr, BM Stein, FM Yatsu (eds), *Stroke: Pathophysiology, Diagnosis, and Management* (2nd ed) (pp. 645–670). New York: Churchill Livingstone.

Naeser MA, Alexander MP, Helm-Estabrooks N, et al. (1982) Aphasia with predominantly subcortical lesion sites. *Archives of Neurology* 39, 2–14.

Newhoff M, Apel K. (1990) Impairments in Pragmatics. In LL LaPointe (ed), *Aphasia and Related Neurogenic Language Disorders* (pp. 221–233). New York: Thieme.

Odell K, McNeil MR, Rosenbek JC, Hunter L. (1990) Perceptual characteristics of consonant production by apraxic speakers. *Journal of Speech and Hearing Disorders* 55, 345–359.

Ommaya AK, Gennarelli TA. (1974) Cerebral concussion and traumatic unconsciousness: correlation of experimental and clinical observations on blunt head injuries. *Brain* 97, 633–654.

Pantel J. (1991) Alzheimer's disease presenting as slowly progressive aphasia and slowly progressive visual agnosia: two early reports. *Archives of Neurology* 52, 10.

Parkin AJ. (1993) Progressive aphasia without dementia—a clinical and cognitive neuropsychological analysis. *Brain and Language* 44, 201–220.

Paquier PF, Van Dongen HR, Loonen CB. (1992) The Landau-Kleffner syndrome or 'acquired aphasia with convulsive disorder': long-term follow-up of six children and a review of the recent literature. *Archives of Neurology* 49, 354–359.

Peach RK. (1992) Factors underlying neuropsychological test performance in chronic severe traumatic brain injury. *Journal of Speech and Hearing Research* 35, 810–818.

Peach RK. (1995) Treating the fluent aphasias. *Topics in Stroke Rehabilitation* 2, 1–14.

Peach RK. (1996) Treatment for aphasic phonological output planning deficits. *Clinical Aphasiology* 24, 109–120.

Peter C, Assal G. (1992) [Atypical verbal behavior in a 30 year follow-up of an acquired aphasia-epilepsy syndrome]. *Psychiatrie de l' Enfant* 35, 109–125.

Pietrini V, Nertempi P, Vaglia A, et al. (1988) Recovery from herpes simplex encephalitis: selective impairment of specific semantic categories with neuroradiological correlation. *Journal of Neurosurgery, Neurology, and Psychiatry* 51, 1284–1293.

Prescott TE, Gruber JL, Olson M, Fuller KC. (1987) Hanoi revisited. *Clinical Aphasiology* 17, 249–259.

Prescott TE, Loverso FL, Selinger M. (1984) Differences between normal and left brain damaged (aphasic) subjects on a nonverbal problem solving task. *Clinical Aphasiology* 14, 235–240.

Raven JC. (1965) *Guide to Using the Coloured Progressive Matrices*. London: H.K. Lewis.

Robin DA, Schienberg S. (1990) Subcortical lesions and aphasia. *Journal of Speech and Hearing Disorders* 55, 90–100.

Rosenbek JC, LaPointe LL, Wertz RT. (1989) *Aphasia: A Clinical Approach*. Austin, TX: PRO-ED.

Salanova V, Andermann F, Rasmussen T, et al. (1995) Parietal lobe epilepsy: clinical manifestations and outcome in 82 patients treated surgically between 1929 and 1988. *Brain* 118, 607–627.

Sambunaris A, Hyde TM. (1994) Stoke-related aphasias mistaken for psychotic speech: two case reports. *Journal of Geriatric Psychiatry & Neurology* 7, 144–147.

Saver JL, Easton JD, Hart RG. (1992) Dissections and Trauma of Cervicocerebral Arteries. In HJM Barnett, JP Mohr, BM Stein, FM Yatsu (eds), *Stroke: Pathophysiology, Diagnosis, and Management* (2nd ed) (pp. 671–688). New York: Churchill Livingstone.

Scheltens P, Vermersch P, Leys D. (1993) Heterogeneite de la maladie d'Alzheimer [Heterogeneity of Alzheimer's disease]. *Revue Neurologique* 149, 14–25.

Schuell H, Jenkins JJ, Jimenez-Pabon E. (1964) *Aphasia in Adults: Diagnosis, Prognosis, and Treatment*. New York: Harper & Row.

Schwartz MF. (1984) What the classical aphasia categories can't do for us, and why. *Brain and Language* 21, 1–8.

Sovilla JY, Despland PA, Bader M. (1988) [Asymmetrical cerebral lesions and subcortical aphasia in carbon monoxide poisoning]. *Revue Medicale de la Suisse Romande* 108, 33–40.

Spatt J, Goldenberg G, Mamoli B. (1994) Simple dysphasic seizures as the sole manifestation of relapse in multiple sclerosis. *Epilepsia* 35, 1342–1345.

Tonkovich J, Peach R. (1989) What to Treat: Apraxia of Speech, Aphasia, or Both. In P Square-Storer (ed), *Acquired Apraxia of Speech in Aphasic Adults* (pp. 115–145). London: Taylor & Francis.

Toole JF. (1990) *Cerebrovascular Disorders* (4th ed). New York: Raven.

Tseng CH, McNeil MR, Milenkovic P. (1993) An investigation of attention allocation deficits in aphasia. *Brain and Language* 45, 276–296.

Van Gorp WG, Miller EN, Satz P, Visscher B. (1989) Neuropsychological performance in HIV-1 immunocompromised patients: a preliminary report. *Journal of Clinical and Experimental Neuropsychology* 11, 763–773.

Wallesch CW, Hundsalz A. (1994) Language function in delirium: a comparison of single word processing in acute confusional states and probable Alzheimer's disease. *Brain and Language* 46, 592–606.

Warrington EK, Shallice T. (1984) Category specific semantic impairments. *Brain* 107, 829–854.

Wechsler D. (1944) *The Measurement of Adult Intelligence* (3rd ed). Baltimore: Williams & Wilkins.

Weintraub S, Mesulam MM. (1993) Four Neuropsychological Profiles in Dementia. In F Boller, J Grafman (eds), *Handbook of Neuropsychology* (Vol. 8) (pp. 253–282). Amsterdam: Elsevier.

Weisberg LA, Shamsnia M, Elliott D. (1991) Nontraumatic posterior temporal lobe hemorrhage: clinical computed tomographic correlations. *Computerized Medical Imaging & Graphics* 15, 355–359.

Wertz RT. (1985) Neuropathologies of Speech and Language: An Introduction to Patient Management. In DF Johns (ed), *Clinical Management of Neurogenic Communicative Disorders* (pp. 1–96). Boston: Little, Brown.

White RF, Feldman RG, Moss MB, Proctor SP. (1993) Magnetic resonance imaging (MRI), neurobehavioral testing, and toxic encephalopathy: two cases. *Environmental Research* 61, 117–123.

Wolfe GR, Davidoff M, Katz R. (1987) Nonverbal problem solving in aphasic and non-aphasic patients with computer presented and actual stimuli. *Clinical Aphasiology* 17, 243–248.

Yesavage JA, Brooks JO III, Taylor J, Tinklenberg J. (1993) Development of aphasia, apraxia, and agnosia and decline in Alzheimer's disease. *American Journal of Psychiatry* 150, 742–747.

Zardini G, Molteni B, Nardocci N, et al. (1995) Linguistic development in a patient with Landau-Kleffner syndrome: a nine year follow-up. *Neuropediatrics* 26, 19–25.

Zhang C. (1991) [The report of organophosphorous pesticides cause delayed nervous system diseases (143 cases)]. *Chung-Hua Shen Ching Ching Shen Ko Tsa Chih* [*Chinese Journal of Neurology and Psychiatry*] 24, 336–338, 383.

Zurif EB. (1990) Language and the Brain. In DN Osherson, H Lasnik (eds), *An Invitation to Cognitive Science* (Vol. 1) (pp. 177–198). Cambridge, MA: MIT Press.

11

Differential Diagnosis of Swallowing Disorders

Jeri A. Logemann

This chapter is designed to review the process of differential diagnosis of dysphagia, including the clinician's data collection from chart review; discussions with family, staff, and the patient; deductive reasoning; and patient testing involved in the differential diagnosis of an oropharyngeal swallowing disorder. The process begins with initial screening and identification of behavioral indications, dysphagic symptoms, or both that may indicate a risk of a swallowing problem. The process then progresses to the identification of the physiologic abnormalities, anatomic abnormalities, or both that cause the behavioral indicators or symptoms; identification of any possible contributing factors; and, in some cases, the identification of an underlying medical etiology for the dysphagia (Logemann 1983, 1993a). For those patients with complaints of dysphagia but no known medical etiology, the speech-language pathologist can play a crucial role in defining the patient's oropharyngeal swallow physiology and in contributing to the identification of the disease process or neural damage of which the swallowing physiology is typical (Robbins 1987; Robbins and Levine 1988; Robbins et al. 1986).

SCREENING TO IDENTIFY POTENTIAL DYSPHAGIC PATIENTS

The initial step in diagnosis of swallowing disorders in the oropharyngeal region is to screen the patient to define the nature of his or her symptoms and indications of an oropharyngeal swallowing disorder. If the screening indicates the possibility of a swallowing disorder, the clinician proceeds to more in-depth diagnosis. Typically, a screening takes

10–15 minutes. The purpose of the screening is to identify patients at highest risk for oropharyngeal dysphagia who require more in-depth physiologic assessment.

Behavioral Indications of Swallowing Disorders

Indications of the presence of swallowing disorders can include slowed eating, coughing while eating or a short time after eating, gurgling voice quality during or immediately after a meal, difficulty managing saliva, a history of pneumonia (especially recurrent), weight loss of no known etiology, bronchitis or continuous increased secretions of no known etiology, visible difficulty initiating the oral stage of swallowing, increased secretions in the chest within 1 hour after eating, and repeated swallows on a single bolus. In addition to these behavioral indicators, patients with certain medical diagnoses are at high risk for dysphagia, including those who have suffered a brainstem stroke and those who have undergone surgical treatment for laryngeal cancer (including supraglottic laryngectomy), anterior floor of mouth cancer, and tonsil base of tongue cancer. Patients who have motor neuron disease, Parkinson's disease, and myasthenia gravis are at high risk for development of dysphagia at some point in their disease progression. Patients who have undergone anterior cervical spinal cord fusions are also at high risk. Patients with any of these diagnoses should be immediately referred for a more in-depth swallowing diagnostic procedure. Though these diagnoses are highly associated with oropharyngeal dysphagia, and many dysphagic patients exhibit the symptoms outlined, it is important to note that some patients with oropharyngeal dysphagia do not exhibit any of the visible or audible symptoms of dysphagia and may lose weight or aspirate on a regular basis.

Differentiation of Dysphagic Symptoms and Swallowing Disorders

There are three major physiologic symptoms of oropharyngeal swallowing disorders: (1) aspiration, (2) penetration, and (3) residue. The behavioral indications of swallowing disorders noted in the previous section are associated with these three major symptoms. For example, if a patient coughs at bedside, it can indicate that there has been aspiration of food or liquid into the trachea. If the patient swallows multiple times on a single bolus, it is an indicator of inefficient swallowing or residual food left behind in the mouth or pharynx. *Aspiration* is defined as food, liquid, or saliva entering the trachea below the true vocal folds. *Penetration* is the entry of food, liquid, or saliva into the entrance of the airway down to but not below the true vocal folds. *Residue* is food that was left in the mouth or pharynx after the swallow. Diagnosis or evaluation of swallowing disorders is designed to define the specific anatomic or physiologic disorders causing the symptoms of aspiration, penetration, or residue. In communicating with the patient's physician, it is critical that the clinician distinguish between the behavioral indicators of a swallowing problem, the physiologic symptoms of a swallowing disorder, and the actual disorder itself. The actual disorder in anatomy or physiology is the entity that is treated. In the course of treatment, the physiologic symptoms and behavioral indicators are eliminated. The physician's understanding of the distinction between the symptoms and the anatomic or physiologic disorders, or both, is critical. If the clinician does not distinguish these terms for the physician, it is possible that when a bedside assessment or screening is completed, and the clinician requests a more in-depth physiologic examination (e.g., videofluorographic study), the physician may respond by denying the more in-depth assessment, stating that now that he or she knows the patient is aspirating no further assessment is needed. The physician may plan to institute symptomatic management such as nonoral feeding or tracheostomy. If the speech-language pathologist communicates the difference between treatment for the physiologic swallowing abnormality and systematic management of symptoms, such as aspiration, the need for the radiographic or other physiologic study is clear. It is also crucial that the clinician explain to the physician that the radiographic study is both a diagnostic and a treatment trial, so that various treatments can be attempted and evaluated to find conditions under which the patient is able to eat successfully with no inefficiency or aspiration (Logemann 1993a, 1993b).

Potential Sequelae of Swallowing Disorders

There are a number of sequelae of chronic oropharyngeal swallowing dysfunctions, including malnutrition, dehydration, weight loss, and pneumonia or other airway problems (Martin et al. 1994; Schmidt et al. 1994). If a patient is chronically dysphagic, he or she may modify his or her diet spontaneously, eliminating those food types, generally according to their viscosity, that are most difficult to swallow. In so doing, the patient may limit nutritional intake and begin to exhibit symptoms of malnutrition or dehydration. For the elderly, dehydration is a particular problem, since it alters alertness and mental abilities. Weight loss can be another symptom of malnutrition. It is not uncommon for some patients with oropharyngeal dysphagia to lose 20–30 pounds over a 2- to 3-month period. Often this symptom is not associated with dysphagia but rather with some other possible medical cause. It is important for the speech-language pathologist to be aware that weight loss can be a sign of dysphagia and that the patient may be malnourished. Patients may not lose weight but instead may have their blood chemistries altered because of dietary changes resulting in dysphagia. Pneumonia, bronchitis, and other airway problems can also result from chronic aspiration. The patient may not get pneumonia but may exhibit what appears to be a low, chronic level of congestion in the chest or in the trachea. Bronchorrhea is a low-level bronchial infection that also can result from chronic aspiration. These sequelae of a swallowing disorder can contribute to the patient's general decline in function over time.

Techniques for Screening

When a consult for a dysphagic patient is received, usually the speech-language pathologist conducts a screening of the patient to identify his or her risk for dysphagia. There are a number of procedures that can be used for screening. Usually the clinical bedside examination is done first. It can include or be followed by the blue-dye test, cervical auscultation (Hamlet et al. 1990), scintigraphy (Espinola 1986), videonasendoscopy (i.e., fiberoptic endoscopic examination of swallowing [FEES]) (Bastian 1989, 1991, 1993; Langmore et al. 1991), or any combination of these. Screening procedures identify the patient's behavioral indications or dysphagic symptoms to determine if there is a high risk of an oral or pharyngeal dysphagia and the need for a study of the patient's pharyngeal anatomy and physiology, esophageal anatomy and physiology, or both. Some of the screening procedures for *pharyngeal* dysphagia are actually in-depth assessment procedures for *oral* dysphagia. For example, the bedside clinical examination can be an in-depth assessment of oral function, identifying oral disorders of swallow. In contrast, the bedside examination cannot identify the pharyngeal-stage swallowing disorders (Logemann 1983; Splaingard et al. 1988). The bedside clinical examination is therefore a screening test for pharyngeal dysphagia, and it can also be a definitive assessment for oral swallowing disorders. The screening test, a relatively short (10- to 15-minute) procedure, leads to the next level of diagnosis (i.e., identification of the particular disorder in swallowing, anatomy, or physiology that causes the symptoms).

Bedside Clinical Observations

Bedside clinical observations can involve observing the patient eating part or all of a meal (if the patient is orally fed) and a brief oral motor assessment of lips, tongue, palate, larynx, and pharynx to define any of the symptoms of a pharyngeal swallowing disorder (e.g., gurgling voice quality after a swallow; difficulty managing oral secretions; coughing or choking before, during, or after any swallows of any foods or saliva; frequent throat clearing after a meal) (Linden and Siebens 1983; Splaingard et al. 1988). Usually, the clinician refers for a radiographic or other instrumental procedure if any of these symptoms are defined during bedside clinical observations.

Blue-Dye Test

The blue-dye test is a screening test used at times with patients who have tracheostomies in place (Thompson-Henry and Braddock 1995). Some amount of blue dye is mixed with food or liquid and presented to the patient for swallowing. As the patient swallows, the clinician looks and suctions for blue-dyed secretions at the tracheostomy site or coughed from the tracheostomy. The test is not definitive for aspiration and certainly is only a screening device to define risk and the need for referral for a radiographic study. A positive blue-dye test, consisting of blue-dyed foods or secretions coming from the tracheostomy, indicates the need for radiographic study or other instrumental procedure. However, the blue-dye test can miss patients who aspirate, if they aspirate small amounts or if a wide variety of food viscosities or volumes are not given. Even if aspiration is detected, the anatomic or physiologic reason for the aspiration is not identified through this test; therefore, the patient requires an instrumental procedure for the next level of diagnosis.

Cervical Auscultation

Cervical auscultation involves listening to the patient's neck sounds during swallowing (Hamlet et al. 1990, 1992, 1994; Logan et al. 1967; Mackowiak et al. 1967; Zenner et al. 1995). Though a number of sounds may be audible through a stethoscope placed against the patient's neck, there is still no clear understanding of what these normal or abnormal sounds represent physiologically, or whether clinicians can differentiate normal and abnormal sounds. Despite this limitation, some clinicians regularly listen to the patient's neck for sounds of residual material in the pharynx or airway during respiration after the swallow. Such sounds indicate the need for an instrumental study to define the physiologic or anatomic abnormality causing the additional sounds.

Videonasendoscopy

Videonasendoscopy, or FEES, involves the nasal placement of a flexible fiberoptic light bundle over the palate and into the pharynx.

Viewing the pharynx from above provides information on pharyngeal anatomy and visualizes the pharynx before and after the swallow. Visualizing the pharynx before the swallow, the clinician can observe premature spillage from the mouth into the pharynx. Delay in triggering the pharyngeal swallow can also be observed as the bolus arriving in the pharynx before the pharyngeal swallow triggering. Differentiating premature spillage and delayed pharyngeal swallow, using videonasendoscopy, can be difficult, however. After the pharyngeal swallow is over, and the pharynx returns to its open respiratory breathing posture, residual food on the pharyngeal walls, in the valleculae, or in the pyriform sinuses can be observed. The location of the residual food can indicate specific swallowing disorders in the pharynx. If the residual food redistributes immediately after the swallow as the pharynx and larynx descend to their resting positions, the clinician can be misled by the relocation of food. Because videonasendoscopy, or FEES, cannot visualize the actual swallow, it can be classified as a screening technique to identify those individuals in need of a radiographic assessment to both define the swallow physiology and anatomy and to identify the efficacy of specific treatment strategies.

At the end of a screening procedure, the clinician should have a good idea of the patient's need for more in-depth testing to define the abnormality or abnormalities causing swallowing symptoms.

THREE LEVELS OF DIFFERENTIAL DIAGNOSIS OF OROPHARYNGEAL DYSPHAGIA

Within the differential diagnosis of oropharyngeal dysphagia, there are three different levels: (1) identification of the physiologic abnormalities, anatomic abnormalities, or both that cause the patient's dysphagic symptoms and management and therapy procedures to improve the swallow; (2) identification of any possible factors contributing to the patient's dysphagia, such as medications, aging, tracheostomy, fatigue, bracing, postural abnormalities, and an improperly placed nasogastric tube; and (3) identification of the underlying medical etiology in those dysphagic patients who do not yet have a medical diagnosis.

Identification of the Anatomic and Physiologic Abnormalities and Therapy Procedures to Improve the Swallow

The most critical aspect of the clinician's diagnosis of dysphagia is the identification of the exact anatomic or physiologic abnormality or abnormalities causing the patient's dysphagic symptoms. Generally, this level of diagnosis begins with careful history taking regarding the patient's prior medical problems, prior and current medications, and behavioral indications and symptoms of the dysphagia. Whether the patient has had respiratory difficulties requiring tracheostomy or mechanical ventilation and for how long is important. The medical diagnosis(es) is an important piece of information. There is a growing body of knowledge regarding the specific types of oral and pharyngeal swallowing disorders that result from specific types of neural or structural damage (Blonsky et al. 1975; Lazarus and Logemann 1987; Robbins 1987; Robbins and Levine 1988). For example, a medullary stroke typically causes unilateral pharyngeal wall paresis, reduced laryngeal and pharyngeal elevation, and unilateral vocal-fold paralysis. Thus, the diagnosis of a medullary stroke should point the clinician toward the specific types of swallowing disorders that can be anticipated. Similarly, a supraglottic laryngectomy that involves removal of the hyoid bone and a small part of the tongue base, the epiglottis, and aryepiglottic folds, as well as the false vocal folds, typically reduces movement of the patient's tongue base during swallow and reduces airway closure. These two swallowing disorders should then be anticipated in these patients.

Oral-Motor Testing

The bedside clinical evaluation typically involves in-depth oral-motor testing of voluntary and involuntary movements of the lips, tongue, palate, pharynx, and larynx. While the bedside clinical evaluation does not define pharyngeal swallowing problems, it can define oral abnormalities and selected pharyngeal wall impairments. At the end of the clinical or bedside evaluation, the clinician should explain the possibility of pharyngeal swallow disorders (e.g., reduced pharyngeal wall contraction, reduced tongue base motion, poor laryngeal elevation) to the patient's physician and, on that basis, request a radiographic study (e.g., modified barium swallow) to define the physiologic disorders and plan appropriate treatment. It is important for the clinician to educate the physician regarding the fact that such a radiographic examination is *not* designed to define whether a patient aspirates but instead to determine the anatomic or physiologic etiology for the aspiration or inefficient swallow and to allow the clinician to define optimal treatment strategies (Logemann 1993a, b, 1997; Logemann et al. 1994). It is important that the physician realize that during the radiographic study, treatment techniques are introduced to define those procedures that are effective immediately, so that the patient can begin to eat safely and efficiently on at least some food viscosities and volumes soon after the radiographic study (Logemann 1993b, 1997; Logemann et al. 1994; Rasley et al. 1993). The goal of the radiographic procedure is to maintain the patient as a safe oral feeder rather than to withdraw oral feeding.

Imaging Procedures

There are several imaging procedures that can contribute to the diagnosis of a specific oropharyngeal dysphagia, including videofluoroscopy and videonasendoscopy (Bastian 1989, 1991, 1993; Kidder et al. 1994; Langmore et al. 1988, 1991). Videonasendoscopy is described in a previous section and serves as a screening tool rather than a definitive procedure for identifying the specific nature of the oropharyngeal dysphagia. In contrast, videofluoroscopy is capable of identifying the particular movement abnormalities causing the behavioral indications and the dysphagic symptoms. It is important during the videofluoroscopic study or any other imaging procedure that the clinician introduce various bolus types, including various volumes of thin liquid, pudding-consistency food, and food requiring mastication (e.g., cookie) (Dodds et al. 1990a, b). Such a protocol usually involves 1 ml, 3 ml, 5 ml, and 10 ml swallows of liquid (two of each), as well as two swallows of 3 ml of barium pudding and a small amount of cookie to be chewed and swallowed. The protocol enables the clinician to observe the normalcy of volume accommodation by the patient, as well as management of various food viscosities and mastication (Logemann 1993a). When any swallowing abnormalities are identified (especially if they cause any severe symptoms such as aspiration or significant residue left in the mouth or pharynx), the clinician should introduce therapy strategies to improve the swallow immediately (Bisch et al. 1994; Ekberg 1986; Logemann 1989; Logemann et al. 1990, 1994). Such strategies include postural changes, which change the pharyngeal dimensions as well as directing the food differently through the oral cavity and pharynx; techniques to enhance sensory input, including changing the taste and temperature of the bolus, thermal and tactile stimulation, and modifications of food placement into the mouth (in terms of its volume, pressure with a spoon, and so on); and, as needed, voluntary swallow maneuvers to modify the actual pharyngeal swallow physiology (Lazarus et al. 1993a, b; Logemann et al. 1989; Sorin et al. 1988; Welch et al. 1993). When the instrumental assessment is completed, the clinician should have identified (1) the anatomic or physiologic abnormality causing the patient's symptoms, (2) the optimum eating strategies that can be used safely, (3) the nature of any swallowing therapy needed, and (4) the scheduling of any follow-up reassessment. This, then, constitutes the first level of differential diagnosis—that is, the identification of the specific physiologic or anatomic abnormality and successful treatment strategies.

Identification of Contributing Factors

The second level of differential diagnosis involves the identification of any factors contributing to the patient's dysphagia. In many cases, elimination of the contributing factors can eliminate the patient's dysphagic symptoms and return the swallow to an efficient and safe level.

Medications can reduce the patient's swallowing function. Antihistamines can dry up secretions and make it difficult for the patient to initiate a swallow. Medications that change the patient's alertness or control behavior (e.g., phenothiazine drugs) can dull the patient's sensory awareness and slow reaction times. There are no controlled studies of medication effects on swallow physiology. However, if the worsening or occurrence of the patient's dysphagia coincides with placement on a particular new medication, eliminating that medication and observing the effects on swallow may be necessary.

Aging can affect the patient's swallow physiology (Logemann 1990; Robbins et al. 1992; Tracy et al. 1989). As individuals reach the age of 60 years, there is a natural prolongation of the pharyngeal swallow delay. As individuals pass the age of 80 years, there tends to be a reduction in maximum laryngeal and hyoid motion, resulting in changes in cricopharyngeal opening. These normal aging effects must be identified and separated from the patient's swallowing abnormalities. These aging effects can interact with swallow disorders, placing an elderly patient at a greater risk for dysphagia than a younger individual with the same medical problem (e.g., stroke, head injury).

Tracheostomy, if in place for more than 6 months or created in such a way that the overlying tissues are sutured to the trachea, can result in swallowing changes, including reduced laryngeal elevation, reduced cricopharyngeal opening diameter, and reduced airway closure. Generally, if the patient lightly covers the end of the tracheostomy tube during the swallow, a relatively new tracheostomy tube with the cuff deflated appears to have little effect on swallow physiology. However, if the tracheostomy cuff is inflated, if the tracheostomy is present for more than 6 months, or if scar tissue has formed, the larynx may be less mobile with a tracheostomy, and the cricopharyngeal sphincter opening may be reduced. It is likely that the effects of tracheostomy are worse in elderly individuals, because laryngeal elevation is already naturally reduced because of age.

Fatigue throughout a meal can change pharyngeal swallow physiology. Clinicians should observe the dysphagic patient as he or she returns to oral intake to assure that he or she does not appear to fatigue from the beginning to the end of the meal.

The effects of neck bracing on swallowing in cervical spinal-cord–injured patients has not been clearly defined. Patients often complain of the discomfort of swallowing while wearing a neck brace, but no studies have examined cervical spinal-cord–injured patients with and without their bracing. A study of normal individuals with and without a sternal-occipital-mandibular immobilizer brace revealed no significant changes in oropharyngeal physiology other than an increased duration of laryngeal closure that may have been a reaction to the discomfort of swallowing with the brace in place (Bisch et al. 1992).

Abnormalities in the cervical spine can create postural changes that change swallow physiology. It is known that voluntary changes in head and neck posture change pharyngeal dimensions in systematic ways. It is possible that arthritis or scoliosis affects swallow physiology in as yet undetected ways.

An improperly placed nasogastric tube can also increase or cause the patient's dysphagia. If the nasogastric tube enters the pharynx and loops around the epiglottis or folds over before proceeding into the esophagus, the presence of the improperly placed tube can create dysphagia.

Identification of the Underlying Medical Diagnosis

The third level of differential diagnosis involves the identification of the underlying medical etiology for the dysphagia in patients who complain of swallowing difficulty but do not have a medical diagnosis. The experience of several swallowing centers, including my own, indicates that patients complaining of dysphagia with no known medical etiology usually have neurologic disease, particularly Parkinson's disease, myasthenia gravis, motor neuron disease, multiple sclerosis, stroke (particularly brainstem), and Guillain-Barré syndrome. When assessing a patient with no known medical etiology and dysphagia complaints, the clinician should observe the patient's gait and fine motor control, including handwriting and presence of tremors in hands, head, or in any structures in the upper aerodigestive tract. Many of these neurologic diseases present with distinctive changes in swallowing. The speech-language pathologist can identify the patient's swallow abnormalities as typical of patients with a particular neurologic condition and refer the patient to a neurologist. With this information, the neurologist makes the diagnosis. In such cases, the speech-language pathologist has efficiently and cost effectively referred the patient into the health care system.

Parkinson's Disease

Patients with Parkinson's disease often exhibit dysphagia characterized by a typical rocking and rolling tongue motion to initiate the oral stage of swallowing, a delay in triggering the pharyngeal swallow, and residual food in the valleculae indicating reduced tongue-base motion (Robbins et al. 1986). These patients are often unaware of their swallowing disorders, which may have caused increased secretions or chronic tracheal or bronchial infection because of chronic aspiration. Patients with Parkinson's disease often exhibit a shuffling gait, rigidity in muscles of the chest, reduced facial expression, and digital tremors. They may also exhibit tremors in structures within the vocal tract. The patient with Parkinson's disease typically shows signs of uneven rate of speech, as well as changes in voice quality (increasing roughness) and reduced precision of articulation, particularly for sounds produced with the back of the tongue (e.g., /k/ and /g/) (Logemann et al. 1978).

Myasthenia Gravis

Myasthenia gravis is characterized by increasing fatigue with use of involved muscles. Cases of myasthenia gravis have exhibited involvement of muscles of mastication alone, so that the patient may become unable to chew over the course of a meal; of muscles of the pharyngeal walls (the pharyngeal constrictors alone); or the larynx alone (Aronson 1981). Typically, these patients fatigue during a meal, finding it difficult to swallow halfway through the meal. Patients may also exhibit a more consistent level of fatigue, if the myasthenia is severe. The patient with myasthenia gravis may exhibit fatiguing in the speech mechanism parallel with changes in swallowing. Usually, but not always, these patients respond positively to a Tensilon test.

Motor Neuron Disease

Patients with motor neuron disease of a bulbar form may exhibit weakness of muscles of the tongue, lips, palate, larynx, pharynx, or any combination of these (Robbins 1987). Most commonly in the early stages of the disease process, fine motor control of the tongue, lips, and palate is reduced, making it difficult for the patient to lateralize food for chewing, and also creating hypernasality of speech and imprecise lingual consonant production. These patients may spontaneously eliminate foods requiring chewing from their diet or toss their head back to facilitate oral transit. As the disease progresses, these patients often display a delay in triggering the pharyngeal swallow and reduced pharyngeal wall contraction. Later in the disease process, laryngeal function is usually reduced. Generally, patients complain of dysphagic symptoms when they are beginning to lose the ability to chew. These patients may or may not exhibit limb and other types of muscle involvement. The patient with motor neuron disease usually exhibits increasing difficulty in swallowing thick foods, because he or she is not able to recruit the additional motor neurons to increase lingual and pharyngeal pressures to drive thicker food through the oral cavity and pharynx.

Multiple Sclerosis

Patients with multiple sclerosis may exhibit swallowing problems, particularly a delay in triggering the pharyngeal swallow and some mild pharyngeal wall impairment (Fabiszak 1987). Usually, these swallowing symptoms are in conjunction with other motor disorders, particularly of the limbs. The patient with multiple sclerosis may exhibit signs of cerebellar involvement in speech, with uneven rate and highly variable use of pitch and loudness. Alternatively, the patient with multiple sclerosis may exhibit reduction in fine motor control characteristic of brainstem damage. However, multiple sclerosis is a highly variable disease in both presentation and course; therefore, diagnosis is often a matter of exclusion of other neurologic damage.

Stroke

Stroke, particularly brain stem stroke, can cause swallowing disorders with no other symptoms. After brainstem stroke, the patient exhibits typical pharyngeal swallow impairments, including delayed pharyngeal swallow, reduced laryngeal elevation, reduced cricopharyngeal opening, and unilateral pharyngeal paresis. It is possible that no lesion will be found with brain-imaging studies. It is also possible to suffer a small stroke in the region of the swallowing center or centers that would only damage swallowing and no other motor function. Patients who have suffered a right or left cortical stroke may also exhibit typical swallow disorders (Robbins and Levine 1988).

Guillain-Barré Syndrome

In its early stages, Guillain-Barré syndrome can affect swallowing. Generally, patients show a weakness in all aspects of the oropharyngeal swallow with no specific single disorder. As paralysis progresses, the severity of the swallowing disorder also progresses.

Patients with No Known Medical Diagnosis

When the swallowing clinician sees a dysphagic patient with no known medical diagnosis, it is important to carefully describe the specific nature of the patient's swallowing disorder(s) and how the disorder(s) compare to those of patients with a known diagnosis of neurologic damage. In this way, the patient's attending physician and neurologist can look for other symptoms of that particular disease entity. While speech-language pathologists do not make the final medical diagnosis, often the speech and swallowing symptoms point directly to the specific neurologic condition. In looking at the patient's swallowing function as a possible indicator of neurologic disease, the speech-language pathologist should also look at the motor control of the same mechanism for speech production and respiration. In some patients, the combination of changes in speech and changes in swallowing point to the differential diagnosis. When doing the radiographic study of oropharyngeal swallow in such a patient, it is often helpful for the clinician to observe speech movements as well as swallowing physiology.

It is possible that the patient with complaints of dysphagia but no known medical etiology has a head-neck tumor. Generally, patients with head-neck tumors exhibit odynophagia (painful swallowing) more frequently than dysphagia. However, patients with tumors on the pharyngeal wall and in the pyriform sinuses may exhibit and complain of difficulty swallowing. Often this is associated with weight loss. The tumor may be visible during a radiographic study, but, in some cases, there is no obvious tumor bulk radiographically during swallow studies. Any patient suspected of having a head-neck tumor should be referred to an otolaryngologist for further assessment.

SUMMARY

The differential diagnosis of dysphagia requires excellent problem-solving skills and deductive reasoning. It involves screening to identify patients at risk for dysphagia based on behavioral indications or dysphagic symptoms and identifying the specific physiologic or anatomic abnormalities causing the patient's signs, symptoms, or both, as well as any possible contributing factors. Finally, using information from the physiologic and anatomic abnormalities in swallowing, the speech-language pathologist may be able to define the underlying medical etiology of the problem, which, in previously undiagnosed patients, is often neurologic damage or disease. The speech-language pathologist can play a crucial role in the definition of the medical diagnosis of the patient and enter the patient into the medical system in a cost-effective and efficient manner.

REFERENCES

Aronson A. (1981) Early motor unit disease masquerading as psychogenic breathy dysphonia: a clinical case presentation. *Journal of Speech and Hearing Disorders* 36, 116–124.

Bastian R. (1989) Videoendoscopic evaluation of dysphagia: comparison with the modified barium swallow [abstract]. *Otolaryngology—Head Neck Surgery* 101, 152.

Bastian RW. (1991) Videoendoscopic evaluation of patients with dysphagia: an adjunct to the modified barium swallow. *Otolaryngology—Head and Neck Surgery* 104, 339–350.

Bastian RW. (1993) The videoendoscopic swallowing study: an alternative and partner to the videofluoroscopic swallowing study. *Dysphagia* 8, 359–367.

Bisch E, Logemann J, Rademaker A, Quigley J. (November 1992) *Swallow effects of the SOMI brace.* Presented at the American Speech-Language Hearing Association annual convention, San Antonio, TX.

Bisch EM, Logemann JA, Rademaker AW, et al. (1994) Pharyngeal effects of bolus volume, viscosity and temperature in patients with dysphagia resulting from neurologic impairment and in normal subjects. *Journal of Speech and Hearing Research* 37, 1041–1049.

Blonsky E, Logemann J, Boshes B, Fisher H. (1975) Comparison of speech and swallowing function in patients with tremor disorders and in normal geriatric patients: a cinefluorographic study. *Journal of Gerontology* 30, 299–303.

Dodds WJ, Logemann JA, Stewart ET. (1990a) Radiological assessment of abnormal oral and pharyngeal phases of swallowing. *American Journal of Roentgenology* 154, 965–974.

Dodds WJ, Stewart ET, Logemann JA. (1990b) Physiology and radiology of the normal oral and pharyngeal phases of swallowing. *American Journal of Roentgenology* 154, 953–965.

Ekberg O. (1986) Posture of the head and pharyngeal swallowing. *Aeta Radiologica* 27, 269–274.

Espinola D. (1986) Radionuclide evaluation of pulmonary aspiration: four birds with one stone—esophageal transit, gastroesophageal reflux, gastric emptying and bronchopulmonary aspiration. *Dysphagia* 1, 101–104.

Fabiszak AJ. (1987) *Swallowing patterns in neurologically normal subjects and two subgroups of multiple sclerosis patients.* Ph.D. diss., Northwestern University.

Hamlet S, Penney DG, Formolo J. (1994) Stethoscope acoustics and cervical auscultation of swallowing. *Dysphagia* 9, 63–68.

Hamlet SL, Nelson RJ, Patterson RL. (1990) Interpreting the sounds of swallowing: fluid flow through the cricopharyngeus. *Annals Otology, Rhinology, and Laryngology* 99, 749–752.

Hamlet SL, Patterson RL, Fleming SM, Jones LA. (1992) Sounds of swallowing following total laryngectomy. *Dysphagia* 7, 160–165.

Kidder TM, Langmore SE, Martin BJW. (1994) Indications and techniques of endoscopy in evaluation of cervical dysphagia: comparison with radiographic techniques. *Dysphagia* 9, 256–261.

Langmore SE, Schatz K, Olson N. (1988) Fiberoptic endoscopic evaluation of swallowing therapy: a new procedure. *Dysphagia* 2, 216–219.

Langmore SE, Schatz K, Olson N. (1991) Endoscopic and videofluoroscopic evaluations of swallowing and aspiration. *Annals Otology, Rhinology, and Laryngology* 100, 678–681.

Lazarus C, Logemann JA. (1987) Swallowing disorders in closed head trauma patients. *Archives of Physical Medicine and Rehabilitation* 68, 79–87.

Lazarus C, Logemann JA, Gibbons P. (1993b) Effects of maneuvers on swallowing function in a dysphagic oral cancer patient. *Head and Neck Surgery* 15, 419–424.

Lazarus CL, Logemann JA, Rademaker AW, et al. (1993a) Effects of bolus volume, viscosity and repeated swallows in non-stroke subjects and stroke patients. *Archives of Physical Medicine and Rehabilitation* 74, 1066–1070.

Linden P, Siebens A. (1983) Dysphagia: predicting laryngeal penetration. *Archives of Physical Medicine and Rehabilitation* 64, 281–284.

Logan WJ, Kavanagh JF, Wornall AW. (1967) Sonic correlates of human deglutition. *Journal of Applied Physiology* 23, 279–284.

Logemann JA. (1983) *Evaluation and Treatment of Swallowing Disorders*. San Diego: College-Hill Press.

Logemann JA. (1989) Evaluation and treatment planning for the head-injured patient with oral intake disorders. *Journal of Head Trauma Rehabilitation* 4, 24–33.

Logemann JA. (1990) Effects of Aging on the Swallowing Mechanism. In G Sisson, H Pelzer (eds), *The Otolaryngologic Clinics of North America:Head & Neck Diseases in the Elderly* (pp. 1045–1056) (Vol. 23, No. 6). Philadelphia: Saunders.

Logemann JA. (1993a) *Manual for the Videofluorographic Study of Swallowing* (2nd ed). Austin, TX: PRO-ED.

Logemann JA. (1993b) The dysphagia diagnostic procedure as a treatment efficacy trial. *Clinics in Communication Disorders* 3, 1–10.

Logemann JA. (1997) *Evaluation and Treatment of Swallowing Disorders* (2nd ed). Austin, TX: PRO-ED.

Logemann JA, Fisher HB, Boshes B, Blonsky ER. (1978) Frequency and co-occurrence of vocal tract dysfunctions in a large sample of Parkinson's patients. *Journal of Speech and Hearing Disorders* 43, 47–57.

Logemann JA, Kahrilas PJ. (1990) Relearning to swallow post CVA: application of maneuvers and indirect biofeedback: a case study. *Neurology* 40, 1136–1138.

Logemann J, Kahrilas P, Kobara M, Vakil N. (1989) The benefit of head rotation on pharyngoesophageal dysphagia. *Archives of Physical Medicine and Rehabilitation* 70, 767–771.

Logemann JA, Pauloski BR, Colangelo L, et al. (1994) Effects of a sour bolus on oropharyngeal swallowing measures in patients with neurogenic dysphagia. *Journal of Speech and Hearing Research* 38, 556–563.

Logemann JA, Rademaker AW, Pauloski BR, Kahrilas PJ. (1994) Effects of postural change on aspiration in head and neck surgical patients. *Otolaryngology—Head and Neck Surgery* 110, 222–227.

Mackowiak RC, Brennan HS, Friedman MHF. (1967) Acoustic profile of deglutition. *Proceedings of the Society for Experimental Biology and Medicine* 125, 1149–1152.

Martin BJ, Corlew M, Wood H, et al. (1994) The association of swallowing dysfunction and aspiration pneumonia. *Dysphagia* 9, 1–6.

Rasley A, Logemann JA, Kahrilas PJ, et al. (1993) Prevention of barium aspiration during videofluoroscopic swallowing studies: value of change in posture. *American Journal of Roentgenology* 160, 1005–1009.

Robbins J, Levine R. (1988) Swallowing after unilateral stroke of the cerebral cortex: preliminary experience. *Dysphagia* 3, 11–17.

Robbins J, Hamilton JW, Lof GL, Kempster GB. (1992) Oropharyngeal swallowing in normal adults of different ages. *Gastroenterology* 103, 823–829.

Robbins JA. (1987) Swallowing in ALS and motor neuron disorders. *Neurologic Clinics* 5, 213–229.

Robbins JA, Logemann JA, Kirshner HS. (1986) Swallowing and speech production in Parkinson's disease. *Annals of Neurology* 19, 283–287.

Schmidt J, Holas M, Halvorson K, Reding M. (1994) Videofluoroscopic evidence of aspiration predicts pneumonia and death but not dehydration following stroke. *Dysphagia* 9, 7–11.

Sorin R, Somers S, Austin W, Bester S. (1988) The influence of videofluoroscopy on the management of the dysphagic patient. *Dysphagia* 2, 127–135.

Splaingard M, Hutchins B, Sulton L, Chaudhuri G. (1988) Aspiration in rehabilitation patients: videofluoroscopy vs. bedside clinical assessment. *Archives of Physical Medicine and Rehabilitation* 69, 637–640.

Thompson-Henry S, Braddock B. (1995) The modified Evan's blue dye procedure fails to detect aspiration in the tracheostomized patient: five case reports. *Dysphagia* 10, 172–174.

Tracy J, Logemann J, Kahrilas P, et al. (1989) Preliminary observations on the effects of age on oropharyngeal deglutition. *Dysphagia* 4, 90–94.

Welch MW, Logemann JA, Rademaker AW, Kahrilas PJ. (1993) Changes in pharyngeal dimensions effected by chin tuck. *Archives of Physical Medicine and Rehabilitation* 74, 178–181.

Zenner PM, Losinski DS, Mills RH. (1995) Using cervical auscultation in the clinical dysphagia examination in long-term care. *Dysphagia* 10, 27–31.

Index

DATE DUE
